Core Concepts in Cardiac Surgery

Core Concepts in Cardiac Surgery

Edited by

David Taggart
Professor of Cardiovascular Surgery, University of Oxford, Oxford, UK

and

Yasir Abu-Omar
Consultant Cardiothoracic and Transplant Surgeon, Royal Papworth
Hospital, Cambridge, UK

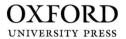
OXFORD
UNIVERSITY PRESS

Great Clarendon Street, Oxford, OX2 6DP,
United Kingdom

Oxford University Press is a department of the University of Oxford.
It furthers the University's objective of excellence in research, scholarship,
and education by publishing worldwide. Oxford is a registered trade mark of
Oxford University Press in the UK and in certain other countries

Published in the United States of America by Oxford University Press
198 Madison Avenue, New York, NY 10016, United States of America

British Library Cataloguing in Publication Data
Data available

Library of Congress Control Number: 2018941854

ISBN 978–0–19–873546–5

Printed and bound by
CPI Group (UK) Ltd, Croydon, CR0 4YY

Contents

List of Abbreviations

ACAB	atraumatic coronary artery bypass		EDHF	endothelium-derived hyperpolarizing factor
ACE	angiotensin-converting-enzyme		ERP	effective refractory period
ACT	activated clotting time		FAA	functional aortic annulus
AF	atrial fibrillation		FDA	Food and Drug Administration
AHA	American Heart Association		FFR	fractional flow reserve
AI	aortic insufficiency		GEA	gastro-epiploic artery
AR	aortic regurgitation		HF	heart failure
AS	aortic valve stenosis		HIFU	high-intensity focused ultrasound
AV	aortic valve		IABP	intra-aortic balloon pump
AVJ	aorto-ventricular junction		ICU	intensive care unit
AVN	atrioventricular node		IEA	inferior epigastric artery
AVR	aortic valve replacement		IEOA	indexed effective orifice area
BAV	bicuspid aortic valve		IMA	internal mammary artery
BH-TECAB	beating heart total endoscopic coronary bypass grafting		IRAD	International Registry of Acute Aortic Dissection
BIMA	bilateral internal mammary artery		ISDN	isosorbide dinitrate
BITA	bilateral internal thoracic artery		ITA	internal thoracic artery
BMI	body mass index		IVC	inferior vena cava
BOS	bronchiolitis obliterans syndrome		LA	left atrium
CABG	coronary artery bypass graft		LAA	left atrial appendage
CAD	coronary artery disease		LAD	left anterior descending artery
CF	continuous flow		LCC	left coronary cusp
CP	chordal procedure		LHB	left-sided heart bypass
CPB	cardiopulmonary bypass		LIMA	left internal mammary artery
CPR	cardiopulmonary resuscitation		LITA	left internal thoracic artery
CT	computed tomography		LRA	leaflet resection with an annuloplasty
DAPT	dual antiplatelet therapy		LV	left ventricular
DCD	donation after cardiac death		LVAD	left ventricular assist devices
DDAVP	desmopressin acetate		LVEDP	left ventricular end diastolic pressure
DES	drug-eluting stent			
DHCA	deep hypothermic circulatory arrest		LVEF	left ventricular ejection fraction
DLCO	diffusing capacity of the lungs for carbon monoxide		MACCE	major adverse cardiac and cerebrovascular events
DT	destination therapy		MCS	mechanical circulatory support
EACTS	European Association for Cardio-Thoracic Surgery		MI	myocardial infarction
ECGI	electrocardiographic imaging		MIDCAB	minimally invasive direct coronary bypass
ECMO	extracorporeal membrane oxygenation			

MIMVS	minimally invasive mitral valve surgery
MLD	minimal lumen diameter
MR	mitral regurgitation
MRA	magnetic resonance angiography
MV	mitral valve
MVST	multivessel small thoracotomy
NC	non-coronary
NCC	non-compaction cardiomyopathy
NIRS	near-infrared spectroscopy
NYHA	New York Heart Association
ONCAB	on-pump coronary artery bypass
OPCAB	off-pump coronary artery bypass
OR	operative room
PA	pulmonary artery
PAU	penetrating atherosclerotic ulcer
PCI	percutaneous coronary intervention
PDA	patent ductus arteriosus
PGD	primary graft dysfunction
PLA	posterolateral artery
PPM	patient–prosthesis mismatch
PTCA	percutaneous transluminal coronary angioplasty
PTFE	polytetrafluoroethylene
PTLD	post-transplantation lymphoproliferative disease
PV	pulmonary vein
PVI	pulmonary vein isolation
PVR	pulmonary vascular resistance
QoL	quality of life
RA	radial artery
RAA	right atrial appendage
RCA	right coronary artery
RCC	right coronary cusp
RCT	randomized controlled trial
RFA	radiofrequency ablation
RGEA	right gastroepiploic artery
RIMA	right internal mammary artery
RITA	right internal thoracic artery
RV	right ventricular
RVAD	right ventricular assist device
SAM	systolic anterior motion
SAN	sinoatrial node
SAVR	surgical aortic valve replacement
SCA	sudden cardiac arrest
STJ	sinotubular junction
STS	Society of Thoracic Surgeons
SV	stroke volume
SVC	superior vena cava
SVG	saphenous vein graft
SVST	single-vessel small thoracotomy direct-vision bypass grafting
TAAA	thoracoabdominal aortic aneurysm
TAVI	transcatheter aortic valve implantation
TECAB	totally endoscopic coronary artery bypass
TEE	transesophageal echocardiography
VAD	ventricular assist device
VAJ	ventriculo-aortic junction
VAS	ventricular assist system

List of Contributors

Ayyaz Ali
Assistant Professor,
Director of Heart Transplantation,
Department of Cardiac Surgery,
Yale School of Medicine,
Connecticut, USA

Johannes Bonatti
Chair of Cardiac Surgery,
Cleveland Clinic,
Abu Dhabi, United Arab Emirates

Munir Boodhwani
Associate Professor in the Division of
Cardiac Surgery at the University of
Ottawa Heart Institute,
Ottowa, Canada

W. Randolph Chitwood, Jr
Emeritus Professor and Founding
Director,
East Carolina Heart Institute,
North Carolina, USA

Joseph S. Coselli
Vice-Chair, Michael E. DeBakey
Department of Surgery,
Professor and Chief, Division of
Cardiothoracic Surgery,
Baylor College of Medicine,
Texas, USA;
Chief, Section of Adult Cardiac Surgery,
Texas Heart Institute,
Texas, USA

Ralph J. Damiano, Jr
Evarts A. Graham Professor and Surgery
Chief,
Division of Cardiothoracic Surgery,
Barnes-Jewish Hospital,
Missouri, USA

A. Marc Gillinov
Chairman,
Department of Thoracic and
Cardiovascular Surgery,
Cleveland Clinic,
Ohio, USA

David Glineur
Cardiac Surgeon,
University of Ottawa Heart Institute,
Ottawa, Canada

Michael E. Halkos
Associate Professor of Surgery,
Chief, Division of Cardiothoracic Surgery,
Emory University School of Medicine,
Georgia, USA

Jörg Kempfert
Consultant Cardiac Surgeon,
German Heart Center,
Berlin, Germany

Suresh Keshavamurthy
Assistant Professor of Surgery,
Temple University Hospital,
Philadelphia, USA

Gebrine El Khoury
Professor,
Department of Cardiac Surgery,
Clinique Saint-Luc,
Brussels, Belgium

Antigone Koliopoulou
Assistant Professor of Surgery,
Division of Cardiothoracic Surgery,
University of Utah,
Salt Lake City, USA

Robert L. Kormos
Brack G. Hattler Professor of
Cardiothoracic Transplantation,
UPMC Presbyterian, Pittsburgh,
Pennsylvania, USA

Stephen H. McKellar
Associate Professor of Surgery,
Division of Cardiothoracic Surgery,
University of Utah,
Salt Lake City, USA

Stephanie Mick
Thoracic and Cardiovascular Surgeon,
Cleveland Clinic,
Ohio, USA

Tomislav Mihaljevic
Department of Cardiothoracic Surgery,
Cleveland Clinic Abu Dhabi,
Abu Dhabi, United Arab Emirates

Emmanuel Moss
Assistant Professor of Surgery,
Jewish General Hospital/McGill
University,
Division of Cardiac Surgery,
Montreal, Canada

G. Alexander Patterson
Joseph Bancroft Professor of Surgery,
Washington University School of
Medicine,
Missouri, USA

Ourania Preventza
Associate Professor,
Michael E. DeBakey Department of
Surgery,
Division of Cardiothoracic Surgery,
Baylor College of Medicine,
Texas, USA;
Cardiac Surgeon,
Department of Cardiovascular Surgery,
Texas Heart Institute,
Texas, USA

Varun Puri
Associate Professor of Surgery,
Washington University School of Medicine,
Missouri, USA

John D. Puskas
Professor of Surgery (Cardiothoracic),
Chair of Cardiovascular Surgery,
Mount Sinai Saint Luke's Hospital,
New York, USA

Jason O. Robertson
Resident, Cardiothoracic Surgery,
Washington University,
St. Louis, Missouri, USA

Evelio Rodriguez
Chief of Cardiac Surgery,
Saint Thomas Health, Nashville,
Tennessee, USA

Lindsey L. Saint
Resident, Cardiothoracic Surgery,
Washington University, St. Louis,
Missouri, USA

Craig H. Selzman
Professor and Chief Division of
Cardiothoracic Surgery,
University of Utah,
Utah, USA

William E. Stansfield
Affiliate Scientist,
Toronto General Hospital Research
Institute,
Toronto, Canada

Thomas Walther
Director of the Department of Cardiac,
Thoracic and Thoracic Vascular Surgery,
Hospital of the Goethe University,
Frankfurt, Germany

Stephen Westaby
Surgeon,
Department of Cardiothoracic Surgery,
John Radcliffe Hospital,
Oxford, UK

Chapter 1

CABG conduits and graft configuration

David Glineur

Coronary artery bypass graft (CABG) conduits

Left internal thoracic artery (LITA)

Anatomy

The internal thoracic artery (ITA) supplies the anterior chest wall; it arises from the sub-clavian artery near its origin and travels downward inside the chest wall, approximately one centimeter from the edges of the sternum. It runs posterior to the internal intercostal muscles, but anterior to the transverse muscles. The ITA divides into the musculophrenic artery and the superior epigastric artery around the sixth intercostal space.

Histology

The major characteristic of the LITA is the presence of more elastic laminae com-pared to gastro-epiploic artery (GEA), inferior epigastric artery (IEA), or radial ar-tery (RA), which contain more smooth muscle cells in their walls and are therefore less elastic.[1]

Intima Both connective tissue and smooth muscle are present in the intima, the border of which is delineated by the internal elastic membrane. The internal elastic membrane may not be conspicuous due to the abundance of elastic material in the tunica media.

Media This is the thickest of the three layers. Smooth muscle cells are arranged in a spiral around the long axis of the vessel, and secrete elastin in the form of lamellae, which are fenestrated to facilitate diffusion. These lamellae, and the large size of the media, are the most striking histological features of elastic arteries. In addition to elastin, the smooth muscle cells of the media secrete reticular and fine collagen fibers and proteoglycans. No fibroblasts are present.

Adventitia This is a relatively thin connective tissue layer. Fibroblasts are the predom-inant cell type, and many macrophages are also present. Collagen fibers predominate and elastic fibers (not lamellae) are also present. The collagen in the adventitia prevents elastic arteries from stretching beyond their physiological limits during systole. Blood vessels supplying the adventitia and outer media, known as the vasa vasorum, are also present.

Endothelium function

Endothelium acts as an antithrombotic barrier as well as a modulator of vascular tone and growth. For these reasons, it is believed to be the milestone of the graft long-term patency. In response to a variety of agonists, endothelial cells generate three major autacoids that regulate vascular relaxation and other endothelium-dependent vascular functions[2]: nitric oxide (NO), prostacyclin (PGI2), and endothelium-derived hyperpolarizing factor (EDHF).

Lüscher and colleagues[3] studied endothelium-dependent relaxation in internal mammary arteries, internal mammary veins, and saphenous veins. Vascular rings with and without endothelium were suspended in organ chambers, and isometric tension was recorded. Acetylcholine, thrombin, and adenosine diphosphate evoked potent endothelium-dependent relaxation in the mammary artery but weak responses in the saphenous vein. In the mammary artery, relaxation was greatest in response to acetylcholine, followed by thrombin and adenosine diphosphate. In the saphenous and mammary veins, relaxation was less than 25%. Relaxation was unaffected by indomethacin but was inhibited by methylene blue and hemoglobin, suggesting that endothelium-derived relaxing factor was the mediator. Endothelium-independent relaxation in response to sodium nitroprusside was similar in arteries and veins. Lüscher concluded that endothelium-dependent relaxation was greater in the mammary artery than in the saphenous vein.

The specificity of the ITA explains why it is less damaged by arteriosclerosis compared to other arteries, a phenomenon that has been studied with an ultrasonic system.[4] This study revealed that the intima-media complex of the ITA is protected from the influence of arteriosclerosis, in comparison with the morphological changes found in the intima-media thickness of the common carotid artery. This demonstrated protective mechanism underlines the widespread use of the ITA as a CABG conduit.

In addition, β-adrenoceptor agonists do not induce a significant relaxation of the ITA, and the use of β-adrenoceptor antagonists do not lead to IMA vasospasm.[5]

Patency

Long-term LITA to the left anterior descending artery (LAD) patency is usually greater than 90% (range 83–98% in historical studies)[6–27] (Table 1.1). Factors known to potentially influence patency include the degree of preoperative proximal coronary stenosis, the time from CABG in non-LAD arteries, sex, date of surgery, target other than LAD, and smoking status.

Degree of coronary stenosis ITA graft patency decreased as proximal coronary stenosis decreased.[28] These findings are consistent with the physiology of arterial grafts. ITAs are able to autoregulate size and blood flow in response to demand. As proximal coronary stenosis decreases, competitive flow increases, and demand for ITA graft flow falls. This cascade of events results in ITA constriction and, over time, increased risk of atrophy and occlusion.[29–32]

Kawasuji and colleagues[33] performed angiography one month after CABG in 100 patients with ITA to LAD grafts; all grafts were patent, but 15% (2/13) of those performed to coronary arteries with 50% or less stenosis were severely constricted. Seki and colleagues[30] observed either severe constriction or occlusion in 9.5% (14/147) of ITA grafts

Table 1.1 Summary of different studies on LITA patency

First author	Year	Studied/ Operated	Percent studied	Interval	Graft patency (%)
Green[6]	1972	70/165	42	2 wk–3 y	97
Kay[7]	1974	91/628	14	19.5 mo	98
Barner[8]	1976	139/307	45	20 days	95
		139/307	45	13 mo	90
Tector[9]	1976	43/275	15	9–24 mo	95
Geha[10]	1979	175/208	82	2 wk	99
		?/208	49	6 mo–5 y	97
Tyras[11]	1980	527/765	69	1 mo	95
		?/765	65	1 y	93
		?/765	63	5 y	90
Lytle[12]	1980	46/100	46	20 mo	91
Tector[13]	1981	88/298	29	60–108 mo	94.40
Singh[14]	1983	34/	NA	3–12 y	94
Grondin[15]	1984	37/40	92	1 mo	97
		32/40	80	1 y	88
		20/40	50	10 y	84
Okies[16]	1984	259/4183	6	5 y, 10 y	83, 70
Lytle[17]	1985	140/?	NA	5 y	97
Loop[18]	1986	855/2306	37	8.7 y	96
Zeff[19]	1988	37/39	92	8.9 y	95
Ivert[20]	1988	91/99	92	2 wk	94
		84/99	85	1 y	90
		66/99	67	5y	89
Goldman[21]	1990	237/670	23	1 y	93
Fiore[22]	1990	182/200	91	13 y	82
Galbut[23]	1990	53/947	6	2 mo–15 y	92
Boylan[24]	1994	57/100	57	<10 y, >10 y	93, 90
Goldman[25]	1994	167/1,031	25	3 y	90
FitzGibbon[26]	1996	456/476	96	6 mo	95
		123/476	26	5 y	80
Gills[27]	1997	25/25	100	4–6 h	96

studied 16 days to 62 months after CABG. Two (14%) of these failed ITA grafts bypassed LADs with more than 50% stenosis, whereas 12 (86%) bypassed LADs with 50% or less proximal stenosis.

Target ITA patency is the most durable of grafts performed to the LAD, possibly because of the ease of anterior coronary arteries grafting, but also because the amount of myocardium supplied by the LAD is greater than that supplied by other coronary arteries, resulting in a larger blood flow demand. ITA grafts with greater blood flow demand are less likely to fail.[34] In contrast, Glineur et al.[35] could not find any significantly difference at 6 months between the right internal thoracic artery (RITA) directed to the lateral wall of the heart versus the LITA to the LAD territory (Table 1.2).

Gender Because of their smaller size, women have smaller coronary arteries than men. Technical difficulties associated with grafting small arteries are one possible cause of the higher operative risk observed in women, and may also be responsible for lower graft patency.[28]

Risk factors Smoking is strongly associated with progression of coronary artery disease (CAD), and patients who continue to smoke after CABG have a higher risk of return of angina, myocardial infarction, and coronary reintervention.[28] In addition, multivariable analysis revealed that a history of smoking decreased ITA graft diameter.[6] These effects on both coronary arteries and ITA grafts probably account for the lower graft patency we observed in smokers.[36]

Right internal thoracic artery (RITA)

Anatomy, histology, endothelium function

There are no significant differences between the left ITA and right ITA in terms of anatomy, histology, and endothelial function.[37] There were also no statistical differences between LITA and RITA concerning mean intimal diameter (1.52 ± 0.24 vs. 1.58 ± 0.28 mm, $P <0.06$), medial diameter (2.21 ± 0.27 vs. 2.52 ± 0.28 mm, $P <0.15$), or wall thickness (0.39 ± 0.12 vs. 0.41 ± 0.16 mm, $P <0.47$). The intimal diameters diminished significantly from the origins (1.69 ± 0.34 and 1.86 ± 0.41 mm, respectively) to the terminations (1.25 ± 0.26 and 1.14 ± 0.25 mm, respectively) of both vessels.

In order to determine whether endothelial function differs between left and right ITA segments in a Y-graft configuration, Glineur et al. studied 11 patients 3 years after surgery.[38] The endothelium-dependent vasodilator substance P was selectively infused (1.4 up to 22.4 pmol/min in doubling dose increments) in the ostium of ITA Y-grafts. A maximal endothelium-independent vasodilatory response was then obtained by intragraft infusion of 2 mg isosorbide dinitrate (ISDN).

A similar dose-dependent vasodilatory response to substance P was observed in the left and in the right ITA (Figure 1.1). No difference in maximal endothelium-dependent response to substance P (7.4 ± 4.3% in left ITA and 8.1 ± 5.3% in right ITA) or in maximal endothelium-independent response to ISDN (12.2 ± 4.4% in left ITA and 10.6 ± 8.1% in right ITA) was observed. The endothelium-dependent and the endothelium-independent

Table 1.2 RITA patency results

Studies cited within Glineur et al. (2008)[35]	Year	n	Methodology	Angiography no.	Mean follow-up	Angiographic patency rate (%)		Actuarial angiographic patency rate (%)	
						LIMA	RIMA	LIMA	RIMA
Dion (49)	1989	231	Retro Seque IMA grafts	157	6 mo	Overall IMA patency of 95%		Overall IMA patency of 95%	
Galbut (50)	1990	1,087	Retro	53	53 mo	92.1	84.9		
Fiore (51)	1990	200	Retro		13 y			82	85
Chocron (52)	1994	80	Retro BIMA Y	62	6–25 mo	97	63		
Tector (53)	1994	486	Retro BIMA T		Perioperative	98.3	86.5		
Barra (54)	1995	80	Retro BIMA Y	80	16 mo	93.4	85.2		
Gerola (55)	1996	201	Retro RIMA TS	36	51.6 mo	94.4	91.6		
					5 y			93.8	84.1
					10 y			93.8	84.1
Pick (56)	1997	320	Retro	84	6.9 y	88	75		
Tatoulis (57)	1997	1,454	Retro free RIMA	71	41.5 mo		94.5		
					5 y	96	89		
Ura (58)	1998	115	Retro RIMA TS	73	59 mo	92.3	89.9		
					6 y			94.5	89.3
Dion (59)	1999	500	Retro Seque IMA grafts	161	7.4 y	94.3% seque IMA anast patent		94.3% seque IMA anast patent	

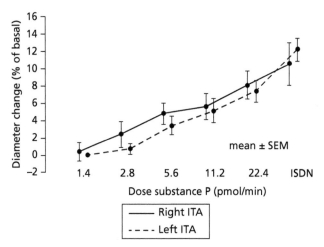

Figure 1.1 Comparison of vasomotion between free right internal thoracic artery (RITA) and *in situ* left internal thoracic artery (LITA).

Reprinted from Glineur D *et al.* (2011) Endothelium-dependent and endothelium-independent vasodilator response of left and right internal mammary and internal thoracic arteries used as a composite Y-graft European Journal of Cardio-Thoracic Surgery 40(2):389–93 with permission from Oxford University Press on behalf of the European Association for Cardio-Thoracic Surgery

vasodilator capacity of the two branches of a Y-graft ITA configuration appear similar 3 years after bypass surgery, suggesting that the preservation of the ITA pedicle did not significantly affect basal vasomotor tone, long-term endothelial function, or vasodilator reserve.

Patency The widely accepted success of the LITA has led to the use of both ITAs, although the RITA, used as an *in situ* or free graft, has never become as popular as the LITA. The apparent difference in the clinical and angiographic performance between the two ITAs was thought to be more related to the technical and flow-dynamic mechanisms than to their intrinsic characteristics.[39–40]

The overall patency of the RITA grafts to the left system is almost identical with that of LITA grafts (Table 1.3).[41–44] This observation is not surprising, considering that both ITAs have identical histopathology.[45–46]

The target artery grafted affected patency of both ITA, with maximum patency when grafted to the LAD. Grafts to the non-LAD arteries were at higher risk with the worst patency seen in the right coronary artery (RCA) territory.

In a recent angiographic study, Glineur *et al.* observed[35] (Table 1.3) an excellent patency rate with no significant difference between the *in situ* or Y-shape use of the RITA. However, there was a significant difference with a larger number of arterial anastomosis allowed by the bilateral internal thoracic artery (BITA) Y-configuration. Long-term follow-up will help determine whether the larger number of ITA distal anastomosis allowed by the use of the Y-graft configuration translates into a superior late clinical outcome.

In a secondary analysis of this population, Glineur *et al.* evaluated the angiographic parameters influencing the function of the RITA used in a Y-graft configuration.[45] In multivariate analysis, the function of the RITA was positively influenced by the number of anastomoses (OR = 0.5, 95% CI: 0.4–0.7), and a severely narrowed first circumflex

Table 1.3 Six-month systematic angiographic control

	BITA Y n = 146	BITA *in situ* n = 126	P value
ITA anastomosis angiographic patency control			
	Patent/total	Patent/total	
LIMA	190/197 (96%)	166/169 (98%)	0.96
Diagonal	49/51	43/43	0.55
LAD	141/146	123/126	0.88
RIMA	260/267 (97%)	121/126 (96%)	0.69
Intermediate	10/10	1/1	
OM1	135/137	120/125	0.37
OM2	81/84		
PLA	17/19		
PDA	17/17		
Total	450/464 (97%)	287/295 (97%)	0.99
Complementary graft anastomosis patency control			
	Patent/total	Patent/total	
RGEA	27/30 (90%)	32/38 (84%)	0.73
SVG	57/59 (97%)	71/76 (93%)	0.66

BITA, bilateral internal thoracic artery; ITA, internal thoracic artery; LIMA, left internal mammary artery; RIMA, right internal mammary artery; RGEA, right gastroepiploic artery; SVG, saphenous vein graft; LAD, left anterior descending artery; OM1, obtuse marginal 1; OM2, obtuse marginal 2; PLA, posterolateral artery; PDA, posterodescending artery

Reprinted from Glineur *et al.* (2008) Comparison of Bilateral Internal Thoracic Artery Revascularization Using In Situ or Y Graft Configurations. *Circulation* 118(14):S216–S221 with permission from the American Heart Association.

(OR = 39.1, CI: 8.1–189.2) and negatively by the presence of a grafted intermediate coronary artery (OR = 0.01, CI: 0.003–0.06), and of a grafted RCA (OR = 0.08, CI: 0.02–0.35). The size of targeted vessel, history of infarction, and regional myocardial function did not influence RITA function.

In a recently published meta-analysis, Yi *et al.*[46] confirmed that use of both mammary arteries in coronary revascularization already allowed survival benefit after 10 years of follow-up. Despite those long-term reported data, RITA remains widely underused.

Right gastroepiploic artery (RGEA)

Anatomy

The RGEA is a branch of the gastro-duodenal artery, which in turn diverges from the common hepatic artery, and thus is the fourth branch of the abdominal aorta. The RGEA runs from right to left along the greater curvature of the stomach, between the layers of the greater omentum, anastomosing with the left gastroepiploic branch of the splenic artery. This vessel gives off numerous branches: the gastric branches that ascend to supply both surfaces of the stomach, and the omental branches that descend to supply the greater omentum and anastomose with branches of the middle colic. This anatomical fact is crucial because coronary blood supply is determined by a pressure gradient between the aorta and the left ventricle; thus, the driving pressure of the RGEA could be lower than other graft (*in situ* ITA or free aorto-coronary graft).

Histology

The RGEA is a more muscular artery than the internal mammary artery (IMA). Smooth muscle fibers are plentiful in the media of the GEA but rare in the IMA, and elastic fibers are more plentiful in the media of the IMA than the GEA. Suma and associates reported that the RGEA has slightly more intimal thickening than the ITA, but significant luminal narrowing caused by arteriosclerosis is rare; however, one RGEA out of 35 (3%) showed overt arteriosclerosis in a patient with associated aortoiliac occlusive disease.[47]

Endothelium function

Experimental data obtained *in vivo* has demonstrated similarities in endothelial function between rings of GEAs and IMAs,[48–50] suggesting that this concept of a protective role of the endothelium contributing to the greater long-term patency rate of mammary arteries may also be applicable to GEAs. Globally similar endothelium-independent and endothelium-dependent relaxation phenomena were observed in response to several substances such as acetylcholine, metacholine, substance P, and histamine, but a much more pronounced contractility was observed in response to norepinephrine or potassium chloride in gastroepiploic than in mammary arteries, which may explain its propensity to spasm.

Cremer *et al.*[51] evaluated endothelium-dependent relaxation *in vivo* by measuring intraoperatively the intraluminal graft pressure at mechanically controlled constant flow rates. They observed a favorable vasodilatory response to acetylcholine in IMAs, but no reaction in GEAs. Hanet *et al.*[52] observed vasoconstriction in GEA grafts in contrast to no vasoconstriction in ITAs in response to methylergometrine.

Patency

The early graft patency rate of the GEA is comparable to that of the ITA, whereas the 10-year patency rate of the GEA is inferior to that of the ITA (Table 1.4).[53–69] Flow competition between the GEA and the coronary artery could be one of the major factors affecting graft patency. The patency rates of the RGEA and the RA are highly dependent on the degree of stenosis of the native vessel, and RGEA use remains limited due to its association with a high risk of graft failure from competitive flow. The flow capacity of the RGEA under maximal stress conditions has also been questioned.[70] For these reasons, the GEA gives an excellent clinical performance when implanted for severe coronary artery stenosis.

Glineur *et al.* reported similar results.[71–72] minimal lumen diameter (MLD) values for RCA stenosis of 0.77–1.4 mm and percent stenosis approximately 48–64% appear to discriminate between functional and non-functional RGEA.

Radial artery (RA)

Anatomy

The radial artery arises from the bifurcation of the brachial artery in the cubital fossa, running distally on the anterior part of the forearm. There, it marks the division between

Table 1.4 Six-month graft function according to approximate quartiles of angiographic characteristics of the grafted coronary vessel

Grafted RCA	RGEA (90 patients)	SVG (82 patients)
MLD (mm)	Functional grafts, n (% of MLD category)	
0	36 (100)	33 (94)
0.01–0.76	7 (88)	7 (78)
0.77–1.40	13 (50)	13 (81)
>1.40	1 (5)	17 (77)
% Stenosis	Functional grafts, n (% of stenosis category)	
100	36 (100)	33 (94)
99–65	11 (92)	7 (88)
64–48	8 (33)	16 (84)
<48	2 (11)	14 (70)

RGEA, Right gastroepiploic artery; SVG, saphenous vein graft; PDA, posterior descending artery; PLA, posterolateral artery; RCA, right coronary artery. Patency grades: 0 = not patent; 1 = balanced: patent but not functioning, when the flow from the native coronary artery is dominant or when flow supply from the native coronary and from the graft is balanced; 2 = fully patent.

Reprinted from Glineur *et al.* (2008) Angiographic Predictors of 6-Month Patency of Bypass Grafts Implanted to the Right Coronary Artery A Prospective Randomized Comparison of Gastroepiploic Artery and Saphenous Vein Grafts. *J Am Coll Cardiol.* 51(2):120–5 with permission from the American Heart Association.

the anterior and posterior compartments of the forearm, with the posterior compartment beginning just lateral to the artery. The artery winds laterally around the wrist, passing through the anatomical snuffbox and between the heads of the first dorsal interosseous muscle. It passes anteriorly between the heads of the adductor pollicis and becomes the deep palmar arch, which joins with the deep branch of the ulnar artery. Along its course, the RA is accompanied by the radial vein.

The most frequently encountered distal anatomical variation of the RA is a rather sizable palmar branch located in a more superficial plane than the tendon of the flexor carpi radialis muscle, situated on its radial side before turning to the dorsum of the hand at the distal extremity of the radius. Their incidence has been reported at between 1% and 15%, depending on their location in the upper or lower forearm, respectively.

Histology

On microscopic analysis, the wall of the RA is significantly thicker than the wall of the ITA, due to an increased thickness of the three layers (intima, media, adventitia).

Intima

The intima of the RA is constituted of one layer of endothelial cells above multiple layers of subendothelial cells. The internal elastic lamina is well-individualized, presenting multiple fenestrations.

Media

The elements found in the media are the same in the RA and ITA: leiomyocytes, elastic fibers, collagen fibers, and few fibroblasts and fibroblast-derived cells. However, architectural differences exist between the media of both arteries; in the RA, the myocytes are organized in multiple tight layers. Due to this dense myocyte architecture, the connective tissue seems rarefied. In the ITA, myocytes are larger and irregular in shape, and are less organized with a loose structure, making the elastic fibers and ground substance appear more abundant. Interestingly, the ratio of the thickness of media/intima is higher in the mammary artery compared to the RA (4 and 3, respectively). The external elastic lamina is identical in both arteries, is less individualized than the internal elastic lamina, and presents large fenestrations.

Adventitia

The adventitia is constituted of connective tissue containing fibroblasts and macrophages. The vasa vasorum accompanied by nerves and lymphatic vessels are exclusively located in the adventitia. This layer is thicker in the RA.

Endothelial function

As a muscular artery, the RA graft is susceptible to vasospasm, which was thought to be the principal cause of early graft failure.[73] Numerous studies have revealed that the RA has a higher receptor-mediated contractility compared with the IMA, and human RA is an α-adrenoceptor dominant artery with weak β-adrenoceptor function.[73-77] In addition, the RA exhibits greater contraction in response to potassium chloride, serotonin, and norepinephrine than the IMA. These aspects of the RA may contribute to its vasospastic characteristics. When a comparison was made of nitric oxide (NO) release and EDHF-mediated hyperpolarization for IMA and RA, the basal and stimulated releases of NO and EDHF-mediated hyperpolarization in the IMA were significantly greater than those in the RA.[78] The lower level of NO basal release, the reduced and shorter period of stimulated NO release, and the lower EDHF-mediated hyperpolarization in the RA may account for the predisposition of RA graft to the perioperative vasospasm, and may have an impact on the early and long-term results of the graft patency.[78]

Patency

Initially described in 1973,[79] RA grafting was soon abandoned because reports documented dismal early angiographic outcomes. However, improvements in graft harvesting techniques, avoidance of mechanical dilation, new preservation methods, and the use of postoperative calcium channel blocker therapy to prevent early vasospasm led to a improvements in RA graft patency and resurgence in the use of the RA as a bypass graft in the 1990s.

Prospective randomized control trials and meta-analyses[80-87] comparing radial and saphenous vein graft (SVG) patency reached the following conclusions: RA patency is comparable to SVG patency in the short term, but is superior over both the medium and long term (Table 1.5).[88] This was most recently demonstrated by Gaudino and the *RADIAL Investigators* (2018), in their landmark patient-level meta-analysis of over 1000 patients. They found that the RA graft occlusion rate of 8.1% was significantly decreased compared to the SVG graft occlusion rate of 19.9% (HR 0.44; 95% CI 0.28–0.70; $P < 0.001$). Finally, a prospective study

Table 1.5 Results of major studies on radial artery patency

Randomized control trial	<1 year	<5 year	>5 year
Desai (2004) RAPS	Occlusion: RA 8.2%, SVG 13.6% ($P = 0.009$)		
Collins (2008) RSVP		Patency: RA 98.3%, SVG 86.4% ($P = 0.04$)	
Hayward (2010) RAPCO			Patency: RA 90.0%, SVG 87.0% ($P = 0.29$)
Goldman (2011)	Patency: RA 89.0%, SVG 89.0% ($P = 0.98$)		
Deb (2012) RAPS			Complete occlusion: RA 8.9%, SVG 18.6% ($P = 0.002$)
Meta-analysis			
Benedetto (2010)		Failure: RA 14.1%, SVG 14.6% ($P = 0.372$)	
Hu (2011)		Occlusion: RA vs. SVG: RR 0.507 (95% CI 0.41–0.63, $P < 0.05$)	
Athanasiou (2011)	Patency: RA vs. SVG: OR 1.04 (95% CI 0.68–1.61, $P = 0.84$)	Patency: RA vs. SVG: OR 2.06 (95% CI 1.29–3.29, $P = 0.002$)	Patency: RA vs. SVG: OR 2.28 (95% CI 1.32–3.94, $P = 0.003$)
Deb (2012)			Occlusion: RA vs. SVG: OR, 0.52 (95% CI, 0.34–0.79; $P = 0.002$)
Cao (2012)	Complete patency: RA 79.2%, SVG 82.5% (OR 0.79, $P = 0.33$)	Complete patency: RA 89.9%, SVG 63.1% (OR 5.19, $P < 0.0001$)	
Gaudino (2018)			Occlusion: RA 8.1%, SVG 19.9% ($P < 0.001$)

Data sourced from Gaudino M, Benedetto U, Fremes S et al. (2018) Radial-Artery or Saphenous-Vein Grafts in Coronary-Artery Bypass Surgery. N Engl J Med. 2018 May 31;378(22):2069–2077. doi: 10.1056/NEJMoa1716026 and Gaudino M, Tondi P, Benedetto U, et al. Radial Artery as a Coronary Artery Bypass Conduit: 20-Year Results. J Am Coll Cardiol. 2016 Aug 9;68(6):603–610. doi: 10.1016/j.jacc.2016.05.062.

with 20-year follow-up by Gaudino and colleagues[88] found a long-term patency of 84.8% with superior patency compared to SVG grafting.

Several factors affect the RA graft patency:

a) The severity of the target coronary artery lesion is a major predictor of RA patency because of its effect on competitive flow. RA patency decreases in correlation with the decrease of the target coronary stenosis. The less stenosed the less patent.[89] The cut off for RA use has been placed above 85% of stenosis.

b) Skeletonization may improve patency at up to 1-year follow-up (96.5–100% vs. 77.5–86.7%).[90] However, this improvement may result from using an ultrasonic scalpel, which has been associated with significantly increased RA blood flow.[91]

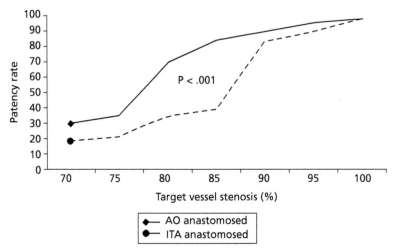

Figure 1.2 Mid-term patency rate of radial artery grafts in relation to the site of proximal anastomosis and the severity of target vessel stenosis.

Reprinted from Gaudino *et al.* (2004) Effect of target artery location and severity of stenosis on mid-term patency of aorta-anastomosed vs. internal thoracic artery-anastomosed radial artery grafts. European Journal of Cardio-Thoracic Surgery 25(3):424–8 with permission from Oxford University Press on behalf of the European Association for Cardio-Thoracic Surgery

c) The proximal site of anastomosis influences the patency of the RA graft. The RA can be anastomosed as an aortocoronary graft or as a composite graft from the LITA. Jung and colleagues[92] stated that increased drive pressure from a direct aortic anastomosis would improve flow through the RA when compared with anastomosis to the left internal mammary artery (LIMA). Gaudino and colleagues[93] studied the same phenomenon. They concluded that ITA-anastomosed RA grafts seem to be more vulnerable to the detrimental effect of chronic native competitive flow than aorta-anastomosed conduits; Y-grafts should then probably be reserved to target vessels with subocclusive stenosis (Figure 1.2).

d) Sequential grafting improves the RA patency,[94-95] especially in coronary targets of less than 1.5 mm diameter and with poor distal runoff.

Saphenous vein graft (SVG)

Since the late 1960s,[96] CABG using saphenous vein conduits has been championed as the solution to CAD. However, it was soon evident that CABG provides only palliation to an ongoing process that is further complicated by the rapid development of vein graft atherosclerosis.

Early thrombosis and neointimal hyperplasia with subsequent atherosclerosis are thought to be the primary causes of graft failure. The cause of this failure may stem from thrombosis within the vein graft, caused by a combination of structural and physiological alterations in the vessel wall.

Neointimal hyperplasia, defined as the accumulation of smooth muscle cells and extracellular matrix in the intimal compartment of the vein, is the major disease process in venous grafts within the first year. Nearly all veins implanted into the arterial circulation develop intimal wall thickening within 4–6 weeks, thereby reducing the lumen size. Smooth muscle cells in the media of normal adult arteries proliferate at a very low rate (<0.1%/day) but can switch very rapidly from quiescence to a proliferative state in response to appropriate stimuli.[97]

Injury to the intima results in migration and proliferation of smooth muscle cells from the media to the intima. The resulting luminal narrowing of the vein graft is not usually flow-limiting in itself. However, over time the area of neointimal hyperplasia may become an atherosclerosis-prone region that may lead to subsequent stenosis (Box 1.1).[98]

Anatomy

The SVG is the large (subcutaneous) superficial vein of the leg and thigh. The SVG originates from the joining of the dorsal vein of the first digit and the dorsal venous arch of the foot. After passing anterior to the medial malleolus (where it often can be visualized and palpated), it runs up the medial side of the leg. At the knee, it runs over the posterior border of the medial epicondyle of the femur bone. The SVG then courses laterally to lie on the anterior surface of the thigh before entering the saphenous opening in the fascia lata. It joins with the femoral vein in the region of the femoral triangle at the saphenofemoral junction.

Histology

Intima This intima consists of the endothelium and a thin subendothelial layer with smooth muscle cells among the connective tissue elements. A thin internal elastic membrane may or may not be present; if present, it is not nearly as prominent as in arteries.

Media This media is much thinner relative to that of an artery, and consists mostly of circularly arranged smooth muscle and collagen fibers. The tunica intima and media therefore tend to be less distinct from one another than is the case in arteries.

Adventitia The adventitia is usually thicker than the media and is made up mostly of collagen fibers. It may contain longitudinally oriented smooth muscle bundles.

Box 1.1 Pathogenesis of venous coronary artery bypass graft (CABG)

Phase I: Acute thrombotic phase (<1 month)

Phase II: Intimal hyperplasia (1–12 months)

- Hyperplasia of smooth muscle cells in the media
- Smooth muscle cell migration from the media to the intima
- Smooth muscle cell proliferation and extracellular matrix production

Phase III: Atherosclerosis (>3 years)

Endothelial function The superiority of the IMA over the SVG is thought to result from favorable biological properties of the endothelium to protect this vessel against vasospasm, thrombus formation, and atherosclerosis.

Unlike ITA grafts, SVGs constrict in response to ergotamine (ERGO) and do not dilate in response to ISDN.[99] These differences in vasomotor response could reflect heterogeneity in the sensitivity of vascular smooth muscle to these agents or differences in the basal level of vasomotor tone.

Patency It is estimated that during the first year after coronary bypass surgery, 10–15% of venous grafts occlude.[100–101] The graft attrition rate has been estimated at 1–2% per year between 1 and 6 years, and at 4% per year between 6 and 10 years after surgery. By 10 years after surgery, approximately 60% of the vein grafts are patent; only 50% of these patent vein grafts remain free of significant stenosis.

The following list describes the relationship of patient variables to graft patency:

1. Younger age and left ventricular ejection fraction <30% significantly reduced graft patency.[102] A possible explanation is that younger patients have a higher prevalence of risk factors (such as smoking and cholesterol) and more severe coronary disease. Reduced ejection fraction may indicate large areas of infarcted myocardium with poor distal runoff.

2. Year of operation significantly affected graft patency. For any given angiogram interval, more recently performed operations were associated with better graft patency. This observation could be due to routine use of aspirin, vigorous treatment with cholesterol-lowering agents, and the improved harvesting, preparation, and storage techniques that have evolved over the last three decades. Aspirin (325 mg/d) is associated with improved SVG patency during the first year after surgery.[103] The Post–coronary Bypass Graft Trial[104] demonstrated that aggressive decreasing of low-density lipoprotein cholesterol to <100 mg/dL decreased obstructive changes in SVGs by 31%. Harvesting, preparation, and storing techniques significantly affect graft patency.[105]

3. The interval from operation to angiogram significantly affected graft patency. Graft patency of angiograms studied at less than 1 year, 1–4 years, 5–9 years, 10–14 years, and >15 years was 78%, 78%, 60%, 50%, and 50%, respectively.

Operative variables were related to graft patency as follows:

1. The target coronary artery grafted significantly affected graft patency. Grafts to the RCA had the worst patency, and those to the LAD had the best patency. The order of increasing patency was RCA > obtuse marginal artery > posterior descending artery > diagonal > LAD.[106]

2. Target coronary artery diameter significantly affected graft patency with endarterectomy presenting the worst patency.[107] The most likely reason is that a large-diameter vessel has a better runoff and, therefore, better graft patency.

3. Conduit diameter significantly affected graft patency.[102] Large-diameter veins were associated with worse graft patency; better graft patency was associated with smaller conduit size.

4. Conduit wall thickness showed a trend toward affecting graft patency.[102] The conduit wall thickness was graded as thick, normal, and thin. A thick wall was defined as >1.5 mm, normal as 1.0–1.5 mm, and thin as <1.0 mm. Thick-walled veins were associated with worst graft patency. Poor results that followed the use of large-diameter and thick-walled saphenous veins may stem from low-velocity flow within the conduit, leading to deposition of oxidized low-density lipoprotein in the graft wall.

5. Target coronary artery stenosis was not significantly associated with graft patency.[108] Venous grafts, as opposed to arterial grafts, are less susceptible to spasm and are less affected by competitive flow and autoregulation.

6. Distal anastomosis type, that is, end to side or side-to-side (sequential), was associated with better graft patency with the latter.[109–110]

Graft configuration

Strategies to revascularize the left coronary system

BITAs have clearly demonstrated their superiority over all other types of grafts in terms of patency, freedom from arteriosclerosis, and survival benefit for revascularization of the left coronary system. Several meta-analyses have demonstrated the benefits of BITA *vs.* single ITA (SITA) grafting. Seven to ten years of follow-up were required before the advantages of BITA grafting were apparent,[111] but from 10 to 20 years, the benefits of BITA are statistically and clinically significant (Figure 1.3). However, even if the ideal graft has clearly been demonstrated, the method of use is still controversial. Therefore, several configurations of BITA have been proposed to achieve complete left-sided myocardial revascularization.

There are two major BITA assembly strategies to revascularize the left coronary system with two ITA: *in situ* and free:

1a. *In situ* LITA to the LAD territory and *in situ* RITA to the circumflex territory through the transverse sinus (Figure 1.4a);

1b. *In situ* RITA to the LAD and *in situ* LITA to the circumflex territory (Figure 1.4b);

2a. *In situ* LITA to the LAD territory and free RITA implanted in a Y or T fashion into the LITA (Figure 1.4c);

2b. *In situ* LITA to the LAD territory and free RITA implanted in the aorta (Figure 1.4d).

1a. *In situ* LITA to the LAD territory and *in situ* RITA to the circumflex territory through the transverse sinus (TS)

Advantages:

a) Each ITA is used *in situ* and therefore is able to consistently provide sufficient blood flow to each target vessel;

b) The RITA does not cross the mid-line of the chest in front of the aorta in case of redo sternotomy or aortic valve surgery.[112–115]

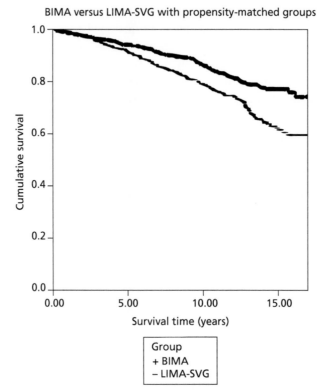

Figure 1.3 Kaplan–Meier survival curves comparing propensity-matched bilateral internal mammary artery (BIMA) and LIMA-SVG patients ($P <0.0001$).

Reprinted from Grau *et al.* (2012) Propensity matched analysis of bilateral internal mammary artery versus single left internal mammary artery grafting at 17-year follow-up: validation of a contemporary surgical experience. European Journal of Cardio-Thoracic Surgery 41(4):770–5 with permission from Oxford University Press on behalf of the European Association for Cardio-Thoracic Surgery

Disadvantages:

a) When using the RITA through the TS, the length used to cross the chest to reach the circumflex territory enables the grafting of medial or distal marginal branches;

b) In order to reach the proximal marginal or intermediate artery, the entire length of the RITA until its distal bifurcation is necessary. Therefore, the RITA anastomotic site is often small and very muscular, which has been identified as a factor leading to worse patency;

c) The possibilities of making sequential anastomosis is poor due to the short RITA length;

d) If multiple marginal branches have to be grafted, it is necessary to use another graft such as the radial graft or SVG. Glineur *et al.*[37] compared *in situ* RITA *vs.* free RITA found that the total number of graft anastomosis performed per patient was similar in both groups. However, the composite BITA Y-configuration allowed the right ITA

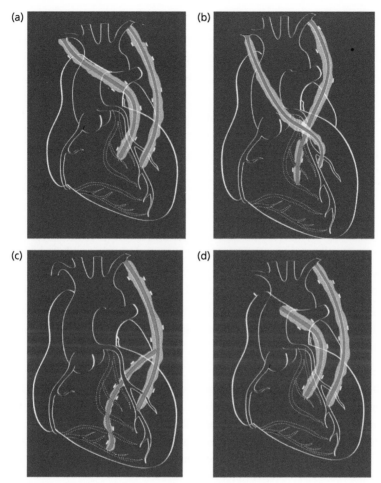

Figure 1.4 Different bilateral internal thoracic artery (BITA) assembling.
Image courtesy of the University of Ottawa Heart Institute

to reach more distal marginal branches and, in some cases, the posterolateral artery (PLA) or the patent ductus arteriosus (PDA); consequently, the number of graft anastomoses performed with ITA was significantly larger in the BITA Y group than in the BITA *in situ* group. Consequently, a larger number of complementary grafts were used in the BITA *in situ* group.

1b. *In situ* RITA to the LAD and *in situ* LITA to the circumflex territory

Advantages:

a) Each ITA is used *in situ* and therefore is able to consistently provide sufficient blood flow to each target vessel;

b) The LITA can revascularize several branches of the circumflex system, avoiding the need for an accessory graft for the circumflex system.

Disadvantages:

a) The RITA crosses the mid-line of the chest in front of the aorta, increasing the risk of graft injury during redo or aortic valve surgery;

b) If the LAD is very diseased and needs to be grafted distally, it is not always possible with the RITA;

c) It is very difficult to perform a sequential grafting of the diagonal and LAD with the RITA used in such configuration because of the shortage of length.

2a. *In situ* LITA to the LAD territory and free RITA implanted in a Y or T fashion into the LITA

Composite Y-graft configurations using the free RITA graft anastomosed proximally to the LITA have been widely used.[116]

Advantages:

a) This assembly allows a complete myocardial revascularization with two ITAs without a complementary graft;

b) RITA does not cross the mid-line in case of redo sternotomy or aortic valve surgery;

c) There is often no need to completely harvest the RITA in this assembly, decreasing the risk of wound complications by keeping a substantial residual blood supply in the lower half of the right hemisternum.

Disadvantages:

a) The ability of this arrangement to completely revascularize the coronary system, including the RCA, has been controversial. It has been questioned whether a single ITA can consistently provide sufficient blood flow, especially in the composite Y-graft to three territories. Royse *et al.*[117] reported that a composite Y-graft configuration led to a 75% increase in the free flow through a single ITA pedicle, and that the composite Y-graft had considerable potential for flow reserve.

b) There is a theoretical possibility of a "steal phenomenon" (the diversion of blood flow from a high resistance to a low resistance branch during hyperemia), resulting in a fall in the perfusion pressure in one branch of the Y assembly during periods of maximal myocardial blood flow demand.

Glineur *et al.* studied the "steal phenomenon" and completeness of revascularization with this configuration by measuring the fractional flow reserve (FFR) and the pressure drops in both branches of the composite configuration at rest and during maximal hyperemia.[118] They demonstrated that a Y-graft arterial configuration with a free RITA attached to an *in situ* LITA allowed adequate revascularization of the entire left coronary system with an even distribution of perfusion pressure in both distal branches, with minimal resistance to maximal blood flow. The resulting gradual decrease in pressure along the graft was negligible under basal conditions, and remained small during maximal hyperemia induced by coronary arteriolar vasodilation. Not surprisingly, most of the pressure drop observed during hyperemia occurred across the common part of the Y-graft where the blood flow is maximal. In addition, the conductance of both branches of the Y-graft, as assessed by FFR, appeared identical, excluding the possibility of a steal phenomenon.

c) A third possible disadvantage of the BITA Y-configuration is the increased risk of competitive flow in the composite graft compared with the *in situ* graft. Indeed, in such assemblies the mechanism of competitive flow is more complex than in the individual graft, where the interaction is only between the proximal inflow and the distal anastomosis outflow. In this sequential composite bypass, the interaction is also between all the anastomosed branches within the composite graft, leading to a phasic delay between the pressure waves in the grafts and in the coronary arteries, especially in the more distant ones such as the RCA. Nakajima *et al.*[119] found that the most significant predictor of competitive flow and graft occlusion was the presence of a moderately stenotic branch in the RCA territory. Glineur *et al.* analyzed the functioning of the right internal mammary artery (RIMA) in a Y-graft assembling, and found that the function of the RITA was significantly improved when used on several branches of the circumflex artery or on a severely narrowed (>70%) first circumflex and negatively by the presence of a grafted RCA.[120]

d) The RITA arrangement for the intermediate branch grafting can be problematic when multiple grafting on the lateral wall of the heart is needed. Indeed, Glineur found that grafting a coronary branch in the intermediate region had a negative prognostic influence on RITA function.[120] Some of these arrangements may cause kinking of the intermediate anastomosis, especially if the proximal Y anastomosis is performed near the pulmonary artery region or inside of the pericardium (Figure 1.5a). As a result of this finding, Glineur proposed several solutions to avoid kinking on the intermediate branch: (a) perform a proximal T anastomoses on the LITA (Figure 1.5b); (b) use a

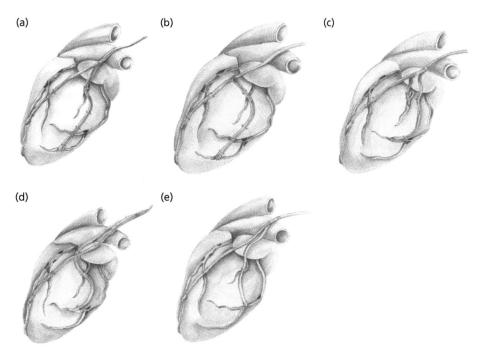

(a) (b) (c)

(d) (e)

Figure 1.5 Different Y-graft composite assembling.
Image courtesy of the University of Ottawa Heart Institute

second small Y-graft to prevent seagull kinking (Figure 1.5c); (c) perform the proximal composite anastomosis of a free RITA on the LITA very high on the LITA in order to obtain a smooth curve of the RITA to the intermediate branch (Figure 1.5d); and (d) perform an L/L anastomosis on the intermediate, and a T anastomosis on the circumflex artery (Figure 1.5e). It must be noted that, the latter three solutions decrease the available length of the RITA to the distal marginal branches or RCA branches.

2b. *In situ* LITA to the LAD territory and free RITA implanted in the aorta:

Advantages:

a) This configuration allows to do multiples anastomosis with the RITA on the lateral wall of the heart;

b) The RITA in this configuration is able to consistently provide sufficient blood flow to each target vessel;

c) The risk of competition flow is decreased in this configuration due to the high pulsatility wave generated by the direct reimplantation in the aorta.

Disadvantages:

a) The reimplantation of the RITA in the aorta requires aortic manipulation;

b) There is often a large discrepancy between the aorta and the RITA. For this reason, some authors have proposed the use of a vein or pericardial patch on the aorta to decrease this mismatch;

C) The patency of RITA reimplanted on the aorta is less than when used *in situ*.[121]

Strategies to revascularize the right coronary system

Left and right coronary systems exhibit distinct physiological flow patterns and different patterns of atheromatous disease, which, for example, may account for poorer patency of an *in situ* RITA grafted to the RCA compared with a left-sided target. Therefore, selection of the optimal conduit for the RCA or its branches cannot simply be extrapolated from data arising from left-sided or mixed targets.

The conduits used for revascularization of the RCA system include the saphenous vein, the RITA *in situ*, or in a Y-composite arrangement, the free RA reimplanted in the aorta or used as a composite graft, and the RGEA. The influence of clinical results on the choice of conduit type remains unclear, and the complementary conduit of choice to this system has yet to be determined. No superior patency rate for any one of these grafts to the RCA has been established.[122–123] The use of the RA or RGEA as the conduit for moderate stenosis of the RCA is limited due to its association with a high risk of graft failure owing to competitive flow. Limited flow capacity of the RGEA has also been reported.[124]

Hadinata and colleagues[125] reported absolute patency rates of 83.6% for the RA and 76.5% for the stroke volume (SV) targeted on the RCA; these patencies are lower than the latest reported patency rates of "Radial Artery Patency and Clinical Outcomes" (RAPCO) patients (90% for RA and 82% for SVG) on a 5-year average follow-up.[126] Possible explanations for these differences include: (a) longer mean duration of follow-up may lead to a later drop off in patency; (b) the RCA is likely a smaller target artery and has a smaller territory of runoff than the majority of the RAPCO study grafts, most of which were directed to the left side (indicating that the RCA was thought by the surgeon to be a lower-order target); (c) competitive flow in native vessel stenosis of at least 80% is a significant risk factor in RA graft failure on the right side[125]; (d) Tatoulis and colleagues[127] demonstrated that competitive flow in native vessel stenosis of at least 80% is a significant risk factor in RA graft failure on the right side, which may be more frequent a problem than on the left side, thereby reducing mean RA patency to the RCA territory; (e) with regards to reporting of results, symptom-directed studies may underestimate overall patency rates compare to protocol-directed angiography.

An important factor in the choice of graft conduit is the analysis of the coronary lesion. In addition to maximal percent stenosis, we use minimum lumen diameter as a surrogate for competitive flow. Maximum percent stenosis is not as good a measure of competitive flow as minimum lumen diameter; competitive flow through a 50% stenosed, 5-mm RCA must be greater than through a similarly stenosed 2-mm artery. Using only maximal coronary artery stenosis does not adjust for coronary artery size, whereas minimum lumen diameter does.

Glineur *et al.* enrolled 172 consecutive patients for coronary revascularization. Revascularization of the RCA was randomly performed with SVG in 82 patients and RGEA in 90 patients. All patients underwent a systematic angiographic control six months after surgery. They found that a measure above a third quartile (0.77–1.4 mm) or a stenosis of less than 55% predicted an unfavorable flow pattern in RGEA but not in SVG at six-month follow-up. In these stenosis of intermediate severity, the SVG is preferred to the RGEA or the RITA (Figure 1.6).

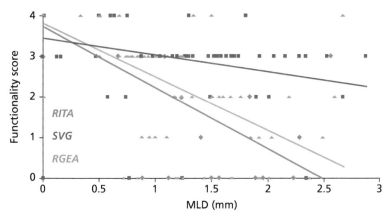

Figure 1.6 In these stenosis of intermediate severity, the saphenous vein graft (SVG, shown in blue) is preferred to the right gastroepiploic artery (RGEA, shown in green) or the right internal thoracic artery (RITA).

Adapted from Glineur *et al.* (2011) Angiographic predictors of 3-year patency of bypass grafts implanted on the right coronary artery system: A prospective randomized comparison of gastroepiploic artery, saphenous vein, and right internal thoracic artery grafts *J Thorac Cardiovasc Surg.* 142(5):980–8 with permission from Elsevier

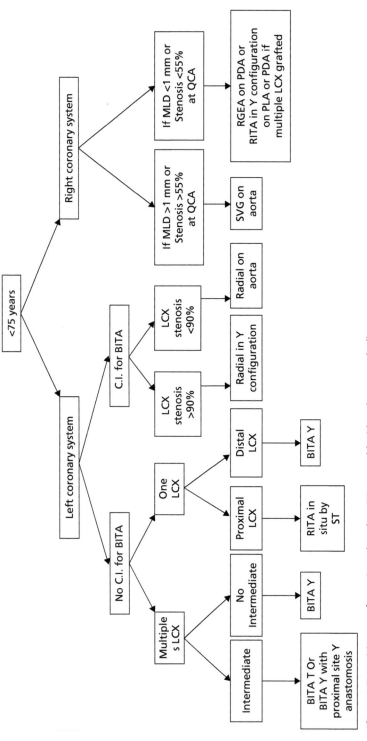

Figure 1.7 Decision tree for patients less than 75 years old with a three-vessels disease.

Reproduced from Glineur D. (2013) Importance of the third arterial graft in multiple arterial grafting strategies, Annals of Cardiothoracic Surgery 2(4):475–480 with permission from the AME publishing company

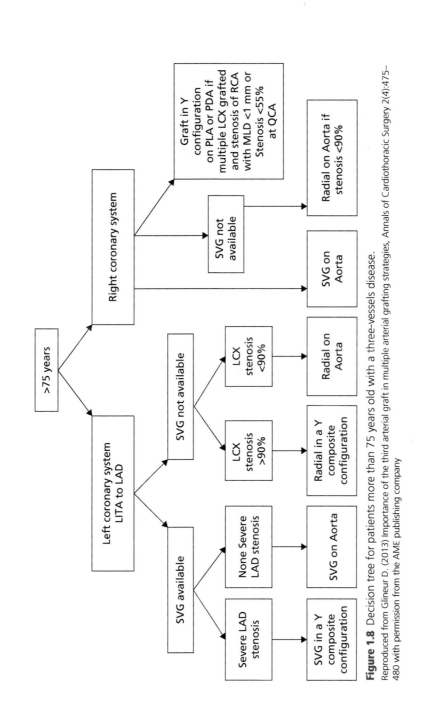

Figure 1.8 Decision tree for patients more than 75 years old with a three-vessels disease.

Summary

This literature review should guide surgeons in their strategies of coronary artery grafting and the manner in which they approach a patient with coronary artery disease. Accurate assessment of the severity of the coronary lesion is paramount. If the severity of the lesion is questionable, then further assessment with FFR is necessary.

Glineur proposed a decisional tree for patients younger than 75 years old (Figure 1.7). They currently use BITAs to revascularize the left coronary system in patients with no contraindications for harvesting of both ITAs. The LITA is systematically used to revascularize the LAD territory. If there is a need to revascularize a diagonal branch, a sequential jump diagonal LAD is then performed. For the lateral wall of the heart, the RITA is used *in situ* or in a composite fashion. If grafting of several marginals is required, the RITA is used in a composite fashion.

If the use of both ITAs is contraindicated, the RA is used for the lateral wall of the heart. Because the RA is much more sensitive to the competition flow than the ITAs, the RA is reimplanted in the aorta if the targeted coronary exhibits less than 90% stenosis. If the stenosis is more the 90%, a composite assembly is performed in the same manner as with the RITA.

For the right coronary system, a RGEA or a RITA is used only if the MLD of the coronary lesion is less than 1 mm or if the stenosis is more than 55%. In all other cases a SVG is used.

For patients older than 75 years[37] (Figure 1.8), the strategy for the LAD territory is the same as just described; for the circumflex territory, a SVG is used. When the quality of the SVG is poor or when there are no available SVGs, a RA is used in the same manner as just described. For the right coronary system, a SVG is systematically used. If there are no SVGs available, a RA is implanted on the aorta.

References

1. **Guo-Wei He** (1999). Arterial grafts for coronary artery bypass grafting: biological characteristics, functional classification, and clinical choice. *Ann Thorac Surg*, **67**, 277–84.

2. **Furchgott RF, Vanhoutte PM** (1989). Endothelium-derived relaxing and contracting factors. *FASEB J*, **3**, 2007–15.

3. **Lüscher TF, Diederich D, Siebenmann R**, *et al.* (1988). Difference between endothelium-dependent relaxation in arterial and venous coronary bypass grafts. *N Engl J Med*, **319**, 462–7.

4. **Marx R, Jax TW, Plehn G**, *et al.* (2001). Morphological differences of the internal thoracic artery in patients with and without coronary artery disease--evaluation by duplex-scanning. *Eur J Cardiothorac Surg*, **20**(4), 755–9.

5. **He G-W, Buxton B, Rosenfeldt F, Wilson AC, Angus JA** (1989). Weak β-adrenoceptor-mediated relaxation in the human internal mammary artery. *J Thorac Cardiovasc Surg*, **97**, 259–66.

6. **Green GE** (1972). Internal mammary artery-to-coronary artery anastomosis. Three-year experience with 165 patients. *Ann Thorac Surg*, **14**(3), 260–71.

7. **Kay EB, Naraghipour H, Beg RA**, *et al.* (1974). Internal mammary artery bypass graft—long-term patency rate and follow-up. *Ann Thorac Surg*, **18**(3), 269–79.

8. Barner HB, Mudd JG, Mark AL, Ahmad N, Dickens JF (1976). Patency of internal mammary-coronary grafts. *Circulation*, **54**(6 Suppl), III70–3.

9. Tector AJ, Davis L, Gabriel R, *et al.* (1976). Experience with internal mammary artery grafts in 298 patients. *Ann Thorac Surg*, **22**(6), 515–9.

10. Geha AS, Krone RJ, McCormick JR, Baue AE (1975). Selection of coronary bypass. Anatomic, physiological, and angiographic considerations of vein and mammary artery grafts. *J Thorac Cardiovasc Surg*, **70**(3), 414–31.

11. Tyras DH, Barner HB, Kaiser GC, Codd JE, Pennington DG, Willman VL (1980). Bypass grafts to the left anterior descending coronary artery: saphenous vein versus internal mammary artery. *J Thorac Cardiovasc Surg*, **80**(3), 327–33.

12. Lytle BW, Loop FD, Thurer RL, *et al.* (1980). Isolated left anterior descending coronary atherosclerosis: long-term comparison of internal mammary artery and venous autografts. *Circulation*, **61**(5), 869–74.

13. Tector AJ, Schmahl TM, Janson B, Kallies JR, Johnson G (1981). The internal mammary artery graft: its longevity after coronary bypass. *JAMA*, **246**(19), 2181–3.

14. Singh RN, Sosa JA, Green GE (1983). Internal mammary artery versus saphenous vein graft. Comparative performance in patients with combined revascularisation. *Br Heart J*, **50**(1), 48–58.

15. Grondin CM, Campeau L, Lespérance J, Enjalbert M, Bourassa MG (1984). Comparison of late changes in internal mammary artery and saphenous vein grafts in two consecutive series of patients 10 years after operation. *Circulation*, **70**(3 Pt 2), I208–12.

16. Okies JE, Page US, Bigelow JC, Krause AH, Salomon NW (1984). The left internal mammary artery: the graft of choice. *Circulation*, **70**(3 Pt 2), I213–21.

17. Lytle BW, Cosgrove DM, Loop FD, *et al.* (1986). Perioperative risk of bilateral internal mammary artery grafting: analysis of 500 cases from 1971 to 1984. *Circulation*, **74**(5 Pt 2), III37–41.

18. Loop FD, Lytle BW, Cosgrove DM, *et al.* (1986). Influence of the internal-mammary-artery graft on 10-year survival and other cardiac events. *N Engl J Med*, **314**(1), 1–6.

19. Zeff RH1, Kongtahworn C, Iannone LA, *et al.* (1988). Internal mammary artery versus saphenous vein graft to the left anterior descending coronary artery: prospective randomized study with 10-year follow-up. *Ann Thorac Surg*, **45**(5), 533–6.

20. Ivert T, Huttunen K, Landou C, Björk VO (1988). Angiographic studies of internal mammary artery grafts 11 years after coronary artery bypass grafting. *J Thorac Cardiovasc Surg*, **96**(1), 1–12.

21. Goldman S, Copeland J, Moritz T, *et al.* (1990). Internal mammary artery and saphenous vein graft patency. Effects of aspirin. *Circulation*, **82**(5 Suppl), IV237–42.

22. Fiore AC, Naunheim KS, Dean P, *et al.* (1990). Results of internal thoracic artery grafting over 15 years: single versus double grafts. *Ann Thorac Surg*, **49**(2), 202–8.

23. Galbut DL, Traad EA, Dorman MJ, *et al.* (1993). Coronary bypass grafting in the elderly. Single versus bilateral internal mammary artery grafts. *J Thorac Cardiovasc Surg*, **106**(1), 128–35; discussion 135–6.

24. Boylan MJ, Lytle BW, Loop FD, *et al.* (1994). Surgical treatment of isolated left anterior descending coronary stenosis. Comparison of left internal mammary artery and venous autograft at 18 to 20 years of follow-up. *J Thorac Cardiovasc Surg*, **107**(3), 657–62.

25. Goldman S, Copeland J, Moritz T, *et al.* (1994). Long-term graft patency (3 years) after coronary artery surgery. Effects of aspirin: results of a VA cooperative study. *Circulation*, **89**(3), 1138–43.

26. Fitzgibbon GM, Kafka HP, Leach AJ, *et al.* (1996). Coronary bypass graft fate and patient outcome: angiographic follow-up of 5,065 grafts related to survival and reoperation in 1,388 patients during 25 years. *J Am Coll Cardiol*, **28**(3), 616–26.

27. Gill IS, FitzGibbon GM, Higginson LA, Valji A, Keon WJ (1997). Minimally invasive coronary artery bypass: a series with early qualitative angiographic follow-up. *Ann Thorac Surg*, **64**(3), 710–4.

28. **Sabik JF 3rd, Lytle BW, Blackstone EH,** *et al.* (2003). Does competitive flow reduce internal thoracic artery graft patency? *Ann Thorac Surg*, **76**, 1490–6; discussion 1497.

29. **Hashimoto H, Isshiki T, Ikari Y,** *et al.* (1996). Effects of competitive blood flow on arterial graft patency and diameter. Medium-term postoperative follow-up. *J Thorac Cardiovasc Surg*, **111**, 399–407.

30. **Seki T, Kitamura S, Kawachi K,** *et al.* (1992). A quantitative study of postoperative luminal narrowing of the internal thoracic artery graft in coronary artery bypass surgery. *J Thorac Cardiovasc Surg*, **104**, 1532–8.

31. **Pagni S, Storey J, Ballen J,** *et al.* (1997). ITA versus SVG: a comparison of instantaneous pressure and flow dynamics during competitive flow. *Eur J Cardiothorac Surg*, **11**, 1086–92.

32. **Shimizu T, Hirayama T, Suesada H,** *et al.* (2000). Effect of flow competition on internal thoracic artery graft: postoperative velocimetric and angiographic study. *J Thorac Cardiovasc Surg*, **120**, 459–65.

33. **Kawasuji M, Sakakibara N, Takemura H,** *et al.* (1996). Is internal thoracic artery grafting suitable for a moderately stenotic coronary artery? *J Thorac Cardiovasc Surg*, **112**, 253–9.

34. **Shaha PJ, Durairaja M, Gordon I,** *et al.* (2004). Factors affecting patency of internal thoracic artery graft: clinical and angiographic study in 1434 symptomatic patients operated between 1982 and 2002. *Eur J Cardiothorac Surg*, **26**(1), 118–24.

35. **Glineur D, Hanet C, Poncelet A,** *et al.* (2008). Comparison of bilateral internal thoracic artery revascularization using *in situ* or Y graft configurations: a prospective randomized clinical, functional, and angiographic midterm evaluation. *Circulation*, **118**(14 Suppl), S216–21.

36. **Voors AA, van Brussel BL, Plokker HW,** *et al.* (1996). Smoking and cardiac events after venous coronary bypass surgery: a 15-year follow-up study. *Circulation*, **93**, 42–7.

37. **Märkl B, Raab S, Arnholdt H, Vicol C** (2003). Morphological and histopathological comparison of left and right internal thoracic artery with implications on their use for coronary surgery. *Interact Cardiovasc Thorac Surg*, **2**(1), 73–6.

38. **Glineur D, Djaoudi S, D'horre W,** *et al.* (2011). Endothelium-dependent and independent vasodilator response of left and right internal thoracic arteries used as a composite Y-graft. *Eur J Cardiothorac Surg*, **40**(2), 38–993.

39. **Chow M, Sim E, Orszulak T, Schaff H** (1994). Patency of internal thoracic artery grafts: comparison of right versus left and importance of vessels grafted. *Circulation*, **90**, II-129-II-32.

40. **Buxton BF, Ruengsakulrach P, Fuller J,** *et al.* (2000). The right internal thoracic artery graft-benefits of grafting the left coronary system and native vessels with a high-grade stenosis. *Eur J Cardiothorac Surg*, **18**, 255–61.

41. **Pick AW, Orszulak TA, Anderson BJ, Schaff HV** (1997). Single versus bilateral internal mammary artery grafts: 10-year outcome analysis. *Ann Thorac Surg*, **64**, 599–605.

42. **Tatoulis J, Buxton BF, Fuller JA** (1997). Results of 1,454 free right internal thoracic artery-to-coronary artery grafts. *Ann Thorac Surg*, **64**(5), 1263–8; discussion 1268–9.

43. **Ura M, Sakata R, Nakayama Y, Arai Y, Saito T** (1998). Long-term patency rate of right internal thoracic artery bypass via the transverse sinus. *Circulation*, **98**(19), 2043–8.

44. **Dion R, Glineur D, Derouck D,** *et al.* (2000). Long-term clinical and angiographic follow-up of sequential internal thoracic artery grafting. *Eur J Cardiothorac Surg*, **17**(4), 407–14.

45. **Glineur D, Hanet C, D'hoore W** *et al.* (2009). Causes of non-functioning right internal mammary used in a Y-graft configuration: insight from a 6-month systematic angiographic trial. *Eur J Cardiothorac Surg*, **36**(1), 129–35.

46. **Yi G, Shine B, Rehman SM, Altman DG, Taggart DP** (2014). Effect of bilateral internal mammary artery on long-term survival: a meta-analysis approach. *Circulation*, **130**(7), 539–45.

47. **Suma H, Takanashi R** (1990). Arteriosclerosis of the gastroepiploic and internal thoracic arteries. *Ann Thorac Surg*, **50**, 413–6.

48. **O'Neil GS, Chester AH, Allen SP**, *et al.* (1993). Endothelial function of human gastroepiploic artery: implications for its use as a bypass graft. *J Thorac Cardiovasc Surg*, **102**, 563–5.

49. **Ochiai M, Ohno M, Taguchi J**, *et al.* (1992). Responses of human gastroepiploic arteries to vasoactive substances: comparison with responses of internal mammary arteries and saphenous veins. *J Thorac Cardiovasc Surg*, **103**, 435–8.

50. **Yang Z, Siebenmann R, Studer M, Egloff L, Lüscher TF** (1992). Similar endothelium-dependent relaxation, but enhanced contractility of the right gastroepiploic artery as compared with the internal mammary artery. *J Thorac Cardiovasc Surg*, **104**, 459–64.

51. **Cremer J, Liesmann T, Wimmer-Greinecker G**, *et al.* (1994). *In vivo* comparison of free coronary grafts using the inferior epigastric, the gastroepiploic and the internal thoracic artery. *Eur J Cardiothorac Surg*, **8**, 240–6.

52. **Hanet C, Seeman C, Khoury G, Dion R, Robert A** (1994). Differences in vasoreactivity between gastroepiploic artery grafts late after bypass surgery and grafted coronary arteries, *Circulation*, **90**(Suppl II), 155–9.

53. **Perrault LP, Carrier M, Hébert Y**, *et al.* (1993). Clinical experience with the right gastroepiploic artery in coronary artery bypass grafting. *Ann Thorac Surg*, **56**(5), 1082–4.

54. **Mills NL, Hockmuth DR, Everson CT, Robart CC** (1993). Right gastroepiploic artery used for coronary artery bypass grafting. Evaluation of flow characteristics and size. *J Thorac Cardiovasc Surg*, **106**(4), 579–85.

55. **Pym J, Brown PM, Charrette EJ, Parker JO, West RO** (1987). Gastroepiploic-coronary anastomosis. A viable alternative bypass graft. *J Thorac Cardiovasc Surg*, **94**(2), 256–9.

56. **Grandjean JG, Boonstra PW, den Heyer P, Ebels T** (1994). Arterial revascularization with the right gastroepiploic artery and internal mammary arteries in 300 patients. *J Thorac Cardiovasc Surg*, **107**(5), 1309–15.

57. **Jegaden O, Eker A, Montagna P**, *et al.* (1995). Technical aspects and late functional results of gastroepiploic bypass grafting (400 cases). *Eur J Cardiothorac Surg*, **9**(10), 575–80.

58. **Albertini A, Lochegnies A, El Khoury G**, *et al.* (1998). Use of the right gastroepiploic artery as a coronary artery bypass graft in 307 patients. *Cardiovasc Surg*, **6**(4), 419–23.

59. **Gagliardotto P, Coste P, Lazreg M, Dor V** (1998). Skeletonized right gastroepiploic artery used for coronary artery bypass grafting. *Ann Thorac Surg*, **66**(1), 240–2.

60. **Suma H, Isomura T, Horii T, Sato T** (2000). Late angiographic result of using the right gastroepiploic artery as a graft. *J Thorac Cardiovasc Surg*, **120**(3), 496–8.

61. **Santos GG, Stolf NA, Moreira LF**, *et al.* (2002). Randomized comparative study of radial artery and right gastroepiploic artery in composite arterial graft for CABG. *Eur J Cardiothorac Surg*, **21**(6), 1009–14.

62. **Takahashi K, Daitoku K, Nakata S, Oikawa S, Minakawa M, Kondo N** (2004). Early and mid-term outcome of anastomosis of gastroepiploic artery to left coronary artery. *Ann Thorac Surg*, **78**(6), 2033–6

63. **Hirose H, Amano A, Takanashi S, Takahashi A** (2002). Coronary artery bypass grafting using the gastroepiploic artery in 1,000 patients. *Ann Thorac Surg*, **73**(5), 1371–9.

64. **Kamiya H, Watanabe G, Takemura H, Tomita S, Nagamine H, Kanamori T** (2004). Total arterial revascularization with composite skeletonized gastroepiploic artery graft in off-pump coronary artery bypass grafting. *J Thorac Cardiovasc Surg*, **127**(4), 1151–7.

65. **Kamiya H, Watanabe G, Takemura H, Tomita S, Nagamine H, Kanamori T** (2004). Skeletonization of gastroepiploic artery graft in off-pump coronary artery bypass grafting: early clinical and angiographic assessment. *Ann Thorac Surg*, **77**(6), 2046–50.

66. **Fukui T, Takanashi S, Hosoda Y, Suehiro S** (2005). Total arterial myocardial revascularization using composite and sequential grafting with the off-pump technique. *Ann Thorac Surg*, **80**(2), 579–85.

67. **Ryu SW1, Ahn BH, Choo SJ**, *et al.* (2005). Skeletonized gastroepiploic artery as a composite graft for total arterial revascularization. *Ann Thorac Surg*, **80**(1), 118–23.

68. **Kim KB, Cho KR, Choi JS, Lee HJ** (2006). Right gastroepiploic artery for revascularization of the right coronary territory in off-pump total arterial revascularization: strategies to improve patency. *Ann Thorac Surg*, **81**(6), 2135–41.

69. **Suma H, Tanabe H, Takahashi A**, *et al.* (2007). Twenty years' experiences with the gastroepiploic artery graft for CABG. *Circulation*, **116**(11 Suppl), I188–91.

70. **Ochi M, Hatori N, Fujii M, Saji Y, Tanaka S, Honma H** (2001). Limited flow capacity of the right gastroepiploic artery graft: postoperative echocardiographic and angiographic evaluation. *Ann Thorac Surg*, **71**, 1210–4.

71. **Glineur D, D'hoore W, El Khoury G**, *et al.* (2008). Angiographic predictors of 6-month patency of bypass grafts implanted to the right coronary artery a prospective randomized comparison of gastroepiploic artery and saphenous vein grafts. *J Am Coll Cardiol*, **51**(2), 120–5.

72. **Glineur D, Hanet C, Poncelet A**, *et al.* (2008). Comparison of saphenous vein graft versus right gastroepiploic artery to revascularize the right coronary artery: a prospective randomized clinical, functional, and angiographic midterm evaluation. *J Thorac Cardiovasc Surg*, **136**(2), 482–8.

73. **Carpentier A** (1975). Discussion of Gaha AS, Krone RJ, McCormic JR, *et al.* Selection of coronary bypass: anatomic, physiological, and angiographic consideration of vein and mammary artery grafts. *J Thorac Cardiovasc Surg*, **70**, 429–30.

74. **Chardigny C, Jebara VA, Acar C**, *et al.* (1993). Vasoreactive of the radial artery comparison with the internal mammary artery and gastroepiploic arteries with implications for coronary artery surgery. *Circulation*, **88**(Suppl II): II–115–II–127; 12.

75. **He G-W, Yang C-Q** (1997). Radial artery has higher receptor-mediated contractility but similar endothelial function compared with mammary artery. *Ann Thorac Surg*, **63**, 1346–52; 13.

76. **Shapira Oz M, Xu A, Aldea GS**, *et al.* (1999). Enhanced nitric oxide-mediated vascular relaxation in radial artery compared with internal mammary artery or saphenous vein. *Circulation*, **100**(Suppl II), II–322–II–327; 14.

77. **Cable DG, Caccitolo JA, Pfeifer EA**, *et al.* (1999). Endothelial regulation of vascular contraction in radial artery and internal mammary arteries. *Ann Thorac Surg*, **67**, 1083–90; 15.

78. **He GW, Liu ZG** (2001). Comparison of nitric oxide release and endothelium-derived hyperpolarizing factor-mediated hyperpolarization between human radial and internal mammary arteries. *Circulation*, **104**(12 Suppl 1), I344–9.

79. **Carpentier A, Guermonprez JL, Deloche A**, *et al.* (1973). The aorta-to-coronary radial artery bypass graft: a technique avoiding pathological changes in grafts. *Ann Thorac Surg*, **16**, 111–121.

80. **Desai ND, Cohen EA, Naylor CD, Fremes SE for the Radial Artery Patency Study Investigators** (2004). A randomized comparison of radial-artery and saphenous-vein coronary bypass grafts. *N Engl J Med*, **351**, 2302–9.

81. **Deb S, Cohen EA, Singh SK**, *et al.*, **RAPS Investigators** (2012). Radial artery and saphenous vein patency more than 5 years after coronary artery bypass surgery: results from RAPS (Radial Artery Patency Study). *J Am Coll Cardiol*, **60**, 28–35.

82. **Collins P, Webb CM, Chong CF, Moat NE; Radial Artery Versus Saphenous Vein Patency (RSVP) Trial Investigators** (2008). Radial artery versus saphenous vein patency randomized trial: five-year angiographic follow-up. *Circulation*, **117**, 2859–64.

83. **Hayward PA, Gordon IR, Hare DL**, *et al.* (2010). Comparable patencies of the radial artery and right internal thoracic artery or saphenous vein beyond 5 years: results from the Radial Artery Patency and Clinical Outcomes trial. *J Thorac Cardiovasc Surg*, **139**, 60–5.

84. Hayward PA, Buxton BF (2011). The Radial Artery Patency and Clinical Outcomes trial: design, intermediate term results and future direction. *Heart Lung Circ*, **20**, 187–92.

85. Athanasiou T, Saso S, Rao C, *et al.* (2011). Radial artery versus saphenous vein conduits for coronary artery bypass surgery: forty years of competition—which conduit offers better patency? A systematic review and meta-analysis. *Eur J Cardiothorac Surg*, **40**, 208–20.

86. Cao C, Manganas C, Horton M, *et al.* (2013). Angiographic outcomes of radial artery versus saphenous vein in coronary artery bypass graft surgery: a meta-analysis of randomized controlled trials. *J Thorac Cardiovasc Surg*, **146**(2), 255–61.

87. Gaudino M, Benedetto U, Fremes S *et al.* (2018). Radial-Artery or Saphenous-Vein Grafts in Coronary-Artery Bypass Surgery. *N Engl J Med*. 2018 May 31;378(22):2069–2077. doi: 10.1056/NEJMoa1716026.

88. Gaudino M, Tondi P, Benedetto U, *et al.* Radial Artery as a Coronary Artery Bypass Conduit: 20-Year Results. *J Am Coll Cardiol*. 2016 Aug 9;68(6):603–610. doi: 10.1016/j.jacc.2016.05.062.

89. Maniar HS, Sundt TM, Barner HB, *et al.* (2002). Effect of target stenosis and location on radial artery graft patency. *J Thorac Cardiovasc Surg*, **123**, 45–52.

90. Amano A, Takahashi A, Hirose H (2002). Skeletonized radial artery grafting: improved angiographic results. *Ann Thorac Surg*, **73**, 1880–7.

91. Fawzy HF (2009). Harvesting of the radial artery for coronary artery bypass grafting: comparison of ultrasonic harmonic scalpel dissector with the conventional technique. *J Card Surg*, **24**, 285–9.

92. Jung SH, Song H, Choo SJ, *et al.* (2009). Comparison of radial artery patency according to proximal anastomosis site: direct aorta to radial artery anastomosis is superior to radial artery composite grafting. *J Thorac Cardiovasc Surg*, **138**, 76–83.

93. Gaudino M, Pragliola F, Cellini C, *et al.* (2004). Effect of target artery location and severity of stenosis on mid-term patency of aorta-anastomosed vs. internal thoracic artery-anastomosed radial artery graft. *Eur J Cardiothorac Surg*, **25**, 424–8.

94. Schwann TA, Zacharias A, Riordan CJ, *et al.* (2009). Sequential radial artery grafts for multivessel coronary artery bypass graft surgery: 10-year survival and angiography results. *Ann Thorac Surg*, **88**, 31–9.

95. Fukui T, Takanashi S, Hosoda Y, Suehiro S (2005). Total arterial myocardial revascularization using composite and sequential grafting with the off-pump technique. *Ann Thorac Surg*, **80**, 579–85.

96. Garret HE, Dennis EW, Debakey ME (1973). Aortocoronary bypass with saphenous vein graft: 7-year follow-up. *J Am Med Assoc*, **223**, 792–4.

97. Majesky MW, Schwartz SM, Clowes MM, Clowes AW (1987). Heparin regulates smooth muscle S-phase entry in the injured rat carotid artery. *Circ Res*, **61**, 296–300.

98. Dollery C, McEwan J, Henney A (1995). Matrix metalloproteinases and cardiovascular disease. *Circ Res*, **77**, 863–8.

99. Hanet C, Robert A, Wijns W (1992). Vasomotor response to ergometrine and nitrates of saphenous vein grafts, internal mammary artery grafts, and grafted coronary arteries late after bypass surgery. *Circulation*, **86**(5 Suppl), II210–6.

100. Bourassa MG (1991). Fate of venous grafts: the past, the present, and the future. *J Am Coll Cardiol*, **5**, 1081–3; Fitzgibbon GM, Kafka HP, Leach AJ, Keon WJ, Hooper D (1996). Coronary bypass graft fate and patient outcome: angiographic follow-up of 5065 grafts related to survival and reoperation in 1388 patients during 25 years. *J Am Coll Cardiol*, **28**, 616–26.

101. Campeau L, Enjalbert M, Lesperance J, *et al.* (1984). The relation risk factor to the development of atherosclerosis in saphenous vein bypass grafts and the progression of disease in the native circulation: a study 10 years after aortocoronary bypass surgery. *N Engl J Med*, **311**, 1329–32.

102. **Shah PJ, Gordon I, Fuller J,** *et al.* (2003). Factors affecting saphenous vein graft patency: clinical and angiographic study in 1402 symptomatic patients operated on between 1977 and 1999. *J Thorac Cardiovasc Surg,* **126**(6), 1972–7.

103. **Goldman S, Copeland J, Moritz T,** *et al.* (1989). Saphenous vein graft patency 1 year after coronary artery bypass surgery and effects of antiplatelet therapy. Results of a Veterans Administration Cooperative Study. *Circulation,* **80**, 1190–7.

104. **The Post Coronary Artery Bypass Graft Trial Investigators** (1997). The effect of aggressive lowering of low-density lipoprotein cholesterol levels and low-dose anticoagulation on obstructive changes in saphenous-vein coronary-artery bypass grafts. *N Engl J Med,* **336**, 153–62.

105. **Souza DS, Dashwood MR, Tusi JCS,** *et al.* (2002). Improved patency in vein grafts harvested with surrounding tissue: results of a randomized study using three harvesting techniques. *Ann Thorac Surg,* **73**, 1189–95.

106. **Roth JA, Cukingnan RA, Brown BG, Gocka E, Carey JS** (1979). Factors influencing patency of saphenous vein grafts. *Ann Thorac Surg,* **28**, 176–9.

107. **Flemma RJ, Johnson WD, Lepley D Jr** (1971). Triple aorto-coronary vein bypass as treatment for coronary insufficiency. *Ann Thorac Surg,* **103**, 82–83.

108. **Glineur D, D'hoore W, de Kerchove L,** *et al.* (2011). Angiographic predictors of 3-year patency of bypass grafts implanted on the right coronary artery system: a prospective randomized comparison of gastroepiploic artery, saphenous vein, and right internal thoracic artery grafts. *J Thorac Cardiovasc Surg,* **142**(5), 980–8.

109. **Jianrong Li** (2011). The patency of sequential and individual vein coronary bypass grafts: a systematic review. *Ann Thorac Surg,* **92**, 1292–8

110. **Weiss AJ, Zhao S, Tian DH, Taggart DP, Yan TD** (2013). A meta-analysis comparing bilateral internal mammary artery with left internal mammary artery for coronary artery bypass grafting. *Ann Cardiothorac Surg,* **2**(4), 390–400.

111. **Grau JB, Ferrari G, Mak AW,** *et al.* (2012). Propensity matched analysis of bilateral internal mammary artery versus single left internal mammary artery grafting at 17-year follow-up: validation of a contemporary surgical experience. *Eur J Cardiothorac Surg,* **41**(4), 770–5.

112. **Follis FM, Pett SB Jr, Miller KB, Wong RS, Temes RT, Wernly JA** (1999). Catastrophic hemorrhage on sternal reentry: still a dreaded complication? *Ann Thorac Surg,* **68**, 2215–9.

113. **Gillinov AM, Casselman FP, Lytle BW,** *et al.* (1999). Injury to a patent left internal thoracic artery graft at coronary reoperation. *Ann Thorac Surg,* **67**, 382–6.

114. **Odell JA, Mullany CJ, Schaff HV,** *et al.* (1996). Aortic valve replacement after previous coronary artery bypass grafting. *Ann Thorac Surg,* **62**, 1424–30.

115. **Roselli E, Pettersson GB, Blackstone EH,** *et al.* (2008). Adverse events during reoperative cardiac surgery: frequency, characterization, and rescue. *J Thorac Cardiovasc Surg,* **135**(2), 316–23.

116. **Imamaki M, Fujita H, Niitsuma Y,** *et al.* (2008). Limitations of right internal thoracic artery to left anterior descending artery bypass: a comparative quantitative study of postoperative angiography of the bilateral internal thoracic artery bypass grafts. *J Card Surg,* **23**(4), 283–7.

117. **Royse AG, Royse CF, Groves KL, Bus B, Yu G** (1999). Blood flow in composite arterial grafts and effect of native coronary flow. *Ann Thorac Surg,* **68**, 1619–22.

118. **Glineur D, Noirhomme P, Reisch J,** *et al.* (2005). Resistance to flow of arterial Y-grafts 6 months after coronary artery bypass surgery. *Circulation,* **112**, I281–5.

119. **Nakajima H, Kobayashi J, Toda K,** *et al.* (2011). A 10-year angiographic follow-up of competitive flow in sequential and composite arterial grafts. *Eur J Cardiothorac Surg,* **40**(2), 399–404.

120. **Glineur D, Hanet C, D'hoore W,** *et al.* (2009). Causes of non-functioning right internal mammary used in a Y-graft configuration: insight from a 6-month systematic angiographic trial. *Eur J Cardiothorac Surg,* **36**(1), 129–35.

121. **Verhelst R, Etienne PY, El Khoury G**, *et al.* (1996). Free internal mammary artery graft in myocardial revascularization. *Cardiovasc Surg*, **4**(2), 212–6.

122. **Diett CA, Benoit CH, Gilbert CL**, *et al.* (1995). Which is the graft of choice for the right coronary and posterior descending arteries? Comparison of the right internal mammary artery and the right gastroepiploic artery. *Circulation*, **92**(9 Suppl), II-92–7.

123. **Buxton BF, Raman JS, Ruengsakulrach P**, *et al.* (2003). Radial artery patency and clinical outcomes: five-year interim results of a randomized trial. *J Thorac Cardiovasc Surg*, **125**, 1363–71.

124. **Voutilainen S, Verkkala K, Jarvinen A, Keto P** (1996). Angiographic 5-year follow-up study of right gastroepiploic artery grafts. *Ann Thorac Surg*, **62**, 501–5.

125. **Hadinata IE, Hayward PA, Hare DL**, *et al.* (2009). Choice of conduit for the right coronary system: 8-year analysis of Radial Artery Patency and Clinical Outcomes trial. *Ann Thorac Surg*, **88**(5), 1404–9.

126. **Hayward PA, Buxton BF** (2007). Contemporary coronary graft patency: 5-year observational data from a randomized trial of conduits. *Ann Thorac Surg*, **84**, 795–9.

127. **Tatoulis J, Buxton BF, Fuller JA** (2004). Patencies of 2127 arterial to coronary conduits over 15 years. *Ann Thorac Surg*, **77**(1), 93–101.

Chapter 2

Off-pump versus on-pump coronary artery bypass grafting

Michael E. Halkos, Emmanuel Moss, and John D. Puskas

Introduction

Coronary artery bypass grafting (CABG) remains the gold standard for multivessel coronary revascularization. Despite advances in percutaneous coronary intervention and medical therapy, CABG continues to play a key role in the treatment of patients with coronary disease. Although an abundance of literature comparing on-pump (ONCAB) versus off-pump (OPCAB) coronary artery bypass grafting exists, the optimal surgical strategy remains controversial. While many centers have adopted off-pump techniques, OPCAB surgery remains in the minority of CABG procedures performed in the United States. Proponents of ONCAB cite the lack of convincing data in randomized trials demonstrating a benefit for OPCAB. Proponents of OPCAB frequently cite large observational and registry data that suggest a reduction in-hospital mortality and morbidity with OPCAB. Even more controversial are the reports of graft patency, completeness of revascularization, and the need for repeat revascularization. Reports from both randomized and observational trials can be found which suggest either equivalent or inferior results with OPCAB. Some studies have suggested that certain high-risk patient subgroups are more likely to benefit from an OPCAB approach. These include patients with advanced ascending aortic atherosclerosis, renal insufficiency, advanced age, ventricular dysfunction, and chronic lung disease, all of which are more common in patients referred for CABG compared to the general population. In these high-risk patients, avoiding the deleterious effects of cardiopulmonary bypass and minimizing or eliminating aortic manipulation may lead to improved short-term outcomes. Thus, it is important for coronary surgeons to be facile with OPCAB techniques in order to be able to implement this strategy when warranted.

Outcomes

Operative mortality

Randomized controlled trials have consistently shown comparable in-hospital mortality rates between OPCAB and ONCAB.[1-17] In the ROOBY trial, the largest randomized trial at the time (2,203 patients), Shroyer and colleagues demonstrated excellent 30-day mortality rates with OPCAB and ONCAB surgery (1.9% *vs.* 1.8%, $P = 0.25$).[15] In a meta-analysis of 37 randomized trials (3,369 predominantly low-risk patients), no significant differences were found for 30-day mortality (odds ratio (OR), 1.02; 95% confidence interval (CI) 0.58–1.80).[18] More recently, the 4,752-patient CORONARY trial compared OPCAB to ONCAB in patients at increased risk of complications following CABG surgery and also showed equivalent 30-day mortality rates (2.5%).[16] OPCAB was, however, beneficial with regard to transfusion rates, reoperation for bleeding, respiratory complications, and acute kidney injury. Another recent randomized controlled trial (RCT) compared the two surgical strategies in patients greater than 75 years of age and found equivalent mortality at 30 days (2.6% *vs.* 2.8% for OPCAB and ONCAB, respectively).[17] In randomized patients undergoing urgent/emergent surgery for ST-segment elevation myocardial infarction, Fattouch and associates demonstrated a reduction of in-hospital mortality with OPCAB compared to ONCAB.[19]

One of the criticisms of earlier randomized trials was the relatively small sample sizes, which increased the probability of type I error, especially when trying to detect differences for an infrequent event (e.g., mortality). The recent RCTs are more robust and, although each has inherent limitations, would appear to more reliably compare rare complications such as mortality, stroke, and renal failure. Several registry studies have been published that are certainly adequately powered to detect differences in mortality outcomes; however, these retrospective studies have their own limitations. In a study by Hannan *et al.*,[20] 49,830 patients from the New York State registry underwent risk-adjusted analysis comparing outcomes after OPCAB versus ONCAB. In this study, OPCAB patients had significantly lower 30-day mortality (adjusted OR 0.81, 95% CI 0.68–0.97, $P = 0.0022$). In a large registry study of California CABG outcomes, Li and colleagues also demonstrated a significant reduction in propensity-adjusted operative mortality with OPCAB compared to ONCAB (OR 2.59% 95% CI 2.52–2.67% *vs.* 3.22%, 95% CI 3.17–3.27%).[21] An intention-to-treat retrospective analysis of 42,477 patients from the Society of Thoracic Surgeons National Database (STS) showed a reduction in risk-adjusted operative mortality (adjusted OR 0.83, $P = 0.03$).[22–25] These studies have demonstrated that operative mortality may be reduced in patients undergoing OPCAB compared to ONCAB. The perceived benefits of OPCAB may become more apparent in high-risk patients, especially those with chronic obstructive pulmonary disease, renal insufficiency, and advanced aortic atheromatous disease where avoiding aortic clamping, as well as the systemic effects of cardiopulmonary bypass being more advantageous than in low-risk patients. In a large retrospective cohort, Puskas and colleagues reported that patients in the highest risk quartile had a significant reduction in-hospital mortality with OPCAB compared to ONCAB (3.2% *vs.* 6.7%, $P < 0.0001$, OR 0.45 95% CI 0.33–0.63, $P < 0.0001$) (Figure 2.1).[26] This study provides further evidence that OPCAB may disproportionately benefit high-risk patients. Additional studies have also reported improved outcomes in high-risk patients such as those with dialysis-dependent renal failure,[27] left ventricular dysfunction,[28] previous sternotomy,[29] advanced age,[29–32] previous stroke,[33] and female patients.[24]

Other studies challenge the aforementioned large registry and STS National Database conclusions. In a study by Chu and associates of 63,000 patients, there was no difference

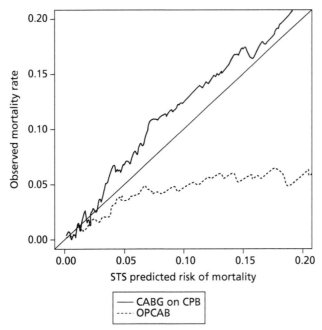

Figure 2.1 Regression curve comparison of observed mortality rates for off-pump coronary artery bypass grafting (OPCAB) and coronary artery bypass grafting (CABG) on cardiopulmonary bypass (CPB) across all levels of predicted risk. (STS = the Society of Thoracic Surgeons.)

Reprinted from Puskas JD *et al.* (2009) Off-pump coronary artery bypass disproportionately benefits high-risk patients. Ann Thorac Surg. 88:1142–1147 with permission from Elsevier.

in-hospital mortality between OPCAB and ONCAB (3.0% *vs.* 3.2%, $P = 0.14$)[34]. In summary, randomized trials have shown comparable in-hospital mortality rates with either strategy, whereas most observational analyses suggest a reduction in-hospital mortality with OPCAB compared to ONCAB.

Emergent conversion from OPCAB to ONCAB has been associated with significantly increased hospital mortality. Patel and colleagues reported an in-hospital mortality rate of 12% in those converted urgently to ONCAB compared to 1.5% in those who did not require urgent conversion ($P = 0.001$)[35]. Similarly, Jin and associates reported results from a large registry of over 70,000 patients. In this cohort, 5.8% of attempted OPCAB patients were converted to ONCAB and hospital mortality was significantly higher in converted patients compared to OPCAB patients or patients initially operated by an on-pump technique (9.9% *vs.* 1.6% *vs.* 3.0%, respectively)[36]. Importantly, there does not appear to be an increased risk of complications in patients who are electively converted to ONCAB. This occurs during a reversible period of hemodynamic instability, which initially manifests during cardiac positioning, displacement, or coronary stabilization. Once these maneuvers are reversed, the clinical condition stabilizes, and commencement of cardiopulmonary bypass can be done under controlled circumstances.

Mid- and long-term mortality

Mid- and long-term survival has been comparable between OPCAB and ONCAB patients.[9,13,20,23,37] In an observational study by Hannan *et al.*, 3-year survival was equivalent in OPCAB versus ONCAB patients (unadjusted 3-year survival 89.4% *vs.* 90.1%, log-rank test, $P = 0.20$). Within our own institutional database, 10-year survival of over 12,000 patients was equivalent between OPCAB and ONCAB groups.[23] In a long-term follow-up (6–8 years) study of two randomized trials, Angelini compared survival outcomes of OPCAB versus ONCAB and found no difference in long-term survival between the two groups (hazard ratio, 1.24; 95% CI 0.72–2.15, $P = 0.44$)[9]. Long-term follow-up of a randomized trial by Puskas and colleagues similarly showed equivalent survival between the two groups at a mean of 7.5 years.[38]

However, the 2009 RCT by Shroyer and colleagues reported a higher 1-year composite outcome of death, repeat revascularization, or non-fatal myocardial infarction for patients undergoing OPCAB compared to ONCAB (9.9% *vs.* 7.4%, $P = 0.04$)[15], although the individual endpoints were not statistically different. With sensitivity analysis, 1-year death from cardiac causes was slightly higher in the OPCAB group compared to the ONCAB group (2.7% *vs.* 1.3%, $P = 0.03$). Therefore, the 1-year results from this multi-institutional randomized trial need to be compared with the aforementioned randomized and observational analyses that have longer follow-up and which have consistently shown comparable mid- and long-term mortality rates.

Neurologic outcomes

There are no prospective randomized trials that have shown a reduction in stroke with OPCAB compared to ONCAB. Large retrospective analyses[20,23,33,39] have shown that OPCAB may be associated with a reduced incidence of stroke compared to ONCAB. Hannan *et al.* reported a risk-adjusted decrease in postoperative stroke with OPCAB compared to ONCAB (adjusted OR 0.70, 95% CI 0.57–0.86, $P = 0.0006$). Nishiyama and colleagues reported that OPCAB was associated with a significant reduction in early stroke compared to ONCAB (0.1% *vs.* 1.1%, $P = 0.0009$). Mishra and colleagues performed a propensity matched comparison of OPCAB versus ONCAB in 6,991 patients with atheromatous aortic disease and found a significant decrease in postoperative stroke, with OPCAB being the only independent predictor of a decreased stroke rate.[40]

Conversely, postoperative stroke was not significantly reduced in two recent meta-analyses of off- versus on-pump CABG among relatively low-risk patients.[41,42] Furthermore, Chu and colleagues did not find any differences in stroke between OPCAB and ONCAB.[34] However, the mechanisms responsible for the observed reduction in postoperative stroke have not been well-defined in most of these studies. OPCAB eliminates the need for aortic cannulation, cardiopulmonary bypass, and application of a cross-clamp but does not eliminate the need for construction of aortocoronary proximal anastomoses. Furthermore, partial aortic clamping for construction of proximal anastomoses is still routinely performed in patients undergoing OPCAB. Thus, the benefits of OPCAB may be attenuated because of aortic manipulation and atheroembolic risk associated with partial aortic clamping. Kim and associates reported a lower incidence of postoperative stroke in patients undergoing OPCAB without any manipulation of the aorta compared to patients undergoing OPCAB with partial clamping and patients undergoing ONCAB.[43] Our group recently published similar findings, showing incremental rise in stroke risk with increased degree of aortic manipulation.[44] Approaches utilized to decrease the incidence of atheroemboli associated with aortic manipulation include avoidance of aortic cannulation for cardiopulmonary bypass, avoidance of aortic clamping, and use of clampless anastomotic devices for proximal anastomoses.[45–47] However, the impact of these different strategies on reducing postoperative stroke has not been investigated in large-scale, prospective trials.

Graft patency and completeness of revascularization

Completeness of revascularization has been critical for the success and durable benefit of coronary artery bypass surgery.[48,49] Evidence from several randomized trials suggests equivalent revascularization with OPCAB compared to ONCAB techniques.[10,11,17,50–51] However, a multicenter study from Veterans Affairs medical centers found that fewer grafts completed than originally planned occurred more frequently in the OPCAB group (17.8% *vs.* 11.1%). A meta-analysis of randomized trials has consistently shown a lower number of grafts per patient in OPCAB versus ONCAB (2.6 *vs.* 2.8, $P < 0.0001$).[24] However, the terms for completeness of revascularization and number of grafts performed should be differentiated. A common formula has been to divide the number of grafts performed by the number of grafts needed (number of graftable vessels with angiographically significant stenosis) by preoperative assessment of the cardiac catheterization. This value gives an index of completeness of revascularization. In a study of the STS National Database by Puskas and colleagues, OPCAB patients had a slightly lower index of complete revascularization than ONCAB patients.[22] In a study by Magee and coworkers, the number of grafts were fewer in the OPCAB group (2.75 ± 1.12) compared to the ONCAB group (3.36 ± 1.01).[52] However, because the OPCAB group needed fewer grafts, the index of complete revascularization was comparable between OPCAB and ONCAB (1.03 and 1.07, respectively). Thus, it appears that selection bias may be partly responsible for this observation, since surgeons may choose to utilize on-pump techniques on patients requiring more than three grafts. Completeness of revascularization should not be compromised when deciding whether to use or avoid cardiopulmonary bypass unless the use of cardiopulmonary bypass poses obvious and significant risk for morbidity or mortality.

Graft patency has been evaluated in five randomized trials from in-hospital to 1 year postoperatively. Puskas demonstrated no difference in graft patency at discharge and at 1 year,[51] whereas Khan showed a decreased graft patency in the off-pump group at 3 months.[10] Similarly, Widimsky and associates demonstrated equivalent arterial but reduced vein graft patency in OPCAB patients compared to ONCAB patients.[8] Shroyer *et al.* found that the overall rate of graft patency (driven by vein graft patency) was lower in the OPCAB group compared to the ONCAB group (82.6% *vs.* 87.8%, $P < 0.001$).[15] Lamy and colleagues found an increased incidence of repeat revascularization at 30 days (0.7 *vs.* 0.2%,

$P = 0.01$), although this was found only to be a significant trend on 1-year analysis.[16,53-60] Three other studies showed no difference in graft patency at 1-year.[11,54,55] Two meta-analyses reported no significant differences between off-pump and on-pump revascularization.[24,56] The largest study to challenge either completeness of revascularization or graft patency is the New York registry data from Hannan *et al.*[20] Although OPCAB was associated with lower in-hospital mortality and morbidity and equivalent long-term outcomes compared to ONCAB, the need for repeat revascularization was slightly greater in the OPCAB group (93.6% *vs.* 89.9%). Because this was a retrospective analysis, this study was unable to differentiate whether this difference was due to incomplete revascularization during OPCAB, reduced graft patency, or due to unrecognized confounding variables.

OPCAB technique

Negotiating the learning curve

Unlike ONCAB, where graft sequence and hemodynamic management are relatively straightforward, OPCAB requires careful consideration of coronary anatomy, confounding patient variables, and attention to hemodynamic fluctuations. Early in a surgeon's experience, patients with difficult lateral wall targets, severe left ventricular dysfunction, left main disease, or other complex cases should be excluded from an OPCAB approach. Ideal early candidates for OPCAB include those undergoing elective primary coronary revascularization with good target anatomy, preserved ventricular function, and one to three grafts with easily accessible lateral wall targets. With increasing experience, OPCAB can be safely and effectively applied to most patients requiring CABG.

Patient variables

The preoperative evaluation of patients for OPCAB demands careful planning and consideration for certain risk factors. It is important to consider the presence of right ventricular dysfunction, valvular regurgitation, or pulmonary hypertension since cardiac positioning and displacement during OPCAB can result in dramatic changes in hemodynamics under these conditions. With lateral displacement and transient lateral wall ischemia, even patients with mild to moderate mitral regurgitation can develop severe mitral regurgitation and pulmonary hypertension, leading to cardiovascular deterioration. Overall, the clinical condition of the patient, the urgency of the operation, and ventricular function need to be carefully assessed to determine whether an off-pump approach is practical. Patients with left ventricular dysfunction from a recent infarct pose a more difficult challenge than those with chronic ventricular dysfunction, with the former being much more sensitive to cardiac manipulation and displacement and more likely to develop intraoperative arrhythmias during transient ischemia.

Anesthesia

As in other cardiac operations, all patients require invasive monitoring. We routinely utilize transesophageal echocardiography to provide valuable information about valvular regurgitation, regional myocardial function, and pulmonary hypertension. Unlike with ONCAB, adequate perfusion pressures are not controlled with cardiopulmonary bypass, careful coordination and communication between the surgeon and anesthesiologist are imperative to avoid hemodynamic demise. Subtle changes in hemodynamic status, gradual elevation in pulmonary artery pressures, frequent boluses or increased requirement of inotropes and vasopressors to maintain hemodynamic stability, and rhythm changes can herald cardiovascular collapse. Therefore, adequate volume-loading and the judicious use of inotropes and vasopressors may be required to ensure stable hemodynamics during cardiac manipulation. To adjust loading conditions, the first maneuver is adjusting the position of the operating table. Autotransfusion of intravascular volume from the lower extremities by Trendelenberg positioning can provide a rapid increase in preload, while reverse Trendelenberg can have the opposite effect. We prefer to avoid giving large volumes of intravenous fluids, which can complicate the postoperative course. If preload conditions have been optimized, then vasopressor agents such as norepinephrine or neosynephrine may be utilized to assist with maintaining adequate blood pressure during distal anastomoses.

Maintaining normothermia is critically important and requires more effort during OPCAB procedures. This can usually be accomplished by infusing intravenous fluids through warmers, warming inhalational anesthetic agents, maintaining warm room temperatures before and during the procedure, and using convective forced-air warming systems.

Anticoagulation

In our practice, patients receive an aspirin rectal suppository (1,000 mg) after induction of anesthesia. Aspirin 81 mg and clopidogrel (150 mg postoperatively, then 75 mg/day) are routinely administered early in the postoperative period after mediastinal drainage decreases below 100 cc/hour for four hours. This has not been associated with an increased risk of mediastinal re-exploration.[57] This regimen is followed due to concerns regarding a relative hypercoagulable state in the early postoperative period. Intraoperative anticoagulation regimens can vary since cardiopulmonary bypass is not required. We routinely administer 5,000 units of heparin prior to the skin incision primarily to prevent thrombus formation within saphenous veins during endoscopic harvest. Prior to coronary anastomosis, some surgeons implement a full dose of heparin with 400 international units/kg to maintain an activated clotting time (ACT) of >400 seconds; others use a half dose or 180 international units/kg while others start with 10,000 units and administer additional doses (3,000 international units every half-hour) to maintain an ACT of 275–300 seconds. Reversal of anticoagulation with protamine is usually administered to facilitate hemostasis.

Exposure

Although OPCAB allows for minimally invasive approaches, the most common approach is via median sternotomy. The pericardium is incised in an inverted T configuration, and then incised laterally along the diaphragm to facilitate cardiac displacement. Unlike ONCAB, the heart is not decompressed and extra conduit length is often necessary to avoid tension on the anastomosis during rightward displacement for lateral wall grafting.

Several pericardial traction sutures are placed to assist with exposure and lateral displacement of the heart. To avoid compression on the right heart during lateral displacement, the right pericardium can be dissected along the diaphragm or the right pleural space opened to allow the heart to fall into the right chest during lateral displacement. Placing rolled towels under the right side of the retractor helps to elevate the right side of the sternum to allow the heart to be displaced into the right chest. An important traction suture is the "deep stitch," which is placed approximately two-thirds of the way between the inferior vena cava and left pulmonary vein at the point where the pericardium reflects over the posterior left atrium (Figure 2.2). Care should be taken with placement of this suture to avoid the underlying descending thoracic aorta, esophagus, left lung, and adjacent inferior pulmonary vein. This suture should be covered with a soft rubber catheter to prevent laceration of the epicardium during retraction. A warm moist laparotomy pad can be placed between the heart and the "deep stitch" to assist with elevating the heart out of the pericardium. Alternatively, a warm laparotomy pad

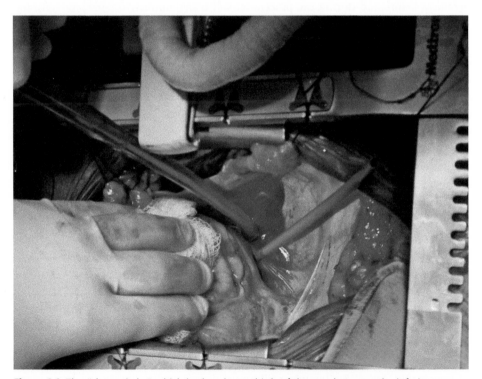

Figure 2.2 The "deep stitch," which is placed two-thirds of the way between the inferior vena cava and inferior left pulmonary vein, allows anterior and lateral displacement with retraction.

can be used alone and the "deep stitch" can be avoided. Retracting on both the left and right sides of the pericardium should not be done simultaneously during cardiac positioning since retracting the right pericardium with lateral displacement of the heart will cause compression of caval inflow. Relaxing the right pericardial sutures while pulling the left-sided sutures and the "deep stitch" taught greatly enhances exposure of the anterior and lateral walls of the heart, while avoiding compression on the right heart. These maneuvers, along with table positioning, facilitate excellent exposure once the cardiac positioner is placed.

Positioning and stabilization

Cardiac positioners and stabilizers have greatly increased the ability to manipulate the heart with minimal hemodynamic compromise. Two such systems include the Medtronic Octopus Tissue Stabilizer and Starfish or Urchin Heart Positioner (Medtronic, Inc, Minneapolis, MN) and the Maquet ACROBAT stabilizer and XPOSE positioner (Maquet, GMBH & Co, Rastatt, Germany). Cardiac positioning devices are frequently placed at the apex or slightly off the apex. Because these suction-based cardiac positioning devices pull the heart in the appropriate direction rather than pushing it, the heart is not compressed, functional geometry is maintained, and hemodynamics remain stable. The current generation of coronary stabilizers relies on epicardial suction rather than compression to maintain epicardial tissue capture and a motionless field in the region of grafting. Aggressive myocardial compression with the stabilizer should be avoided, since this will compromise ventricular function and lead to a paradoxical increase in motion in the target region. Instead, gentle traction on the epicardium provides for an area of stabilization. The anterior wall vessels often require only the coronary stabilizer for adequate exposure (Figure 2.3). The stabilizer is positioned along the caudal aspect of the retractor toward the left, with the retractor arm placed out of the way to prevent interference during the anastomosis. For the lateral and inferior wall vessels, the cardiac positioner is usually placed on the surgeon's side at the most cephalad location of the retractor. The coronary stabilizers can then be placed on either side (Figure 2.4). A general rule is to put the stabilizer in the assistant's way instead of the surgeon's, to prevent these devices from obstructing the surgeon's view or interfering with hand positioning during suturing.

In preparation for distal anastomosis, a soft silastic retractor tape mounted on a blunt needle (Retract-o-tape, Quest Medical, Inc, Allen, TX) is placed widely around the proximal vessel for transient occlusion (Figure 2.5). For inferior wall vessels, this suture can be displaced posteriorly and caudally by tying a more posterior pericardial suture loosely around the Retract-o-tape. The pericardial retraction suture serves as a "pulley," which not only enhances coronary exposure and the surgeon's view but also keeps this retraction stitch from interfering with the sutures during the anastomosis (Figure 2.6). Similarly, this maneuver can be employed for lateral wall targets. If there are concerns about hemodynamic stability during regional ischemia, the proximal vessel can be test occluded for 2–5 minutes. This gives the surgeon some assurance before committing to

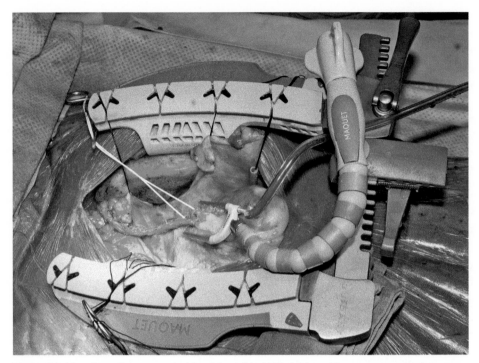

Figure 2.3 View from the surgeon's side of the table. With LAD grafting, exposure can be obtained with lateral traction of the "deep stitch" and the coronary stabilizer. A wet laparotomy pad placed between the "deep stitch" and the heart can provide additional displacement.

the anastomosis by creating an arteriotomy. After a brief period of reperfusion of 2–3 minutes, the vessel can be reoccluded and the artery prepared for anastomosis. The field is kept free of blood with a humidified CO_2 blower (DLP, Medtronic, Inc, Minneapolis, MN), which is managed by the scrub nurse or second assistant (Figure 2.7). During the inferior wall or lateral wall targets, the second assistant may occasionally provide better exposure by standing at the head of the bed, to the surgeon's left. In chronically occluded vessels that have collateral and/or retrograde flow, bleeding into the field can be controlled with another Retract-o-tape distally, a MyOcclude device (United States Surgical Corporation, Norwalk CT), or an intracoronary shunt.[58] A final preparatory measure is to place temporary atrial or ventricular pacing cables prior to positioning the heart.

Coronary grafting

Careful attention must be paid to the sequence of grafting since regional myocardial perfusion is temporarily interrupted in the beating heart. As a general rule, the collateralized vessel is grafted first, and the collateralizing vessel grafted last. For example, in patients with an occluded right coronary artery with a posterior descending artery supplied by collaterals from the left anterior descending artery, grafting the left anterior

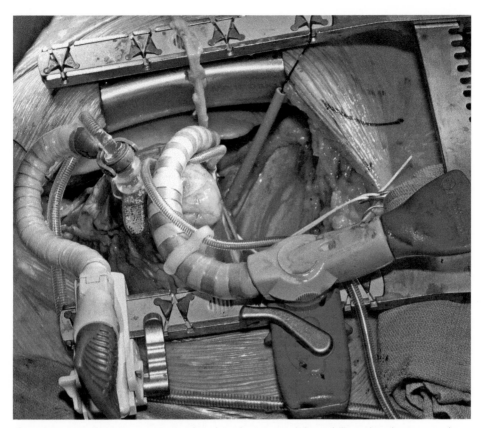

Figure 2.4 With a cardiac positioner placed on the apex and the stabilizer placed to expose the posterior descending coronary artery, excellent exposure can be obtained of the inferior wall vessels. Placing the patient in the Trendelenberg position with the table rotated slightly to the right will also facilitate exposure. The right pericardial traction sutures are relaxed, and the "deep stitch" is retracted infero-laterally. The positioner and the stabilizer are placed on the right side of the retractor.

descending first would not only leave the anterior wall ischemic, but also disrupt flow to the septum, inferior wall, and right ventricle. Thus, a more reasonable approach would involve grafting the posterior descending artery first, then performing a proximal anastomosis to ensure adequate flow while the proximal left anterior descending is occluded during construction of the left anterior descending artery (LAD) anastomosis. Another scenario that may pose problems is a large moderately (60–70%) stenotic right coronary artery. Not uncommonly, temporary occlusion of this artery will result in profound bradycardia and hypotension. In these circumstances, the surgeon must be prepared to use an intracoronary shunt or provide temporary epicardial pacing. A "proximals first" approach has been advocated by some OPCAB surgeons to allow adequate regional perfusion following completion of each distal anastomosis. With this approach, the left internal mammary artery/left anterior descending artery (LIMA-LAD) anastomosis can

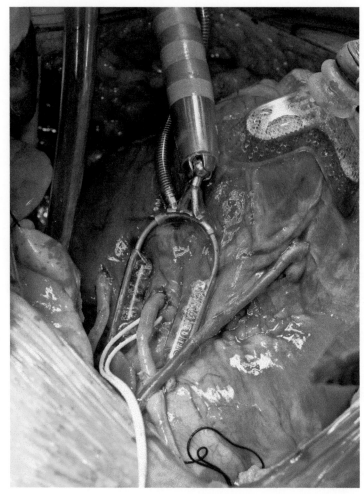

Figure 2.5 With the cardiac positioner and coronary stabilizer, the obtuse marginal vessels can be exposed. The right pericardial sutures should be relaxed to allow the heart to rotate into the right chest. After positioning the coronary stabilizer, a Retract-o-tape is doubly-looped around the proximal coronary artery to allow transient occlusion during the anastomosis.

be performed after the other territories have been revascularized which minimizes subsequent cardiac and LIMA pedicle manipulation after completion of this anastomosis. During the anastomosis, it is important for the surgeon and anesthesiologist to communicate any hemodynamic alterations that occur. If hemodynamics become compromised, gently relaxing the cardiac positioner or coronary stabilizer can often ameliorate the situation. Optimizing table positioning, fluid boluses, inotropes, vasopressors, or pacing, may also help. However, if it appears that hemodynamic conditions are deteriorating, then the safe next step is to place an intracoronary shunt,[58] relax and release both the

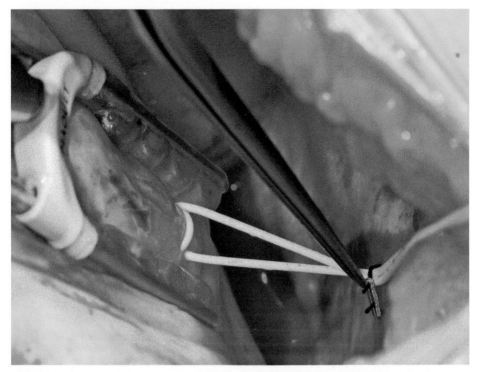

Figure 2.6 The Retract-o-tape is positioned as a "pulley" by placing a superficial pericardial traction suture posteriorly (below) to the placement of the Retract-o-tape around the coronary artery. A medium clip secures the suture and Retract-o-tape in place which can then be retracted to transiently occlude the artery.

stabilizer and positioner, and allow the heart to recover. At this point a decision must be made to convert "electively" to an on-pump procedure or to complete the procedure off-pump.

Proximal anastomoses

Epiaortic ultrasononography is utilized in all our patients undergoing cardiac surgery. It adds only 2–3 minutes to the procedure and provides both the surgeon and the anesthesiologist a simple, non-invasive, and inexpensive tool for assessing the extent of atheromatous disease in the ascending aorta in preparation for aortic clamping[59] or selection of an alternative clampless technique. The 8.5 MHz linear array probe is placed inside a sterile sleeve filled with sterile saline to act as a medium between the probe and the surface of the aorta (Figure 2.8). This information allows the surgeon to individualize placement of aortic clamps and proximal anastomotic devices to minimize the risk of atheroembolism.

Traditionally, proximal anastomoses during OPCAB have been performed with the use of an aortic partial-occluding clamp. Unlike on-pump coronary artery bypass,

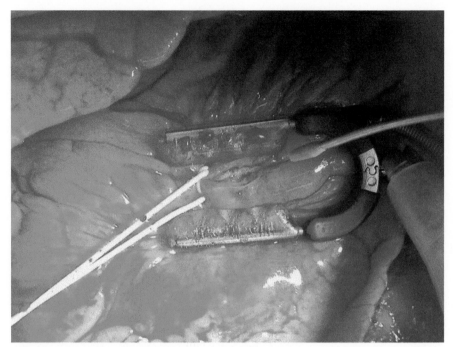

Figure 2.7 The coronary vessel is exposed and occluded proximally using the Retract-o-tape. The humidified CO_2 blower is shown maintaining a blood-free field.

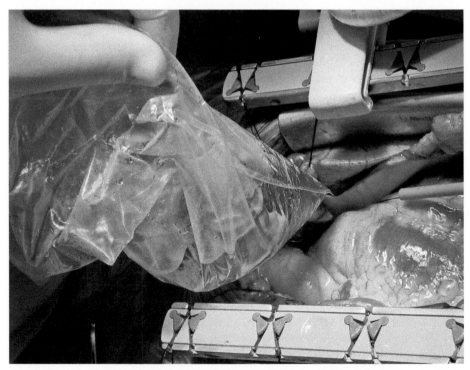

Figure 2.8 The epiaortic ultrasound probe can be seen in a sterile saline-filled bag, being positioned over the aorta. Ascending aortic atherosclerotic burden can be adequately assessed, allowing safety of partial aortic clamping, and optimal location of proximal anastomoses, to be determined.

OPCAB provides the opportunity to completely avoid manipulation of the aorta. Avoiding partial clamping during proximal anastomoses can be achieved by performing proximal anastomoses to *in situ* arterial grafts, or using proximal automated anastomotic connectors or facilitating devices.[47,60–62] Commercially available devices available for clampless proximal anastomoses include the Heartstring III™ (Maquet Cardiovascular LLC, San Jose, CA) or the PAS-Port™ Proximal Anastomosis System (Cardica Inc, Redwood City, CA). The Heartstring device creates a hemostatic seal with the inner surface of the ascending aorta that allows the creation of a hand-sewn anastomosis with a relatively bloodless field. The PAS-Port Proximal Anastomosis System was specifically designed to create an automated anastomosis between a saphenous vein graft and the aorta.

Conclusions

In conclusion, OPCAB provides surgeons with a valuable tool to enable coronary revascularization without the use of cardiopulmonary bypass or aortic clamping. This technique requires a unique skill set that can be mastered with careful patient selection and experience. While it is readily apparent that either an on- or off-pump approach can yield excellent in-hospital outcomes, there is some data suggesting that OPCAB may be advantageous in certain high-risk subgroups. Although technically more demanding than ONCAB, OPCAB allows the surgeon to avoid the potentially deleterious consequences of extracorporeal circulation and aortic manipulation, which is clearly beneficial in select circumstances. Conversely, several reports about incomplete revascularization and inferior graft patency plague the otherwise comparable mid- and long-term outcomes seen with OPCAB. Regardless of the approach selected, patients referred for surgery should undergo complete revascularization, and the precision and quality of the anastomosis must not be compromised in an effort to avoid the pump. With modern cardiac stabilizers and positioners, and with the techniques described here, excellent surgical outcomes can be expected in patients undergoing off-pump coronary artery bypass surgery.

Acknowledgments

The authors would like to thank David J. Fary, CCP for his assistance with digital photography.

References

1. **Moller CH, Perko MJ, Lund JT**, *et al.* (2010). No major differences in 30-day outcomes in high-risk patients randomized to off-pump versus on-pump coronary bypass surgery: the best bypass surgery trial. *Circulation*, **121**, 498–504.

2. **Gerola LR, Buffolo E, Jasbik W**, *et al.* (2004). Off-pump versus on-pump myocardial revascularization in low-risk patients with one or two vessel disease: perioperative results in a multicenter randomized controlled trial. *Ann Thorac Surg*, **77**, 569–73.

3. **Puskas JD, Williams WH, Duke PG**, *et al*. (2003). Off-pump coronary artery bypass grafting provides complete revascularization with reduced myocardial injury, transfusion requirements, and length of stay: a prospective randomized comparison of two hundred unselected patients undergoing off-pump versus conventional coronary artery bypass grafting. *J Thorac Cardiovasc Surg*, **125**, 797–808.

4. **Angelini GD, Taylor FC, Reeves BC, Ascione R** (2002). Early and midterm outcome after off-pump and on-pump surgery in beating heart against cardioplegic arrest studies (bhacas 1 and 2): a pooled analysis of two randomised controlled trials. *Lancet*, **359**, 1194–9.

5. **Kobayashi J, Tashiro T, Ochi M**, *et al*. (2005). Early outcome of a randomized comparison of off-pump and on-pump multiple arterial coronary revascularization. *Circulation*, **112**, I338–43.

6. **Muneretto C, Bisleri G, Negri A**, *et al*. (2003). Off-pump coronary artery bypass surgery technique for total arterial myocardial revascularization: a prospective randomized study. *Ann Thorac Surg*, **76**, 778–82; discussion 783.

7. **van Dijk D, Nierich AP, Jansen EW**, *et al*. (2001). Early outcome after off-pump versus on-pump coronary bypass surgery: results from a randomized study. *Circulation*, **104**, 1761–6.

8. **Widimsky P, Straka Z, Stros P**, *et al*. (2004). One-year coronary bypass graft patency: a randomized comparison between off-pump and on-pump surgery angiographic results of the prague-4 trial. *Circulation*, **110**, 3418–23.

9. **Angelini GD, Culliford L, Smith DK**, *et al*. (2009). Effects of on- and off-pump coronary artery surgery on graft patency, survival, and health-related quality of life: long-term follow-up of 2 randomized controlled trials. *J Thorac Cardiovasc Surg*, **137**, 295–303.

10. **Khan NE, De Souza A, Mister R**, *et al*. (2004). A randomized comparison of off-pump and on-pump multivessel coronary-artery bypass surgery. *N Engl J Med*, **350**, 21–8.

11. **Nathoe HM, van Dijk D, Jansen EW**, *et al*. (2003). A comparison of on-pump and off-pump coronary bypass surgery in low-risk patients. *N Engl J Med*, **348**, 394–402.

12. **Ascione R, Williams S, Lloyd CT**, *et al*. (2001). Reduced postoperative blood loss and transfusion requirement after beating-heart coronary operations: a prospective randomized study. *J Thorac Cardiovasc Surg*, **121**, 689–96.

13. **Karolak W, Hirsch G, Buth K, Legare JF** (2007). Medium-term outcomes of coronary artery bypass graft surgery on pump versus off pump: results from a randomized controlled trial. *Am Heart J*, **153**, 689–95.

14. **Fu SP, Zheng Z, Yuan X**, *et al*. (2009). Impact of off-pump techniques on sex differences in early and late outcomes after isolated coronary artery bypass grafts. *Ann Thorac Surg*, **87**, 1090–6

15. **Shroyer AL, Grover FL, Hattler B**, *et al*. (2009). On-pump versus off-pump coronary-artery bypass surgery. *N Engl J Med*, **361**, 1827–37.

16. **Lamy A, Devereaux PJ, Prabhakaran D**, *et al*. (2012). Off-pump or on-pump coronary-artery bypass grafting at 30 days. *N Engl J Med*, **366**, 1489–97.

17. **Diegeler A, Borgermann J, Kappert U**, *et al*. (2013). Off-pump versus on-pump coronary-artery bypass grafting in elderly patients. *N Engl J Med*, **368**, 1189–98.

18. **Cheng DC, Bainbridge D, Martin JE, Novick RJ** (2005). Does off-pump coronary artery bypass reduce mortality, morbidity, and resource utilization when compared with conventional coronary artery bypass? A meta-analysis of randomized trials. *Anesthesiology*, **102**, 188–203.

19. **Fattouch K, Guccione F, Dioguardi P**, *et al*. (2009). Off-pump versus on-pump myocardial revascularization in patients with ST-segment elevation myocardial infarction: a randomized trial. *J Thorac Cardiovasc Surg*, **137**, 650–6; discussion 656–7.

20. **Hannan EL, Wu C, Smith CR**, *et al*. (2007). Off-pump versus on-pump coronary artery bypass graft surgery: differences in short-term outcomes and in long-term mortality and need for subsequent revascularization. *Circulation*, **116**, 1145–52.

21. Li Z, Yeo KK, Parker JP, *et al.* (2008). Off-pump coronary artery bypass graft surgery in california, 2003 to 2005. *Am Heart J*, **156**, 1095–102.

22. Puskas JD, Edwards FH, Pappas PA, *et al.* (2007). Off-pump techniques benefit men and women and narrow the disparity in mortality after coronary bypass grafting. *Ann Thorac Surg*, **84**, 1447–54; discussion 1454–46.

23. Puskas JD, Kilgo PD, Lattouf OM, *et al.* (2008). Off-pump coronary bypass provides reduced mortality and morbidity and equivalent 10-year survival. *Ann Thorac Surg*, **86**, 1139–46; discussion 1146.

24. Puskas JD, Kilgo PD, Kutner M, *et al.* (2007). Off-pump techniques disproportionately benefit women and narrow the gender disparity in outcomes after coronary artery bypass surgery. *Circulation*, **116**, I192–99.

25. Puskas J, Cheng D, Knight J, *et al.* (2005). Off-pump versus conventional coronary artery bypass grafting: a meta-analysis and consensus statement from the 2004 ismics consensus conference. *Innovations*, **1**, 3–27.

26. Puskas JD, Thourani VH, Kilgo P, *et al.* (2009). Off-pump coronary artery bypass disproportionately benefits high-risk patients. *Ann Thorac Surg*, **88**, 1142–7.

27. Dewey TM, Herbert MA, Prince SL, *et al.* (2006). Does coronary artery bypass graft surgery improve survival among patients with end-stage renal disease? *Ann Thorac Surg*, **81**, 591–8; discussion 598.

28. Darwazah AK, Abu Sham'a RA, Hussein E, Hawari MH, Ismail H (2006). Myocardial revascularization in patients with low ejection fraction < or = 35%: effect of pump technique on early morbidity and mortality. *J Card Surg*, **21**, 22–7.

29. Mishra YK, Collison SP, Malhotra R, Kohli V, Mehta Y, Trehan N (2008). Ten-year experience with single-vessel and multivessel reoperative off-pump coronary artery bypass grafting. *J Thorac Cardiovasc Surg*, **135**, 527–32.

30. Panesar SS, Athanasiou T, Nair S, *et al.* (2006). Early outcomes in the elderly: a meta-analysis of 4921 patients undergoing coronary artery bypass grafting—comparison between off-pump and on-pump techniques. *Heart*, **92**, 1808–16.

31. Morris CD, Puskas JD, Pusca SV, *et al.* (2007). Outcomes after off-pump reoperative coronary artery bypass grafting. *Innovations*, **2**, 29–32.

32. Vohra HA, Bahrami T, Farid S, *et al.* (2008). Propensity score analysis of early and late outcome after redo off-pump and on-pump coronary artery bypass grafting. *Eur J Cardiothorac Surg*, **33**, 209–14.

33. Halkos ME, Puskas JD, Lattouf OM, *et al.* (2008). Impact of preoperative neurologic events on outcomes after coronary artery bypass grafting. *Ann Thorac Surg*, **86**, 504–10; discussion 510.

34. Chu D, Bakaeen FG, Dao TK, *et al.* (2009). On-pump versus off-pump coronary artery bypass grafting in a cohort of 63,000 patients. *Ann Thorac Surg*, **87**, 1820–6; discussion 1826–7.

35. Patel NC, Patel NU, Loulmet DF, McCabe JC, Subramanian VA (2004). Emergency conversion to cardiopulmonary bypass during attempted off-pump revascularization results in increased morbidity and mortality. *J Thorac Cardiovasc Surg*, **128**, 655–61.

36. Jin R, Hiratzka LF, Grunkemeier GL, Krause A, Page US, 3rd (2005). Aborted off-pump coronary artery bypass patients have much worse outcomes than on-pump or successful off-pump patients. *Circulation*, **112**, I332–7.

37. Motallebzadeh R, Bland JM, Markus HS, Kaski JC, Jahangiri M (2006). Health-related quality of life outcome after on-pump versus off-pump coronary artery bypass graft surgery: a prospective randomized study. *Ann Thorac Surg*, **82**, 615–9.

38. Puskas JD, Williams WH, O'Donnell R, *et al.* (2011). Off-pump and on-pump coronary artery bypass grafting are associated with similar graft patency, myocardial ischemia, and freedom from

reintervention: long-term follow-up of a randomized trial. *Ann Thorac Surg*, **91**, 1836–42; discussion 1842–33.

39. Sharony R, Grossi EA, Saunders PC, *et al.* (2004). Propensity case-matched analysis of off-pump coronary artery bypass grafting in patients with atheromatous aortic disease. *J Thorac Cardiovasc Surg*, **127**, 406–13.

40. Mishra M, Malhotra R, Karlekar A, Mishra Y, Trehan N (2006). Propensity case-matched analysis of off-pump versus on-pump coronary artery bypass grafting in patients with atheromatous aorta. *Ann Thorac Surg*, **82**, 608–14.

41. Czerny M, Baumer H, Kilo J, *et al.* (2001). Complete revascularization in coronary artery bypass grafting with and without cardiopulmonary bypass. *Ann Thorac Surg*, **71**, 165–9.

42. Alamanni F, Dainese L, Naliato M, *et al.* (2008). On- and off-pump coronary surgery and perioperative myocardial infarction: an issue between incomplete and extensive revascularization. *Eur J Cardiothorac Surg*, **34**, 118–26.

43. Kim KB, Kang CH, Chang WI, *et al.* (2002). Off-pump coronary artery bypass with complete avoidance of aortic manipulation. *Ann Thorac Surg*, **74**, S1377–82.

44. Daniel WT 3rd, Kilgo P, Puskas JD, *et al.* (2014). Trends in aortic clamp use during coronary artery bypass surgery: effect of aortic clamping strategies on neurologic outcomes. *J Thorac Cardiovasc Surg*, **147**, 652–7.

45. Hammon JW, Stump DA, Butterworth JF, *et al.* (2006). Single crossclamp improves 6-month cognitive outcome in high-risk coronary bypass patients: the effect of reduced aortic manipulation. *J Thorac Cardiovasc Surg*, **131**, 114–21.

46. Scarborough JE, White W, Derilus FE, *et al.* (2003). Combined use of off-pump techniques and a sutureless proximal aortic anastomotic device reduces cerebral microemboli generation during coronary artery bypass grafting. *J Thorac Cardiovasc Surg*, **126**, 1561–7.

47. Guerrieri Wolf L, Abu-Omar Y, Choudhary BP, Pigott D, Taggart DP (2007). Gaseous and solid cerebral microembolization during proximal aortic anastomoses in off-pump coronary surgery: the effect of an aortic side-biting clamp and two clampless devices. *J Thorac Cardiovasc Surg*, **133**, 485–93.

48. Jones EL, Weintraub WS (1996). The importance of completeness of revascularization during long-term follow-up after coronary artery operations. *J Thorac Cardiovasc Surg*, **112**, 227–37.

49. Synnergren MJ, Ekroth R, Oden A, Rexius H, Wiklund L (2008). Incomplete revascularization reduces survival benefit of coronary artery bypass grafting: role of off-pump surgery. *J Thorac Cardiovasc Surg*, **136**, 29–36.

50. Legare JF, Buth KJ, King S, *et al.* (2004). Coronary bypass surgery performed off pump does not result in lower in-hospital morbidity than coronary artery bypass grafting performed on pump. *Circulation*, **109**, 887–92.

51. Puskas JD, Williams WH, Mahoney EM, *et al.* (2004). Off-pump vs conventional coronary artery bypass grafting: early and 1-year graft patency, cost, and quality-of-life outcomes: a randomized trial. *JAMA*, **291**, 1841–9.

52. Magee MJ, Hebert E, Herbert MA, *et al.* (2009). Fewer grafts performed in off-pump bypass surgery: patient selection or incomplete revascularization? *Ann Thorac Surg*, **87**, 1113–8; discussion 1118.

53. Lamy A, Devereaux PJ, Prabhakaran D, *et al.* (2013). Effects of off-pump and on-pump coronary-artery bypass grafting at 1 year. *N Engl J Med*, **368**, 1179–88.

54. Magee MJ, Alexander JH, Hafley G, *et al.* (2008). Coronary artery bypass graft failure after on-pump and off-pump coronary artery bypass: findings from prevent iv. *Ann Thorac Surg*, **85**, 494–9; discussion 499–500.

55. **Lingaas PS, Hol PK, Lundblad R,** *et al.* (2006). Clinical and radiologic outcome of off-pump coronary surgery at 12 months follow-up: a prospective randomized trial. *Ann Thorac Surg,* **81,** 2089–95.

56. **Parolari A, Alamanni F, Polvani G,** *et al.* (2005). Meta-analysis of randomized trials comparing off-pump with on-pump coronary artery bypass graft patency. *Ann Thorac Surg,* **80,** 2121–5.

57. **Halkos ME, Cooper WA, Petersen R,** *et al.* (2006). Early administration of clopidogrel is safe after off-pump coronary artery bypass surgery. *Ann Thorac Surg,* **81,** 815–9.

58. **Bergsland J, Lingaas PS, Skulstad H,** *et al.* (2009). Intracoronary shunt prevents ischemia in off-pump coronary artery bypass surgery. *Ann Thorac Surg,* **87,** 54–60.

59. **Whitley WS, Glas KE** (2008). An argument for routine ultrasound screening of the thoracic aorta in the cardiac surgery population. *Semin Cardiothorac Vasc Anesth,* **12,** 290–7.

60. **Medalion B, Meirson D, Hauptman E, Sasson L, Schachner A** (2004). Initial experience with the heartstring proximal anastomotic system. *J Thorac Cardiovasc Surg,* **128,** 273–7.

61. **Akpinar B, Guden M, Sagbas E,** *et al.* (2005). Clinical experience with the novare enclose ii manual proximal anastomotic device during off-pump coronary artery surgery. *Eur J Cardiothorac Surg,* **27,** 1070–3.

62. **Puskas JD, Halkos ME, Balkhy H,** *et al.* (2009). Evaluation of the pas-port proximal anastomosis system in coronary artery bypass surgery (the epic trial). *J Thorac Cardiovasc Surg,* **138,** 125–32.

Chapter 3

Current status of minimally invasive, robotic and hybrid coronary artery bypass surgery

Stephanie Mick, Suresh Keshavamurthy, and Johannes Bonatti

Minimally invasive direct coronary bypass (MIDCAB)

MIDCAB surgery (also referred to as single-vessel small thoracotomy direct-vision bypass grafting, or SVST) uses an anterior, medially placed, mini-thoracotomy incision for both direct-vision left internal mammary (LIMA) harvest and creation of an anastomosis of the LIMA to a coronary artery in off-pump fashion.[1] It requires the use of a stabilizer placed directly through the operative (or separate port) incision.

Due to limited access to the lateral and posterior surfaces of the heart, revascularization using MIDCAB is generally limited to the left anterior descending artery (LAD) or the diagonal vessels. Specially designed retractors are available for internal mammary artery (IMA) harvesting. Originally described in 1965 by Kolessov,[2] the MIDCAB procedure was reintroduced in the mid-1990s and was adopted at many centers. In comparison to conventional coronary artery bypass grafting (CABG), its decreased utilization of resources, earlier return to full activity, reduced transfusion requirement, and initially acceptable graft patency were demonstrated in many early series.[3] Studies have also suggested decrease in duration of ventilation and hospital stay.[4]

Pain due to chest wall retraction may be experienced following MIDCAB[1] and this may have contributed to the decreased popularity. Nevertheless, experienced centers continue to successfully perform large numbers of MIDCAB procedures.[5] The significant learning curve[5,6] and less than optimal graft patency at some centers are probable causes for the low general acceptance of MIDCAB.

Technical details

Preoperative considerations

As in standard CABG, all patients should undergo a complete preoperative work-up, and body mass index and body habitus are to be noted. Obesity is considered a relative contraindication for MIDCAB as it may predispose to wound infection; this concern is primarily due to tissue necrosis caused due to the pressure on the wound edges by the retractor during LIMA harvest. For similar reasons, female patients with large breasts may be at increased risk for wound-related complications.[7] With regard to preoperative imaging, taking note of the heart position relative to the interspaces on chest X-ray can be helpful in determining the optimal placement of the access incision.

Conduct of operation

The patient is positioned supine with the left side up. Optimally, single lung ventilation is employed, however this is not absolutely necessary (if not utilized, reduction in tidal volume and packing of the lung away from the field are helpful maneuvers). The incision is placed in the left submammary area approximately at the mid-clavicular line in either the fourth or fifth intercostal space[8,9] (Figure 3.1). The level of incision constitutes the lower limit of LIMA harvesting as the chest wall caudal to the incision cannot be visualized. Some surgeons use the fifth interspace approach in order to obtain maximal conduit length.[8] Extending the LIMA using a segment of an additional arterial conduit to reach distal LAD targets and to avoid graft tension have been described.[10]

Retractors utilized for LIMA harvesting (e.g., Medtronic Inc, Minneapolis, MN) have an elongated superior blade designed to retract the upper ribs out of the line of vision, preventing them from acting as a shelf, thereby limiting exposure (Figure 3.2). The LIMA is preferably taken down in a skeletonized fashion or as a thin pedicle,[8] and is divided

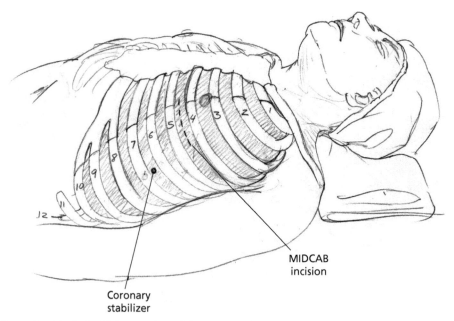

Coronary
stabilizer

MIDCAB
incision

Figure 3.1 The limited left anterolateral thoracotomy for minimally invasive direct coronary bypass (MIDCAB) is ~5–7 cm commencing in the mid-clavicular line in the fourth intercostal space. Also shown is the port placement for the endo stabilizer which can later be used for insertion of a chest tube.

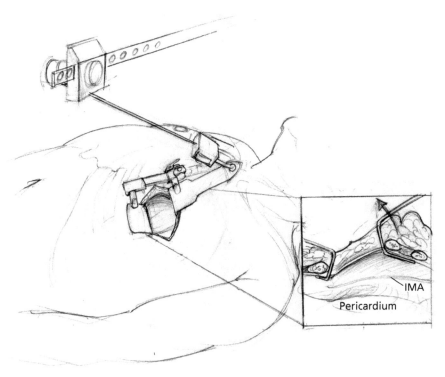

Figure 3.2 Specialized retractor setup for left internal mammary artery (LIMA) harvest in MIDCAB.
Reprinted with permission, Cleveland Clinic Center for Medical Art & Photography © 2015–2016. All Rights Reserved

following systemic anticoagulation (to ACT levels of 300 s). The LIMA retractor is then replaced with a standard thoracotomy retractor. The pericardial fat pad is then resected.

Prior to incising the pericardium, the phrenic nerve should be identified. The pericardium is incised longitudinally anterior to the phrenic to the level of the base of the heart. Stay sutures are useful in positioning the heart. The apex is first identified and then the LAD, which is situated to its right and courses parallel to the sternum. A diagonal artery may be the first vessel visualized and it is important not to mistake this for the LAD.[7] Once the LAD has been identified, a stabilizer is positioned (Figure 3.3). Silastic loops are placed proximally and distally if necessary (note that distal snares are preferably avoided as they may lead to scar lesions and impaired flow). Premedication with lidocaine or another antiarrhythmic should be employed prior to vessel occlusion. Should hemodynamic compromise be encountered following occlusion, the use of an intracoronary shunt may be employed with the vessel occluders released while performing the anastomosis. Whether shunted or not, the anastomosis is created with continuous 7-0 Prolene if the artery is fragile or small. Assessment of flow is recommended using transit time ultrasound.

After heparin reversal and confirmation of hemostasis, the pericardium is loosely reapproximated to prevent heart herniation and adherence of the apex to the intercostal

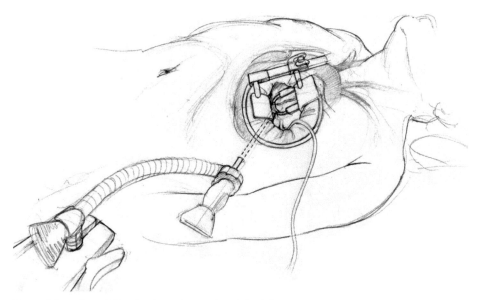

Figure 3.3 Endo stabilizer has been inserted and the left anterior descending artery (LAD) is exposed for grafting. Note the presence of a soft tissue retractor to optimize visibility.
Reprinted with permission, Cleveland Clinic Center for Medical Art & Photography © 2015–2016. All Rights Reserved

space (some authors recommend using a patch of bovine pericardium).[7] It is important to ensure the LIMA does not kink, particularly as it passes through the pericardium. A nerve block may be achieved by direct infiltration of 0.25% bupivacaine into the posterior intercostal spaces from ribs four to six. A single chest tube is placed and the ribs, pectoral muscle, and skin closed in a standard fashion.

Thoracoscopic MIDCAB

The LIMA is harvested thoracoscopically via port access incisions and the LIMA to LAD anastomosis is created through a mini-thoracotomy with minimal rib spreading.

The largest series of thoracoscopic MIDCAB was reported by Vassiliades *et al.* in 2007 who termed this approach "endoscopic atraumatic coronary artery bypass" (endo-ACAB) and reported a 3.6% conversion to sternotomy/thoracotomy rate, a 1% postoperative mortality rate (compared to the Society of Thoracic Surgeons (STS) National Database-predicted 30-day mortality of 2.7%), and a 0.3% stroke rate. These authors report a 96% LIMA to LAD patency rate at a mean follow-up of 18 months. The mean length of stay in the intensive care unit was 11.2 ± 9.9 hours, and hospital stay an impressive 2.4 ± 1.3 days.[10]

With an estimated 50-case learning curve required for mastery of the technique,[11] the thoracoscopic MIDCAB has not achieved widespread adoption at this time; however, centers with expertise in the technique have shown good results. Robotically assisted MIDCAB represents an alternative and will be discussed here in conjunction with other robotic techniques.

Technical details

Preoperative considerations

In general, patients with body mass index less than 30 are selected for surgeons early into their learning curve. Women with large breasts may be challenging as a larger submammary incision may be required or ports may need to pass through breast tissue. Thoracoscopic LIMA takedown requires hemithorax insufflation with CO_2 and the ability to tolerate single lung ventilation should be assessed preoperatively[1]—FEV1 less than 1 L on spirometry is usually the cutoff value.[12]

Conduct of operation

The patient is positioned supine as with MIDCAB. Using single lung ventilation, three ports are placed in the left mid-axillary line in the third, fifth, and seventh interspaces (some recommend the fifth interspace port be placed in the anterior axillary line.[13]). Standard thoracoscopic instruments are used. A 30-degree (either 5 mm or 10 mm) thoracoscope is placed via the fifth space and carbon dioxide insufflation is initiated to a target pressure of 8 mmHg. If hemodynamic compromise occurs, it may be due to hypertensive pneumothorax (especially in patients with compromised left ventricular function). Decreasing the rate of insufflation or evacuating some of the carbon dioxide from the thoracic space should rapidly improve the hemodynamics.

Next, a grasper and electrocautery or harmonic scalpel via the third and seventh interspaces are inserted. Gentle spatulation with the electrocautery or harmonic scalpel should be used to identify the side branches of the IMA. The entire IMA can be harvested from the subclavian vein to the level of the xiphoid process (clips are seldom used) in a pedicled fashion.[7,13] Care should be taken to avoid damage to the phrenic nerve and subclavian vein

Anastomosis creation proceeds in a manner similar to that described for MIDCAB.

Multivessel minimally invasive procedures

The benefits of the MIDCAB can be extended to those patients with multivessel disease by combining it with percutaneous coronary intervention (PCI) for lesions on the posterior and lateral surfaces of the heart in a hybrid approach when the non-LAD lesions are amenable to PCI.

The use of bilateral MIDCABs involving the use of bilateral anterior (medially placed) mini-thoracotomies and bilateral direct-vision internal mammary (as well as radial artery) conduits use has been reported.[14] The use of bilateral thoracoscopic IMA harvesting followed by right anterior thoracotomy for the bypass of right coronary artery and LAD territories has also been described. However, bypassing the posterolateral surface requires bilateral thoracotomies.[15]

One procedure, termed the "anterolateral thoracotomy/coronary artery bypass" (ALT-CAB) uses a larger left thoracotomy to harvest both the LIMA and right internal mammary artery (RIMA) under direct vision and all territories of the heart may be bypassed.

In a series of 255 patients, complete revascularization was achieved in all patients with no conversions to cardiopulmonary bypass (CPB). The mortality and stroke rate in this series was 1.2% and 0.8%, respectively, and 65.1% of patients were discharged within 48 hours.[16]

The most recent non-robotic minimally invasive option for multivessel disease (introduced in 2005) is termed "minimally invasive coronary artery bypass grafting" (MICS-CABG)[15] (also referred to as "multivessel small thoracotomy," MVST).[17] The MICS-CABG technique uses a more laterally placed thoracotomy than open MIDCAB and employs a specialized pivoting retractor that allows harvesting of the full-length of the LIMA. Two additional port-site incisions allow for the use of an epicardial stabilizer and an apical positioner. MICS-CABG is performed off-pump and does not require the use of thoracoscopic or robotic equipment and essentially amounts to a multivessel off-pump coronary artery bypass (OPCAB) performed through small non-sternotomy incisions. One limitation of the MICS-CABG is that RIMA takedown is not possible without using a larger incision, thoracoscopic or robotic assistance[18]; however, this limitation is in part offset by the use of saphenous vein grafts with proximal anastomoses to the ascending aorta.[15]

A dual center series of 450 patients over 3.5 years was reported for the MICS-CABG technique and showed encouraging results. A 3.8% conversion to sternotomy was reported and conversion to on-pump procedure (via peripheral cannulation) was reported in 7.6%. Proponents of MICS-CABG assert that it has a greater potential for wider adoption as it does not require the costly infrastructure associated with robotic or thoracoscopic procedures.[17]

MICS-CABG was compared to standard OPCAB using case-matching of a single surgeon's practice. There were no differences in mortality or rate of atrial fibrillation between groups, however a higher rate of pleural effusion in the MICS-CABG group was observed (15% *vs.* 4%, $P = 0.002$).[19] There is no long-term data available on graft patency, but early studies suggest acceptable short-term patency rates (92% for all grafts and 100% for LIMA grafts at 6 months).[20]

Robotically assisted revascularization

Robotic surgical systems are telemanipulators in which a surgeon controls microinstruments remotely from a console. The most widely used system is the da Vinci Si (Intuitive Surgical, Mountain View, CA). The system conveys high definition three-dimensional imaging to the surgeon at the console and sensors register finger and wrist movements and translate them, tremor-free, into the motion of the microinstruments in the operative field. Around 2,000 robotic cardiac operations are performed in the United States per year and the number is increasing modestly.[21]

There are several ways in which robots are used in CABG. These include robotically assisted MIDCAB (robotic IMA harvest with hand-sewn anastomosis via anterior thoracotomy) to totally intrathoracic revascularization performed solely through small port-site incisions (totally endoscopic CABG, or totally endoscopic coronary artery bypass (TECAB)). TECAB can be performed with or without use of CPB and cardioplegic arrest. When cardioplegic arrest is used, the term arrested heart TECAB (AH-TECAB) is used. When the heart is not arrested, the procedure is referred to as beating-heart TECAB (BH-TECAB).

Robotically assisted IMA harvest is followed by single hand-sewn anterior anastomosis via a small thoracotomy in an off-pump fashion. When compared with a single-vessel OPCAB, robotically assisted MIDCAB has been shown to result in shorter hospital stay and quicker return to work.[22] Robotically assisted MIDCAB has also been utilized as part of hybrid revascularization. TECAB may be used for single or multiple vessel bypasses (generally utilizing bilateral IMAs) and is the least physically invasive means of coronary revascularization. In contrast to other minimally invasive approaches, TECAB does not involve the use of incisions larger than port sites. First performed in 1998,[23] proponents of TECAB cite minimal surgical trauma and rapid recovery as the major advantages to this procedure. As no rib spreading is involved, there is minimal intercostal nerve trauma and less postoperative pain.

A recent review on TECAB[24] showed results that compare favorably with conventional approaches with the exception of reoperation for bleeding. The early patency rate was 96.4% (in the 253 patients who had some form of early imaging study). Five-year data on 62 single-vessel disease patients undergoing TECAB demonstrate 95.8% survival, 83.1% freedom from major adverse cardiac and cerebrovascular events (MACCE), and 91.1% freedom from angina.[24] Long-term follow-up on graft patency comes from Currie et al.,[25] who reported a 92.7% overall patency rate at 8 years in a mixed on- and off-pump practice.

Technical details

Preoperative evaluation

We recommend preoperative computed tomography (CT) angiography of the chest, abdomen, and pelvis to assess for the size of the heart and its relation to the chest wall, size of the pericardial fatpad, and relation of the internal mammary arteries to the target vessels. In our experience, a distance of less than 25 mm from the left heart border to the chest wall can lead to significant technical challenges owing to insufficient working space. Additionally, the course (intramyocardial *vs.* epicardial) of the target vessels should be noted along with the ascending aortic diameter and grade of aortoiliac atherosclerosis. We also recommend pulmonary function testing in all patients being considered for TECAB with the FEV1 and diffusing capacity of the lungs for carbon monoxide (DLCO) values, which are important not only for determining the patient's ability to tolerate single lung ventilation during IMA takedown but also to obtain a sense of intrathoracic volume. We have observed intraoperative technical difficulties (related to space limitations), and postoperative morbidity to increase in patients with an FEV1 of less than 2.5 L.

The role of cardiopulmonary bypass and cardioplegic arrest in TECAB

TECAB can be performed with or without the use of CPB. Endoscopic suturing is technically challenging and we strongly advise gaining experience with arrested heart TECAB prior to undertaking BH-TECABs. We recommend prophylactic peripheral cannulation under all circumstances, even if BH-TECAB is planned, to be prepared for "worst case scenarios" (e.g., ventricular fibrillation with the robot docked). Without prior cannulation and the ability to immediately initiate CPB, such situations can rapidly grow dire, with potential for great harm to the patient and the TECAB program at the surgeon's institution. Therefore, we reiterate our recommendation to prophylactically cannulate *all* cases under controlled conditions. It is to be noted that going on bypass and deflating both lungs can also provide significant additional space inside the chest if needed in a BH-TECAB.

Arrested heart TECAB requires specific perfusion and cardioplegia skills. Surgeons are strongly advised to develop remote access perfusion techniques in other minimally invasive cardiac cases before attempting TECAB. Remote access CPB and the use of ascending aortic balloon occlusion is technically challenging and requires discipline in patient selection. Femoral cannulation and endoballoon should only be used in patients *without* aortoiliac atherosclerosis (~2/3 of patients in our experience). Axillary antegrade perfusion and femoral insertion of the endoballoon is the best option for patients with moderate grades of aortoiliac atherosclerosis. Transthoracic clamping and direct aortic root cannulation for cardioplegia is in its early stages of development; challenges associated with this technique include transthoracic puncture of the ascending aorta, as well endoscopic robotic control of bleeding after catheter removal.

Technical considerations in cannulation

If there is no aortoiliac atherosclerosis, femoro-femoral CPB and use of an endoaortic balloon is standard. It is possible for all cannulation maneuvers including exposure of femoral vessels to be performed by one team member as another harvests the IMA. We also recommend use of a distal perfusion cannula via superficial femoral artery in all cases to ensure adequate limb perfusion. The aortic endoballoon catheter is inserted into the sidearm of an arterial perfusion cannula and advanced into the aortic root over a guidewire. We recommend cardioplegia induction with 6 mg adenosine after cross-clamping to induce prompt arrest. Use of a percutaneous coronary sinus cannula allows a standard protocol of antegrade and retrograde cardioplegia administration.

If mild to moderate aortoiliac atherosclerosis is present, femoral arterial retroperfusion is avoided and perfusion through the left axillary (via an 8-mm Dacron sidearm) and a non-perfusing endoballoon is used. Axillary exposure and anastomosis of the sidearm should be completed before docking of the robot. In these cases, the aortic endoballoon is inserted through a separate 19 F cannula in the femoral artery.

In case preoperative CT shows significant aortoiliac atherosclerosis, we forgo endoballoon use and operate on the beating heart with prophylactic peripheral cannulation. An ACT level of ≥300 sec is used for cannulation and before starting the anastomosis with cardioplegia, the ACT is increased to ≥480 s.

Procedural details

Single lung ventilation is mandatory as is transesophageal echo (TEE) monitoring throughout the entire procedure. R2 defibrillator patches are placed in positions that allow sternotomy. An endovent and/or percutaneous coronary sinus cannula are placed if arrested heart TECAB is planned.

The patient is placed on the operating table (Figure 3.4) in the supine position with arms tucked and left chest slightly elevated (Figure 3.5). The patient is prepped and draped as for open CABG and all equipment for conversion to full sternotomy should be immediately available.

Correct port insertion is a step that significantly influences the whole procedure and should be performed by the most experienced team member. First, a 12.5 mm camera port is inserted (gently and cautiously so as to avoid injury to the heart or mediastinum) into the fifth intercostal space in the anterior axillary line after deflation of the left lung. Carbon dioxide insufflation (at pressures of 8 mmHg) is then initiated and an angled camera inserted. Under direct videoscopic vision, the left and right instrument ports are then placed into the third and seventh intercostal spaces, slightly anterior to the camera port. During this phase, the surgical team should remain focused on the patient's hemodynamics as increase in intrathoracic pressure may cause hemodynamic compromise. Communication with the anesthesia team is critical; if hypotension develops during insufflation, the first attempts at correction should be lowering the CO_2 pressure or evacuating intrathoracic CO_2 (via one of the ports) rather than fluid or inotrope administration.

Following port placement, the robotic system is docked and the internal mammary artery is harvested in skeletonized fashion with the angled camera view in the "up" position using the robotic electrocautery spatula (on low-power setting) and a DeBakey forceps. Most side branches can be cauterized and clips used only for larger branches. Dissection should proceed primarily via cautery tip spatulation of surrounding tissue (Figure 3.6). It should be noted that both the left and right IMA can be taken down using the aforementioned technique. To access the right IMA, the retrosternal tissue is divided and the right pleura is entered. When bilateral conduits are used, the right IMA is harvested prior to the left. Approximately midway through IMA takedown, we fully heparinize to allow bypass to be started expeditiously should technical difficulties occur as the case proceeds.

A 5 mm assistance port is placed after IMA harvesting in the left parasternal region. This port allows insertion of material needed throughout the procedure such as bulldogs, suture material, silastic tapes, and suction tubing.

The pericardial fatpad is removed and pericardiotomy performed with the angled camera view "down" using robotic longtip forceps and electrocautery at 30 Watts. The pericardium is opened slightly lateral to the right ventricular outflow tract and extended all the way down to its reflection and then taken laterally in the caudal and cranial part, so

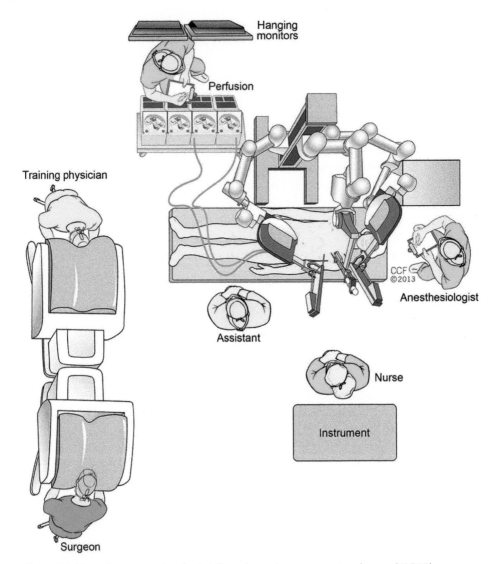

Figure 3.4 Operating room setup for totally endoscopic coronary artery bypass (TECAB).
Reprinted with permission, Cleveland Clinic Center for Medical Art & Photography © 2015–2016. All Rights Reserved

that a pericardial flap is created which falls into the left pleural space. This step is significantly easier on CPB (especially in obese patients and those with cardiomegaly).

Exposure of target vessels

The LAD can be visualized and accessed without difficulties using the aforementioned port arrangement. In beating-heart TECAB and arrested heart cases with lateral target vessels, vessel exposure is facilitated with an endostabilizer (brought in through a

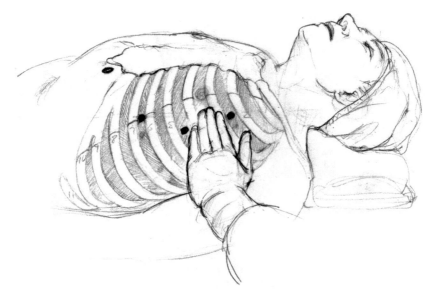

Figure 3.5 Patient positioning for TECAB with port placement sites. Ports are placed four fingerbreadths apart.

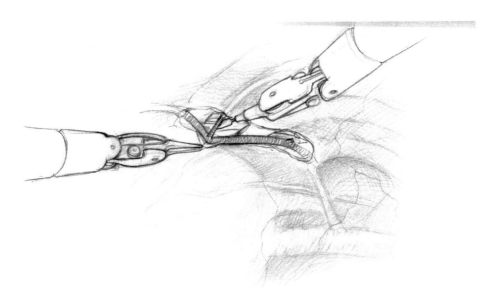

Figure 3.6 Robotic internal mammary artery (IMA) take-down.

subcostal port inserted two finger breaths left lateral to the xiphoid angle) docked to the fourth arm of the robotic system.

In using the endostabilizer to access obtuse marginal branches, the operator should steer the endostabilizer gently over the left ventricle and then lift the lateral wall. In beating-heart TECAB, this maneuver can lead to hemodynamic compromise and ischemic changes and CPB could be used to obviate this problem.

The right coronary artery system may also be accessed from the patient's left side. In this case, the endostabilizer is inserted through the left instrument port (change to a 12-mm port is necessary) and the left robotic instrument is inserted through a subcostal port. The acute margin can be lifted so that the posterior descending artery and the posterolateral branch are easily visible and accessible for anastomosis, taking great care not to injure the right ventricular epimyocardium. It should be noted that we have only utilized this technique on the arrested heart.

Once the target coronary artery is properly located and exposed, a robotic DeBakey forceps and robotic Pott's scissors are used to incise the epicardium. The target vessel is then incised using robotic lancet beaver knife. This can be challenging at first due to the lack of tactile feedback (Figures 3.7 and 3.8). For anastomosis creation, bilateral robotic black diamond microforceps are used as needle drivers of a 7 cm 7-0 double armed polypropylene suture. The first stitch is inside-to-out on the coronary artery, forming the first bite of the first stitch of the back wall of the anastomosis close to the toe. This needle is then "parked" at a distance from the anastomosis and the anastomosis is continued with the other arm of the stich, suturing the whole back wall going inside-to-out on the graft and outside-in on the target vessel. The graft parachuted to the coronary artery wall following the first three bites and the operator gently pulls on both suture ends frequently to ensure adequate suture tension (Figure 3.9). Suturing then continues around the heel of the anastomosis, again suturing inside-to-out on the graft and outside-to-in on the

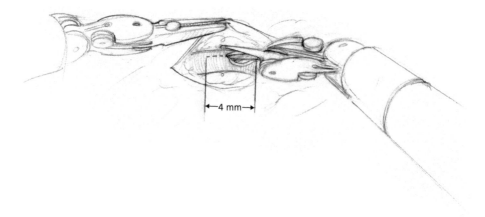

Figure 3.7 Exposure of the LAD and completion of a 4 mm arteriotomy.

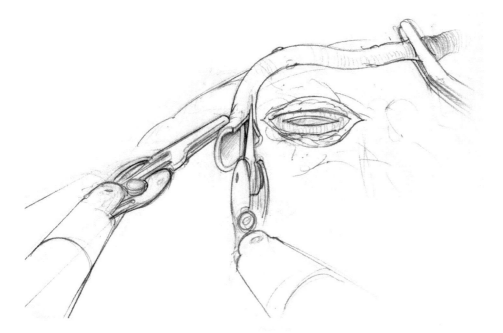

Figure 3.8 Preparation of the conduit for grafting.

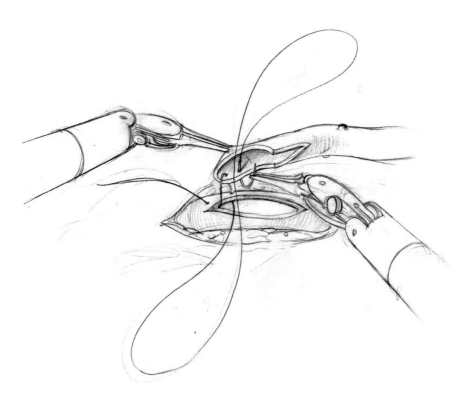

Figure 3.9 Technique of anastomosis starting at the "toe": note "inside-out" bites on both the coronary artery and the conduit.

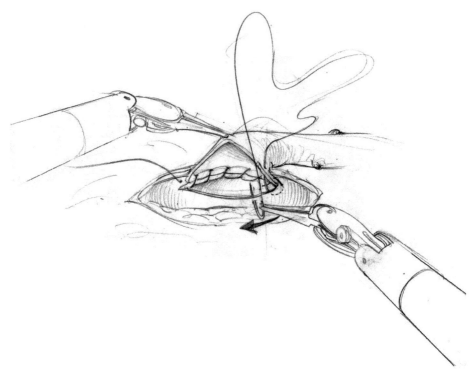

Figure 3.10 Progression of TECAB anastomosis; note completion of the 'heel' and the direction of suturing.

Reprinted with permission, Cleveland Clinic Center for Medical Art & Photography © 2015–2016. All Rights Reserved

target coronary artery (Figure 3.10). This needle is then "parked" and the previously used needle is used to suture the toe and rest of the anterior wall of the anastomosis (Figure 3.11).

Tips on anastomotic creation in arrested heart TECAB

The coronary artery should be incised during administration of antegrade cardioplegia to fill the vessel and reduce the risk of back wall injury. The use of silastic vessel occluding loops can be very helpful in cases of target vessel backflow. All foreign material should be removed from the chest before the aortic endoballoon is deflated. The heart may later on become hyperdynamic and these maneuvers will be difficult.

Tips on anastomotic creation in beating-heart TECAB

Silastic loops should be placed both proximally and distally to the anastomotic site (although usually only the proximal needs to be occluded) and suturing is carried out around an intraluminal shunt. All stitches require an extra degree of gentleness in order to avoid injury to vessel walls. The magnified bouncing operative field is challenging until experience has been gained.

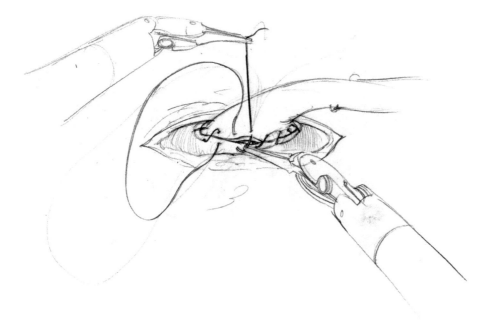

Figure 3.11 Completed anastomosis; note last few bites using the first needle that had previously been "parked."

Multivessel TECAB

Multivessel TECAB may be achieved using bilateral *in situ* mammary artery grafts, sequential grafting, or Y-grafts constructed with the contralateral IMA or radial artery. Use of a vein graft with proximal anastomosis creation to the left axillary artery is also possible.[26]

Post-anastomosis procedures

In the robotic setting with high magnification, any needed repair sutures can be placed with excellent visualization. We recommend intraoperative flow measurements using a transit time flowprobe. Residual blood in the left pleural space may be evacuated using a tracheal suction tube brought through the parasternal assistance port. After confirmation of hemostasis, the robotic system is undocked but all ports are left in place, to be removed under direct videoscopic vision. A chest tube is inserted through the camera port *with the left lung inflated* so as to avoid injuries to the graft during tube insertion.

Postoperative considerations

There are currently no temporary pacing wires which can be placed endoscopically; other methods of temporary pacing (e.g., endovenous, transthoracic, pacing Swan Ganz) are used if necessary. Special attention (neurovascular checks) should be paid to peripheral pulses following cannulation in arrested heart TECAB. Owing to single-lung ventilation during the case, respiratory compromise can occur, and the postoperative chest X-ray may show a degree of atelectasis. The camera port site is usually the most painful area until the chest tube is removed. No sternal precautions are required. MIDCAB and thoracoscopic MIDCAB patients can be extubated in the operating room (OR). We recommend initiation of dual antiplatelet therapy (DAPT: aspirin and clodipogrel) after six hours (or once chest tube drainage is minimal).

Hybrid coronary revascularization

Introduction and definition

Hybrid coronary revascularization combines surgical and catheter-based therapies for the treatment of coronary artery disease (CAD). Usually, a LIMA to the LAD is placed with PCI to the non-LAD targets.

Rationale and background

The hybrid approach is an effort to bring "the best of both worlds" of cardiac surgery and interventional cardiology together for the treatment of multivessel CAD.

Angelini and colleagues reported the first series of six patients, treated with a MIDCAB LIMA to LAD and percutaneous transluminal coronary angioplasty (PTCA) or PTCA and stent in 1996. A decade later, a multicenter trial showed the basic feasibility of combining robotic TECAB and PCI.[27] Twenty-seven patients requiring double vessel revascularization were treated with TECAB LIMA-LAD, and PCI to non-LAD targets. Three-month follow-up angiography showed an excellent LIMA-LAD patency of 96.3% but lower than expected PCI patency of 66.7%. One patient suffered perioperative myocardial infarction (MI). The early reintervention rate, primarily due to stent failures, was 29.3%.

Current state of hybrid revascularization

Experience with this technique remains limited. No prospective randomized trials on hybrid revascularization have been published and only three series with large numbers of patients have been reported.

Available data show a low mortality (0–2%) and low morbidity overall (average of ~4.7% in hospital morbidity across all studies), with shorter hospital and intensive care unit (ICU) stays than would be expected with conventional CABG.[28] Immediate LIMA to LAD patency rates range from 92% to 100%. With respect to restenosis rates, the data are mixed. Earlier series, which made use of bare metal stents or angioplasty without stenting, revealed higher 6-month stent restenosis rates, so that in the entire experience thus far, these rates range from 2.3% to 23%, with an average of 11% across all of the literature. When only drug-eluting stents were used in procedures combining MIDCAB and PCI, 97% 1-year patency rates were reported.[28]

In the largest reported series of 226 patients with five-year follow-up, 1.3% hospital mortality, average hospital stay of 6 days and 92.9% 5-year survival rate were found. Five-year freedom from MACCE was 75.2% and reintervention rates were 2.7% with respect to bypass grafts and 14.2% with respect to PCI targets.[29]

Technical and timing considerations

The timing of the surgical procedure in relation to the PCI has been a subject of some discussion. All hybrid procedures are staged; only the duration between procedures and the order in which they are performed is varied. "Two-staged" hybrid procedures are those in which PCI and CABG are performed in separate operative locations, separated by hours, days, or weeks. "One-stop" procedures are performed in one setting, separated by minutes in a hybrid operating room.[27] In a two-stage hybrid procedure, either the surgical or percutaneous intervention can be performed first. In a simultaneous procedure, the surgical intervention is usually performed first.

Percutaneous intervention prior to surgical intervention

Most patients who are treated with a "PCI first" approach undergo acute percutaneous intervention of the culprit lesion for acute coronary syndrome and the LIMA to LAD graft is placed later. Disadvantages of this approach include: the need for antiplatelet agents following PCI necessitates performing the surgical revascularization on DAPT with a slightly increased risk of bleeding[1]; PCI is performed in a setting in which no protection is afforded by a LIMA to LAD graft; and unless a third procedure (completion angiogram) is performed after the surgical procedure, no imaging of the LIMA-LAD graft is afforded at time of PCI.

Potential advantages to this approach include the decreased risk of ischemia if LAD occlusion is used in a beating-heart surgical approach (due to collateral circulation from the revascularized non-LAD targets). Additionally, there is the opportunity for aggressive multivessel PCI since if a complication occurs or PCI is not successful, surgical revascularization can be performed later.

Surgical intervention prior to percutaneous intervention

Performing PCI after LIMA-LAD grafting allows one to avoid possible DAPT related bleeding complications during the surgical procedure; DAPT can be started after surgery and continued long-term. Additionally, the percutaneous interventions are performed under the protection of a revascularized LAD and affords the opportunity for angiographic evaluation of the LIMA-LAD anastomosis.[1]

The optimal duration of time between the two interventions is unclear. Patients should at least be able to tolerate lying flat on the angiography table (this may take several days due to postoperative respiratory compromise). It also seems reasonable to delay PCI until the inflammatory milieu following surgery resolves, by perhaps 3–5 days. Additionally, patients may wish for 7–10 days of mental/physical recovery following surgery. Ideally, PCI is completed at the index hospitalization so that the patient is not discharged without being fully revascularized.[1]

Simultaneous procedures

Two-staged procedures involve more resources (two teams, logistical challenges, costs associated with two separate procedures and possible hospitalization between the procedures) and many patients prefer the simplicity of one inclusive procedure. In centers with hybrid operating rooms, a "one-stop" procedure is possible.

Attractive features about this approach include: monitoring throughout the procedure under general anesthesia so that any complications can be resolved in one setting; a completion angiogram can be done to evaluate the LIMA-LAD graft; and the patient experiences the emotional/psychological benefit of a complete "fix" in one setting.[1] Drawbacks include the need for specialized facilities, increased procedural times, and cost. At this point, the data regarding the effect of DAPT on bleeding in patients undergoing hybrid procedure are mixed (with some reporting increased bleeding and others reporting no such increase[28–30]; and the effects of protamine reversal on stent patency are unknown).

Srivastava *et al.* investigated the timing of PCI related to TECAB in hybrid procedure.[31] Most patients (73%) in their study underwent TECAB before PCI and they concluded that the timing of interventions should be individually tailored to the patient's needs.

Conclusion

Improvements in technology and imaging have made a variety of minimally invasive approaches to coronary revascularization available. Despite market forces and financial considerations, it should be emphasized that the procedure is tailored to the individual patient. This is an exciting phase of reinvention for the "Heart Team" concept and it remains to be seen which of these procedures gains momentum in the community at large.

References

1. DeRose JJ (2009). Current state of integrated "hybrid" coronary revascularization. *Semin Thorac Cardiovasc Surg*, **21**(3), 229–36.
2. Kolessov VI (1967). Mammary artery-coronary artery anastomosis as method of treatment for angina pectoris. *J Thorac Cardiovasc Surg*, **54**(4), 535–44.
3. Sellke FW, Chu LM, Cohn WE (2010). Current state of surgical myocardial revascularization. *Circ J*, **74**(6), 1031–7.
4. Karpuzoglu OE, Ozay B, Sener T, *et al.* (2009). Comparison of minimally invasive direct coronary artery bypass and off-pump coronary artery bypass in single-vessel disease. *Heart Surg Forum*, **12**(1), E39–43.
5. Holzhey DM, Cornely JP, Rastan AJ, Davierwala P, Mohr FW (2012). Review of a 13-year single-center experience with minimally invasive direct coronary artery bypass as the primary surgical treatment of coronary artery disease. *Heart Surg Forum*, **15**(2), E61–8.

6. Holzhey DM, Jacobs S, Mochalski M, *et al.* (2007). Seven-year follow-up after minimally invasive direct coronary artery bypass: experience with more than 1300 patients. *Ann Thorac Surg,* **83,** 108–14.

7. Reddy RC (2011). Minimally invasive direct coronary artery bypass: technical considerations. *Semin Thorac Cardiovasc Surg,* **23**(3), 216–9.

8. Itagaki S, Reddy RC (2013). Options for left internal mammary harvest in minimal access coronary surgery. *J Thorac Dis,* **5**(Suppl 6), S638–S40.

9. Subramanian VA (1996). Clinical experience with minimally invasive reoperative coronary bypass surgery. *Eur J Cardiothorac Surg,* **10**(12), 1058–62; discussion 1062–3.

10. Vassiliades TA Jr, Reddy VS, Puskas JD, Guyton RA (2007). Long-term results of the endoscopic atraumatic coronary artery bypass. *Ann Thorac Surg,* **83**(3), 979–84; discussion 984–5.

11. Vassiliades TA Jr (2002). Technical aids to performing thoracoscopic robotically-assisted internal mammary artery harvesting. *Heart Surg Forum,* **5**(2), 119–24.

12. Sellke FW, Ruel ME (2010). *Atlas of Cardiac Surgical Techniques.* Townsend C, Evers BM (eds). Philadelphia, PA: Elsevier.

13. Hrapkowicz T, Bisleri G (2013). Endoscopic harvesting of the left internal mammary artery. *Ann Cardiothorac Surg,* **2**(4), 565–9.

14. Weerasinghe A, Bahrami T (2005). Bilateral MIDCAB for triple vessel coronary disease. *Interact Cardiovasc Thorac Surg,* **4**(6), 523–5.

15. McGinn JT Jr, Usman S, Lapierre H, *et al.* (2009). Minimally invasive coronary artery bypass grafting: dual-center experience in 450 consecutive patients. *Circulation,* **120**(11 Suppl), S78–84.

16. Guida MC, Pecora G, Bacalao A, *et al.* (2006). Multivessel revascularization on the beating heart by anterolateral left thoracotomy. *Ann Thorac Surg,* **81**(6), 2142–6.

17. Lapierre H, Chan V, Ruel M (2006). Off-pump coronary surgery through mini-incisions: is it reasonable? *Curr Opin Cardiol,* **21**(6), 578–83.

18. Ruel M, Une D, Bonatti J, McGinn JT (2013). Minimally invasive coronary artery bypass grafting: is it time for the robot? *Curr Opin Cardiol,* **28**(6), 639–45.

19. Lapierre H, Chan V, Sohmer B, Mesana TG, Ruel M (2011). Minimally invasive coronary artery bypass grafting via a small thoracotomy versus off-pump: a case-matched study. *Eur J Cardiothorac Surg,* **40**(4), 804–10.

20. Ruel M, Shariff MA, Lapierre H, *et al.* (2014). Results of the minimally invasive coronary artery bypass grafting angiographic patency study. *J Thorac Cardiovasc Surg,* **147**(1), 203–9.

21. Robicsek F (2008). Robotic cardiac surgery: time told! *J Thorac Cardiovasc Surg,* **135**(2), 243–6.

22. Martens TP, Argenziano M, Oz MC (2006). New technology for surgical coronary revascularization. *Circulation,* **114**(6), 606–14.

23. Loulmet D, Carpentier A, d'Attellis N, *et al.* (1999). Endoscopic coronary artery bypass grafting with the aid of robotic assisted instruments. *J Thorac Cardiovasc Surg,* **118**(1), 4–10.

24. Bonatti J, Lehr EJ, Schachner T, *et al.* (2012). Robotic total endoscopic double-vessel coronary artery bypass grafting--state of procedure development. *J Thorac Cardiovasc Surg,* **144**(5), 1061–6.

25. Currie ME, Romsa J, Fox SA, *et al.* (2012). Long-term angiographic follow-up of robotic-assisted coronary artery revascularization. *Ann Thorac Surg,* **93**(5), 1426–31.

26. Bonatti J, Lee JD, Bonaros N, Schachner T, Lehr EJ (2012). Robotic totally endoscopic multivessel coronary artery bypass grafting: procedure development, challenges, results. *Innovations (Phila),* **7**(1), 3–8.

27. Katz MR, Van Praet F, de Canniere D, *et al.* (2006). Integrated coronary revascularization: percutaneous coronary intervention plus robotic totally endoscopic coronary artery bypass. *Circulation,* **114**(1 Suppl), I473–6.

28. **Bonatti J, Schachner T, Bonaros N**, *et al.* (2008). Simultaneous hybrid coronary revascularization using totally endoscopic left internal mammary artery bypass grafting and placement of rapamycin eluting stents in the same interventional session. The COMBINATION pilot study. *Cardiology*, **110**(2), 92–5.

29. **Bonatti JO, Zimrin D, Lehr EJ**, *et al.* (2012). Hybrid coronary revascularization using robotic totally endoscopic surgery: perioperative outcomes and 5-year results. *Ann Thorac Surg*, **94**(6), 1920–6.

30. **Kon ZN, Brown EN, Tran R**, *et al.* (2008). Simultaneous hybrid coronary revascularization reduces postoperative morbidity compared with results from conventional off-pump coronary artery bypass. *J Thorac Cardiovasc Surg*, **135**(2), 367–75.

31. **Srivastava MC, Vesely MR, Lee JD**, *et al.* (2013). Robotically assisted hybrid coronary revascularization: does sequence of intervention matter? *Innovations (Phila)*, **8**(3), 177–83.

Chapter 4

Aortic valve repair

Munir Boodhwani and Gebrine El Khoury

Introduction

Aortic valve replacement remains the gold standard treatment for severe aortic valve disease. However, valve repair is emerging as a feasible and attractive alternative to valve replacement in selected patients. Valve repair can reduce or eliminate the risks of prosthesis-related complications including thromboembolism, endocarditis, anticoagulant related hemorrhage, and reoperation due to structural valve deterioration among others. Analogous to the mitral valve, a reconstructive approach to the aortic valve requires a thorough and detailed understanding of the valve anatomy, valve function, assessment and classification of pathologic lesions, and treatment of all affected components of the valve. In this chapter, we review the key features of aortic valve and root anatomy, an approach to valve assessment and lesion classification, and a demonstration of commonly used reparative techniques for aortic valve repair. Furthermore, we review the outcomes of aortic valve repair in unselected cohorts as well as distinct subsets of patients undergoing aortic valve preservation and repair.

Aortic valve anatomy and function

The anatomy of the aortic valve and root is familiar to cardiac surgeons.[1] However, there are some features outlined next that are particularly relevant to aortic valve preserving and repair surgery.[2] Like the mitral valve, aortic valve function involves an important interaction between the valve annulus and leaflets. Importantly, however, the annulus of the aortic valve is not a single structure but rather consists of three different components namely, the sinotubular junction, the ventriculo-aortic junction, and the anatomic crown-shaped annulus which serves as the insertion point of the aortic valve cusps (Figure 4.1).[3] These components work together to facilitate normal valve function and together are termed the "functional aortic annulus." The atrioventricular (AV) leaflets insert into the aortic annulus proximally at the aorto-ventricular junction (AVJ) and distally at the sinotubular junction (STJ). In a normal AV, the cusps coapt at the center of the AV orifice with a coaptation height that is approximately at the mid-level between the AVJ and the STJ. The height of the sinuses of Valsalva (from the AVJ to the STJ) corresponds to the external diameter of the STJ, which can be useful to size prostheses for aortic root replacement and to assess cusp geometry after AV repair.

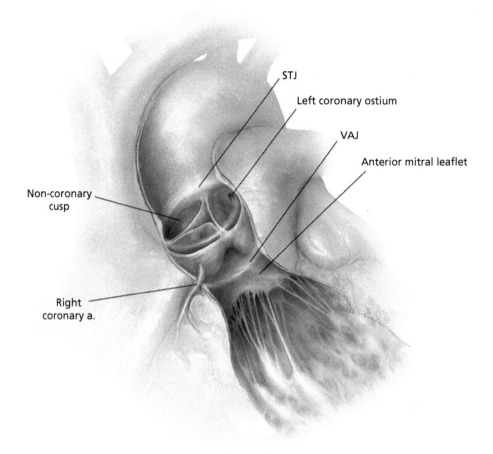

Figure 4.1 Anatomy of the aortic valve and the functional aortic annulus (FAA). Anatomy of the subvalvular region of the aortic valve. The dotted line marks the limits of external dissection of the aortic root and the proximal suture line for a valve-sparing root replacement procedure using the reimplantation technique.

STJ, sinotubular junction; VAJ, ventriculo-aortic junction.

Adapted from Boodhwani M and El Khoury G (2009) Aortic Valve Repair, Operative Techniques in Thoracic and Cardiovascular Surgery 14(4):266–280 with permission from Elsevier

As a functional entity, the AV consists of the functional aortic annulus (FAA) and the valve cusps. The integrity of these two functional components (i.e., the cusps and FAA) is the basis for good valvular function, and alteration in one of these components is frequently associated with alteration in the other. Thus, a fundamental principle in AV repair is that lesions of the cusps *and* the FAA should both be addressed at the time of valve repair.

The anatomy of the subvalvular region of the aortic valve and its surrounding structures also has important implications for aortic valve repair[4] (Figure 4.1). An important observation is that external dissection of the aortic root from its surrounding structures

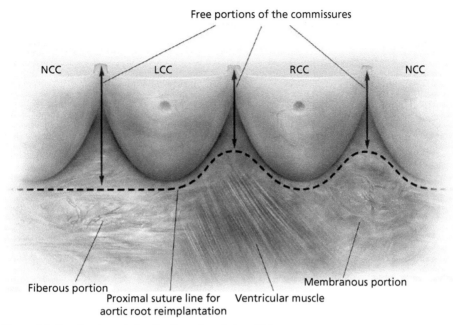

Figure 4.2 Repair-oriented classification of aortic insufficiency.
NCC, non-compaction cardiomyopathy; LCC, left coronary cusp; RCC, right coronary cusp.
Adapted from Boodhwani M and El Khoury G (2009) Aortic Valve Repair, Operative Techniques in Thoracic and Cardiovascular Surgery 14(4):266–280 with permission from Elsevier

is limited by the membranous septum (at the junction of the non-coronary and right coronary cusps) and by ventricular muscle (at the junction of the left and right coronary cusps) whereas at all other points, external dissection down to the level of the anatomic valve annulus is possible and necessary when valve-sparing root replacement is performed using the reimplantation technique. Thus, the proximal suture line for the aortic valve reimplantation procedure follows these external limitations in a curvilinear fashion.

Classification of aortic insufficiency

Until recently, a major limitation to the more generalized application of aortic valve repair techniques was the absence of a common framework for valve assessment to help guide the approach to valve repair. Important lessons in this regard may be learned from the development of mitral valve repair. The Carpentier classification[5] of mitral valve insufficiency was responsible, in large part, for the development and generalized dissemination of repair techniques for the mitral valve because it provided a common language for cardiologists, anesthesiologists, and surgeons to communicate about disease mechanisms and pathology. Key characteristics of that classification system were that it encompassed the entire spectrum of disease; it clarified and provided insight into the mechanism of insufficiency; it could be consistently applied using different assessment modalities (i.e., echocardiography

AI class	Type I Normal cusp motion with FAA dilatation or cusp perforation				Type II cusp prolapse	Type III cusp restriction
	Ia	Ib	Ic	Id		
Mechanism	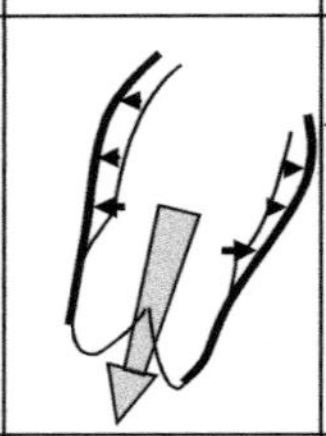	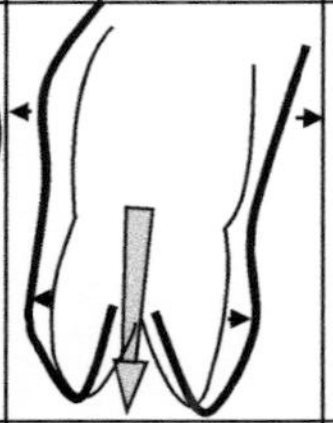	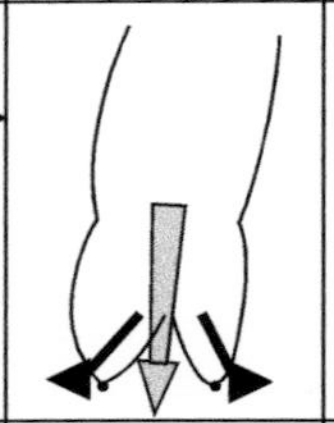	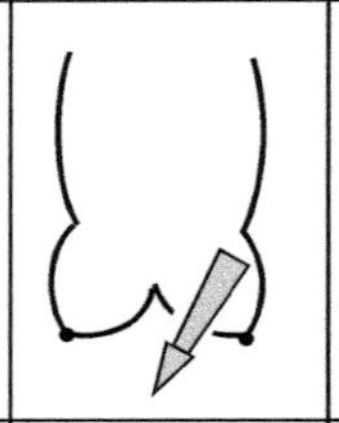	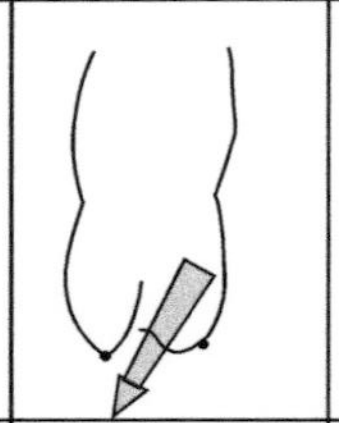	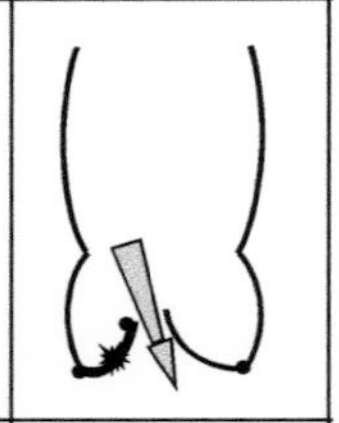
Repair techniques (Primary)	STJ remodeling *Ascending aortic graft*	Aortic Valve sparing: *Reimplantation or Remodeling with SCA*	SCA	Patch repair *Autologous or bovine pericardium*	Prolapse repair *Plication Triangular resection Free margin resuspension Patch*	Leaflet repair *Shaving decalcification patch*
(Secondary)	SCA		STJ annuloplasty	SCA	SCA	SCA

Figure 4.3 Classification of aortic insufficiency.

AI, aortic insufficiency; FAA, functional aortic annulus; SCA, sudden cardiac arrest; STJ, sinotubular junction.

Adapted from Boodhwani M and El Khoury G (2009) Aortic Valve Repair, Operative Techniques in Thoracic and Cardiovascular Surgery 14(4):266–280 with permission from Elsevier

and surgical assessment); it guided the repair techniques; and lastly, it provided a framework for the assessment of long-term outcome for differing mitral valve pathologies.

Over the past decade, we have developed a similar classification of aortic valve insufficiency with the aforementioned characteristics in mind[6] (Figure 4.3). This classification centers around the idea that the aortic valve, much like the mitral valve consists of two major components, namely the aortic annulus and the valve leaflets. Contrary to the mitral valve, however, the annulus of the aortic valve is not a single anatomic structure. The functional aortic annulus, rather, consists of two separate components, namely the ventriculo-aortic junction and the sinotubular junction. As in Carpentier's classification of mitral valve disease, regurgitation associated with normal leaflet motion is designated as type I. This is largely due to lesions of the FAA with type Ia aortic insufficiency (AI) due to sinotubular junction enlargement and dilatation of the ascending aorta, type Ib due to dilatation of the sinuses of Valsalva and the sinotubular junction, type Ic due to dilatation of the ventriculo-aortic junction, and lastly type Id due to cusp perforation without a primary FAA lesion. Type II AI is due to leaflet prolapse secondary to excessive cusp tissue or due to commissural disruption. Type III AI is due to leaflet restriction, which may be found in bicuspid, degenerative, or rheumatic valvular disease due to calcification, thickening, and fibrosis of the aortic valve leaflets.

Patients can present with either single or multiple lesions contributing to their aortic insufficiency. For example, patients with isolated type Ib AI (due to dilatation of the sinuses of Valsalva) are expected to have a central regurgitant jet. Thus, the presence of a sinus of Valsalva aneurysm with an eccentric AI jet suggests concomitant leaflet prolapse (type II) or restriction (type III). Further assessment of leaflet anatomy can help to better delineate the different mechanisms contributing to AI. Once the mechanism of AI is well understood, the classification system can help to guide the surgeon in the choice of surgical techniques for correction of the pathology.

Surgical techniques

Exposure and assessment

Aortic valve repair procedures are generally performed through a median sternotomy. Arterial cannulation is performed distal to any diseased aortic segments, typically in the distal ascending aorta or aortic arch. Alternatively, axillary artery cannulation may be performed in the setting of aortic arch pathology. A single, two-venous cannula is inserted through the right atrial appendage. Following cardioplegic arrest, a transverse aortotomy is performed ~1 cm above the sinotubular junction starting above the non-coronary sinus and the posterior 2–3 cm of aortic wall is left intact. The distal aorta is retracted cephalad. Full thickness 4-0 polypropylene traction sutures are placed at the three commissures and retracted using clamps but not tied in order to permit a dynamic assessment of valve anatomy. Axial traction is applied (perpendicular to the level of the annular plane) on the commissural traction sutures. This maneuver demonstrates physiological aortic valve closure position and the area and height of coaptation

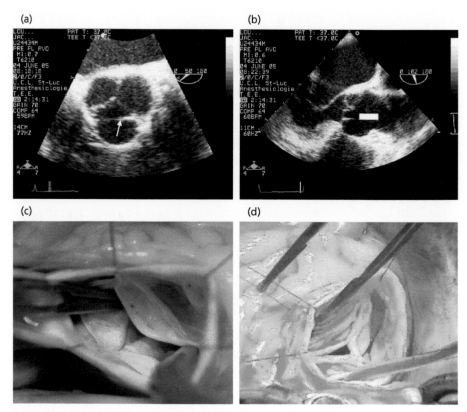

Figure 4.4 A transverse fibrous band is typically visible on echocardiography (a, b) and surgical inspection (c, d) in the setting cusp prolapse in trileaflet aortic valves and may help in the detection and localization of cusp prolapse.

Adapted from Boodhwani et al. (2011) Assessment and repair of aortic valve cusp prolapse: Implications for valve-sparing procedures, the Journal of Thoracic and Cardiovascular Surgery 4(9):917–25 with permission from Elsevier

is observed. Leaflets are inspected to assess mobility, restriction, calcification, and prolapse. A prolapsing cusp will exhibit a transverse fibrous band at this time, also visible on echocardiography[7] (Figure 4.4).

Interventions on the aortic root and annulus

Type 1 lesions are most frequently due to dilatation of the various components of the FAA and may occur in isolation or in association with cusp disease. A type 1a lesion occurs due to a supracoronary ascending aortic aneurysm with concomitant dilatation of the STJ. This is corrected by replacing the ascending aorta and remodeling the STJ using a Dacron tube graft. When significant associated AI is present, subcommissural annuloplasty is also performed. Aneurysms of the aortic root (type 1b) are frequently associated with dilatation of the STJ and the AVJ. These are treated using valve-sparing root replacement, preferentially using the reimplantation technique[8] because it provides better stabilization

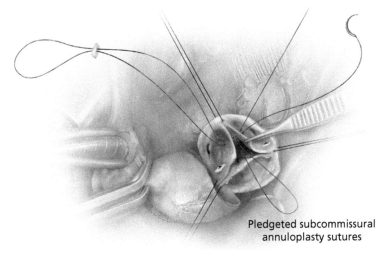

Pledgeted subcommissural
annuloplasty sutures

Figure 4.5 Subcommissural annuloplasty.
Reprinted from Boodhwani M and El Khoury G (2009) Aortic Valve Repair, Operative Techniques in Thoracic and
Cardiovascular Surgery 14(4):266–280 with permission from Elsevier

of the ventriculo-aortic junction (VAJ). Aortic root remodeling[9] may also be used to treat
aneurysms of the aortic root and is particularly useful when only one or two sinuses are
involved.

Subcommissural annuloplasty

Subcommissural annuloplasty is typically performed at mid-commissural height, except
at the non-coronary/right coronary commissure where it should be performed higher in
order to avoid the membranous septum and conduction tissue (Figure 4.5). Care should
also be taken in this area when tying the suture in order to avoid a tear in the septum.
At the other two commissures, the subcommissural annuloplasty may be performed at
a lower level if greater increase in the coaptation surface is desired. A subcommissural
annuloplasty reduces the width of the interleaflet triangle, improves cusp coaptation, and
may help to stabilize the ventriculo-aortic junction. In the setting of a bicuspid aortic
valve, however, subcommissural is not always sufficient for the prevention of future VAJ
dilatation. Alternative approaches to annuloplasty of the aortic valve, without root replacement, are currently under development.[10,11]

Valve-sparing root replacement—reimplantation technique

A valve-sparing root replacement using the reimplantation technique provides the most
stable form of functional aortic annuloplasty. In addition to patients with aortic root aneurysms, this technique can also facilitate aortic valve repair in patients with moderate
root dilatation in the setting of bicuspid aortic valves. The important steps of this procedure are described next.[12]

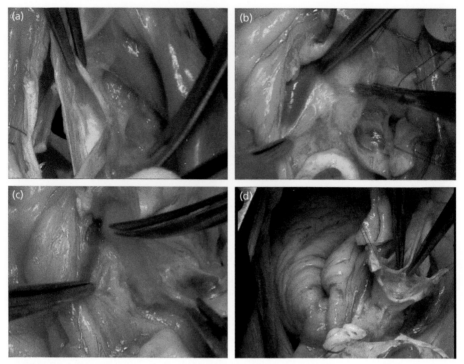

Figure 4.6 (a to d) External dissection for a valve-sparing root replacement procedure using the reimplantation technique.

Aortic root preparation

The key principle is to externally dissect the aortic root as low as possible, given the natural anatomic limitations (i.e., where the root inserts into ventricular muscle). The root dissection is started along the non-coronary (NC) sinus and continued toward the left coronary (LC)/NC commissure. In this area, the subannular region of the AV is fibrous and dissection can therefore be carried to below the level of insertion of the leaflets. Moving toward the right coronary (RC)/NC commissure as well as along the right sinus and the RC/LC commissure, the dissection is limited by non-fibrous portions of the annulus (Figure 4.6). The sinuses of Valsalva are then resected, leaving approximately 5 mm of aortic wall attached and the coronary buttons are harvested.

Prosthesis sizing

The three commissural traction sutures are pulled perpendicular to the annular plane with a slight inward motion to ensure good leaflet coaptation. When the leaflets are coapting adequately, a Hagar dilator is used to size the circle that includes the three commissures and a graft 4 mm larger is chosen, as this graft will sit outside the commissural posts. An alternative approach to prosthesis sizing takes advantage of the principle that in a normally

Height of the commissure

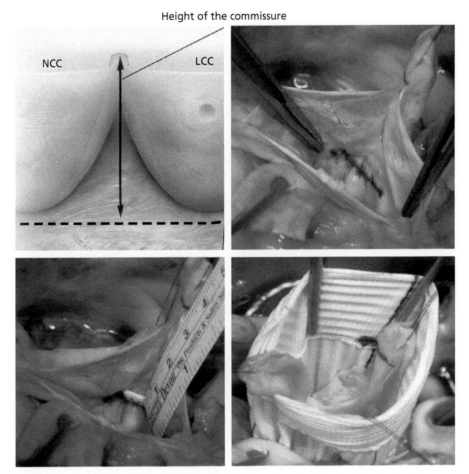

Figure 4.7 A novel method for prosthesis sizing when using the reimplantation technique.
NCC, non-compaction cardiomyopathy; LCC, left coronary cusp.

functioning aortic valve, the height of the commissure (measured from the base of the interleaflet triangle to the top of the commissure) is equal to the external diameter of the sinotubular junction[13] (Figure 4.7). Although various components of the aortic root and the FAA may dilate in the setting of root aneurysms, the height of the commissure remains relatively constant. The height of the commissure is most easily measured at the non-coronary/left-coronary commissure by first drawing a connecting line between the nadirs of the two adjacent cusps (base of interleaflet triangle) and measuring the distance between this line and the top of the commissure. This height corresponds to the diameter of the graft chosen.

Proximal suture line

2-0 Tycron sutures with pledgets are passed from inside to outside the aorta with the pledgets on the inside, starting from the NC/LC commissure and moving clockwise.

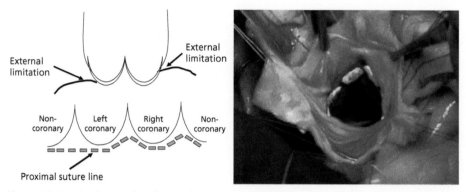

Figure 4.8 Proximal suture line for a valve-sparing root replacement procedure using the reimplantation technique.

Reproduced from Boodhwani M and de Kerchove L (2009) Aortic root replacement using the reimplantation technique: tips and tricks, Interactive Cardiovascular and Thoracic Surgery 8(5): 584–586 with permission from Oxford University Press

Along the fibrous portion of the aortic annulus, these sutures are inserted along the horizontal plane formed by the base of the interleaflet triangles. Importantly, however, along the non-fibrous portions of the annulus where the external dissection of the aortic root is limited by muscle, these sutures are inserted along the lowest portion of the freely dissected aortic root making the proximal suture line slightly higher at the RC/NC and RC/LC commissures compared to the LC/NC commissure (Figure 4.8).

Prosthesis preparation and fixation

A Dacron prosthesis with or without built-in neo-aortic sinuses may be used. To prevent AI, the three commissures must be attached to the prosthesis along the same plane, the new sinotubular junction. Due to external limitations of root dissection, the graft has to be tailored. First, the distance from the base of the interleaflet triangle to top of the commissure is measured at the LC/NC commissure and marked on the graft. Then, at the RC/NC and RC/LC commissures, the distance from the proximal suture to the top of the commissure is measured and used to determine the amount of graft material that needs to be trimmed (Figure 4.9). Thus, the height of the trimmed portion is the difference between height of the unrestricted LC/NC commissure and the distance from the proximal suture line to the top of the respective commissure. The exact shape of the trimmed portion is less important as the prosthesis will accommodate to the external limitations of the aortic root. The pledgeted sutures are then passed through the base of the prosthesis, respecting the spaces between sutures and importantly, the curvilinear contour of the suture line. The commissural traction sutures are pulled up together while tying down the prosthesis to ensure appropriate seating around the aortic annulus.

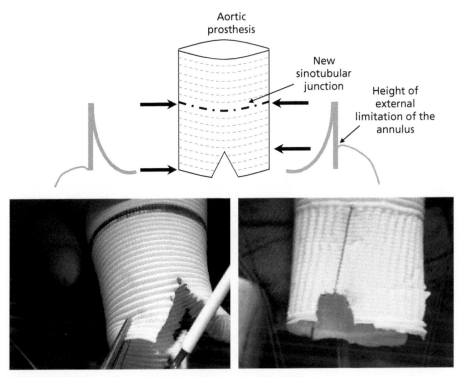

Figure 4.9 Tailoring of the prosthesis for the reimplantation technique.
Reproduced from Boodhwani M and de Kerchove L (2009) Aortic root replacement using the reimplantation technique: tips and tricks, Interactive Cardiovascular and Thoracic Surgery 8(5): 584–586 with permission from Oxford University Press

Valve reimplantation

The commissures are reimplanted first using 4-0 polypropylene sutures while pulling up on the prosthesis and the native commissure and then tied into place. Radial traction is then applied on two adjacent commissural sutures and this clearly delineates the "line of implantation." This running suture line is performed in small regular steps passing the suture from outside the prosthesis to inside and through the aortic wall, staying close to the annulus, and then back out of the prosthesis.

Leaflet assessment and repair

After valve reimplantation, it is critical to re-examine the leaflets for any unmasked prolapse, symmetry, and the height and depth of coaptation. Prolapse can be repaired using a variety of techniques described next. Cardioplegia is administered through the distal end of the graft with partial clamping to distend the new aortic root, assess root pressure, and signs of left ventricular (LV) dilatation. A limited echocardiographic view may be obtained at this time. The cardioplegia solution is then slowly aspirated out of the prosthesis without distorting the leaflets. This gives another visual assessment of AV in its physiologic closed state as well as the area and height of coaptation. Coronary ostia are then reimplanted on the graft and the distal anastomosis is performed at the level of normal aorta.

Cusp repair techniques

Cusp prolapse correction

Cusp prolapse is associated with excess length of the free margin, which can be corrected using either central free margin plication or free margin resuspension. When a single cusp is prolapsing, the two non-prolapsing cusps serve as the reference and are used to estimate the required reduction in the free margin length. When two cusps are prolapsing, the third non-prolapsing cusp is used as a reference to indicate the desired height of coaptation. In the rare instance that all the cusps are prolapsing, the goal is to achieve a cusp coaptation height at the mid-level of the sinuses of Valsalva.

Free margin plication

The technique for central free margin plication has been previously described[14] (Figure 4.10). A 7-0 polypropylene suture is passed through the center of the two non-prolapsing reference cusps and gentle axial traction is applied. The prolapsing cusp is

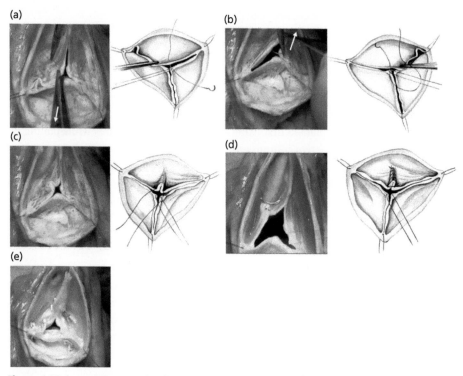

Figure 4.10 (a to e) Free margin plication technique for the correction of cusp prolapse.
Adapted from Boodhwani M and El Khoury G (2009) Aortic Valve Repair, Operative Techniques in Thoracic and Cardiovascular Surgery 14(4):266–280 with permission from Elsevier

gently pulled parallel to the reference cusp and a 6-0 polypropylene suture is passed through the prolapsing cusp, from the aortic to ventricular side, at the point at which it meets the center of the reference cusp. Next, the direction of traction on the pro-lapsing cusp is reversed and the same suture is passed from the ventricular to the aortic side of the cusp where it meets the middle of the reference cusp. The length of cusp-free margin between the two ends of this 6-0 suture represents the quantity of excess-free margin which is then plicated by tying this suture with the excess tissue on the aortic side.

The plication is extended by about 5–10 mm onto the body of the aortic cusp by adding interrupted or running locked 6-0 polypropylene sutures. If there is significant excessive tissue, it can be shaved off using a scalpel or scissors keeping sufficient tissue to bring the edges together.

Free margin resuspension

Excess length of the cusp free margin may also be corrected using resuspension with polytetrafluoroethylene (PTFE) suture[15,16] (Figure 4.11). A 7-0 polypropylene suture is first passed through the center (nodule of Arantis) of the two non-prolapsing cusps, which serves as a reference. A 7-0 PTFE suture is passed twice at the top of the commis-sure. Next, one arm of the suture is passed over and over the length of the free margin in a running fashion. The suture is locked at the other commissure. A second 7-0 PTFE is then passed in the same fashion along the cusp free margin. The length of the free margin is reduced by applying gentle traction on each branch of the PTFE sutures and applying opposite resistance with forceps at the middle of the free margin. This maneuver is used to plicate and shorten the free margin until it reaches the same length as the ad-jacent reference cusp-free margin. The same maneuver is applied for the second half of the free margin. This two-step technique for free margin resuspension allows symmetric and homogenous shortening. When the appropriate amount of free margin shortening is achieved, the two suture ends at each commissure are tied.

This technique may be used in isolation or in combination with other cusp repair tech-niques and is particularly useful in the setting of a fragile free margin with multiple fen-estrations or to homogenize the free margin when a pericardial patch is used for cusp augmentation.

Approach and techniques for bicuspid aortic valves

Bicuspid aortic valve disease affects not only the valve cusps, but also the FAA. Bicuspid AV may be divided into two general types[17,18] (Figure 4.12). Type 0 bicuspid AV do not contain a median raphé, have two symmetric aortic sinuses, two commissures, and a sym-metric base of leaflet implantation of the two cusps. This configuration is present in a minority of cases. The mechanism of AI in this setting is usually cusp prolapse of one or both cusps due to the presence of excess cusp tissue.

Type 1 bicuspid AVs, which are significantly more prevalent, have a median raphé on the conjoint cusp and an asymmetric distribution of the aortic sinuses with a large aortic sinus accompanying a large non-conjoint cusp and two smaller cusps fused together

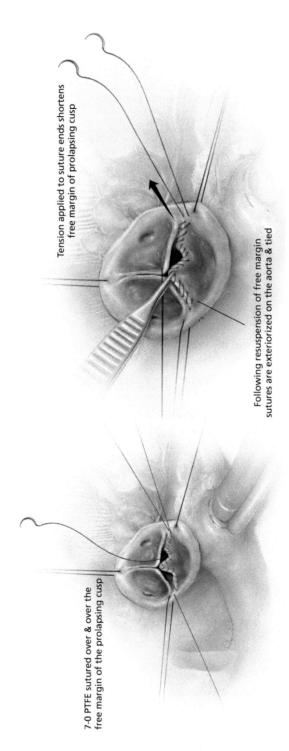

Tension applied to suture ends shortens
free margin of prolapsing cusp

Following resuspension of free margin
sutures are exteriorized on the aorta & tied

7-0 PTFE sutured over & over the
free margin of the prolapsing cusp

Figure 4.11 Free margin resuspension technique using polytetrafluoroethylene (Gore-Tex) suture for cusp prolapse correction.

Reprinted from Boodhwani M and El Khoury G (2009) Aortic Valve Repair, Operative Techniques in Thoracic and Cardiovascular Surgery 14(4):266–280 with permission from Elsevier

(a)   (b)   (c)

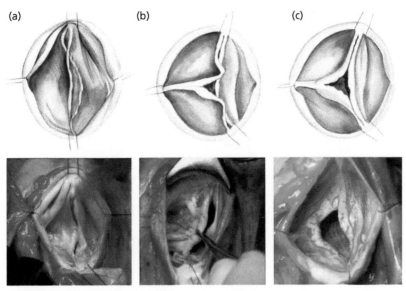

Figure 4.12 (a to c) Cusp anatomy in bicuspid aortic valves.

Reprinted from Boodhwani *et al.* (2010) Repair of regurgitant bicuspid aortic valves: a systematic approach, The Journal of Thoracic and Cardiovascular Surgery 140(2):276–284 with permission from Elsevier

with a median raphé. The raphé often attaches to the cusp base in the form of a "pseudo-commissure," which has a height lower than that of the true commissures. The raphé may be restrictive, fibrotic, calcified, or prolapsing. Furthermore, the base of leaflet implantation is typically larger (i.e., occupying a greater proportion of valve circumference) and higher on the conjoint cusp compared to the non-conjoint cusp. The mechanisms of AI in type 1 valves can be due to a rigid and restrictive raphé associated with small fused cusps resulting in a triangular coaptation defect. Alternatively, the raphé may be short and non-restrictive with well-developed cusps and associated prolapse of the conjoint cusp. Bicuspid valve anatomy can be anywhere along a spectrum between type 0 and type 1. The general algorithm for the repair of bicuspid aortic valves is presented in Figure 4.13.

In type 0 valves, the degree of prolapse is assessed by comparing the prolapsing cusp to the non-prolapsing cusp, similar to trileaflet valves. In the case where both cusps are prolapsing, the goal is to restore the height of coaptation to the mid-point of the sinuses of Valsalva. This may be performed using either free margin plication, free margin resuspension with 7-0 PTFE suture, or both as previously described for trileaflet valves. Thickened, fibrotic areas of the leaflet (typically central aspect of the free margin) are shaved and localized decalcification is performed if calcium is present.

In type 1 valves, the median raphé is addressed first. If the raphé is relatively mobile and only mildly thickened and fibrosed, it is preserved and shaved using a combination of a scalpel and scissors (Figure 4.14). When a severely restrictive or calcified raphé is present, a parsimonious triangular resection of this tissue is performed (Figure 4.15). Next, the

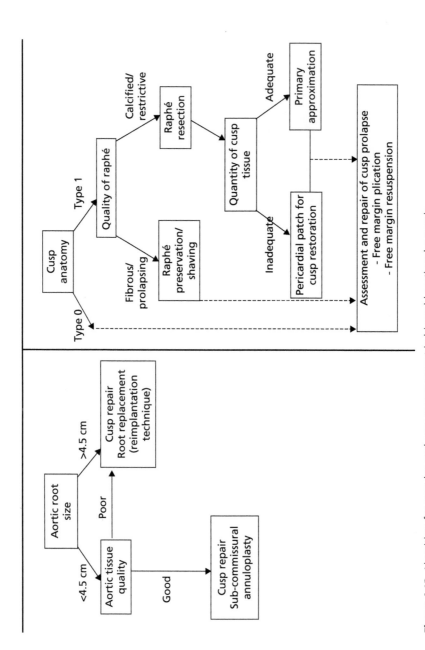

Figure 4.13 Algorithm for annulus and cusp management in bicuspid aortic valve repair.

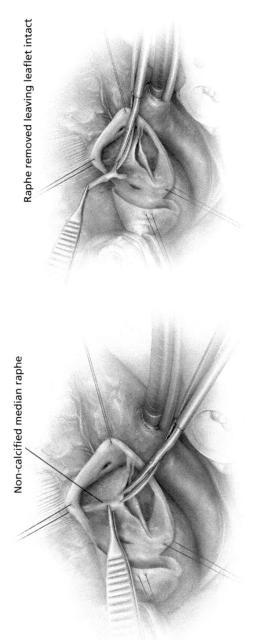

Figure 4.14 Shaving of a non-calcified, fibrous raphé.

Adapted from Boodhwani M and El Khoury G (2009) Aortic Valve Repair, Operative Techniques in Thoracic and Cardiovascular Surgery 14(4):266–280 with permission from Elsevier

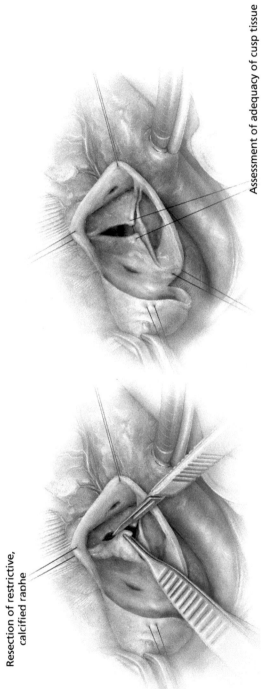

Resection of restrictive, calcified raphe

Assessment of adequacy of cusp tissue

Figure 4.15 Resection of a restrictive or calcified raphé (left) and assessment of the quantity of available tissue (right).

Adapted from Boodhwani M and El Khoury G (2009) Aortic Valve Repair, Operative Techniques in Thoracic and Cardiovascular Surgery 14(4):266–280 with permission from Elsevier

quantity of remaining cusp tissue is assessed by putting the two arms of a 6-0 polypropylene suture on the free margin of the conjoint cusp, on either side of the resected raphé. At this point, lack of cusp restriction and good valve opening are signs of the presence of adequate cusp tissue. The leaflet edges are reapproximated primarily when adequate cusp tissue is present using running locked or interrupted 6-0 polypropylene sutures. In the absence of adequate tissue, a triangular autologous treated or bovine pericardial patch is used for cusp restoration (Figure 4.16).

Next, the free margins of both cusps are compared for the presence of any prolapse, which is corrected using free margin plication or resuspension with PTFE.

Intraoperative echocardiography

In addition to providing important information regarding valve anatomy and mechanism of valve dysfunction, post-repair transesophageal echocardiography is mandatory in patients undergoing aortic valve repair.[19] More than trivial to mild residual aortic insufficiency (particularly eccentric jets), coaptation height below the aortic annulus, and coaptation length <5 mm have been shown to be important predictors of late repair failure and warrant aortic valve re-exploration.[20]

Outcomes

There are no randomized controlled trials comparing the outcomes of aortic valve repair versus replacement. Data on the durability of AV repair techniques are currently limited to single-center series that are small to moderate in size, with a mean follow-up time of 5–10 years.

Overall, there are few studies reporting the outcome of unselected patients referred for aortic valve repair surgery. The success rate of valve preservation and repair in this context is rarely reported. The patients presenting for aortic valve repair are typically a heterogenous group and span the spectrum from young patients with congenital valve disease to elderly patients with degenerative aortic aneurysms and concomitant AI. As such, outcomes are frequently reported for specific subsets of patients undergoing aortic valve repair.

In a study examining the role of AI classification on surgical techniques and outcome, we evaluated 264 unselected patients undergoing AV repair (mean age 54 ± 16 years, 80% male).[6] Approximately two-thirds of patients were identified as having a single lesion causing AI. Two lesions were identified in 30% and three in 6% of patients. Fifty percent of lesions were type I, 35% were type II, and 15% were type III. The most common set of multiple lesions were prolapse of AV leaflet in combination with type Ia (STJ dilatation, n = 14) or type Ib (aortic root aneurysm, n = 38) disease. The classification of AI correctly predicted the surgical technique utilized in the vast majority of patients (82–100%). Overall survival in this cohort was 95 ± 3% at 5 years and 87 ± 8% at 8 years. Freedom from cardiac death was 95 ± 5% at 8 years. Freedom from aortic valve reoperation and replacement at 8 years was 91 ± 5% and 93 ± 4%, respectively. Importantly, classification of

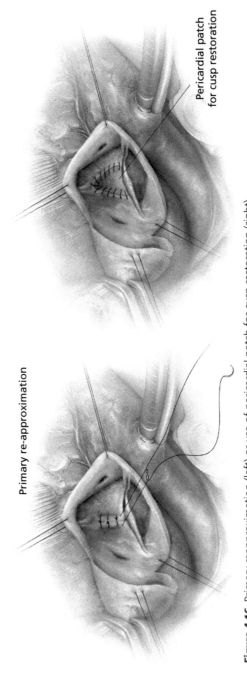

Primary re-approximation

Pericardial patch
for cusp restoration

Figure 4.16 Primary reapproximation (left) or use of pericardial patch for cusp restoration (right).

Adapted from Boodhwani M and El Khoury G (2009) Aortic Valve Repair, Operative Techniques in Thoracic and Cardiovascular Surgery 14(4):266–280 with permission from Elsevier

AI was also predictive of late outcome with patients with type III demonstrating increased late AV reoperation and recurrent AI.

Valve-sparing aortic replacement

Results from large cohorts of patients performed in centers with experience with this technique generally show similar outcomes. David *et al.*, pioneers of the reimplantation technique, reported their experience in 289 patients, 228 of which underwent the reimplantation technique and 61 underwent the remodeling technique.[21,22] Early mortality was 1.7% and 12-year survival was 83%. Late freedom from reoperation at 12 years was 90% with the remodeling technique and 97% with the reimplantation technique ($P = 0.09$). Freedom from recurrent AI at 12 years was 83% after remodeling and 91% after reimplantation ($P = 0.035$). The authors concluded that the reimplantation technique provides more durable outcome.

Schafers *et al.* reported the outcome of the remodeling approach in 274 patients and found that early mortality was 3.6%, freedom from reoperation was 96% at 10 years, and freedom from recurrent AI was 87% at 10 years.[23]

Our group has reported outcome in 164 consecutive patients who underwent valve-sparing aortic root replacement (74% reimplantation, 26% remodeling) looking specifically at the presence of preoperative aortic insufficiency on late outcome.[24] Severe preoperative AI was present in 57% of patients. In this cohort, early mortality was 0.6% and late survival was 88% at 8 years. Freedom from reoperation was 90% at 8 years and freedom from recurrent AI was 90% at 5 years, and both were independent of preoperative AI severity.

Bicuspid AV repair

Unlike the results of valve-sparing aortic root replacement, results of bicuspid aortic valve repair reported in the literature have been quite variable between groups. These differences are largely due to the heterogeneity in the surgical techniques employed, particularly the degree of annular stabilization. Schafers *et al.* reported freedom from reoperation of 97% at 5 years in those undergoing the remodeling approach, but was only 53% in those not undergoing root replacement for bicuspid valve repair.[25] A more recent update of their experience in 316 patients showed a 10-year survival of 92% and a 10-year freedom from reoperation of 81%. Absence of root replacement was predictive of repair failure.[26] David *et al.*[27] reported outcome following bicuspid aortic valve repair in 71 patients. Despite low early and late mortality, freedom from reoperation and recurrent AI at 8 years were 82% and 44%, respectively.

In our cohort of 122 patients undergoing bicuspid aortic valve repair, there was no early mortality and late survival was 97% at 8 years.[17] Freedom from late AV reoperation was 98% and 87% at 5 and 8 years, respectively, and freedom from recurrent AI was 94% at 5 years. In our experience, root replacement led to a more durable outcome compared with subcommissural annuloplasty alone. A follow-up study was performed comparing patients undergoing valve-sparing root replacement using the reimplantation technique to all other forms of annular stabilization in a matched cohort of patients. Patients undergoing the reimplantation technique had significantly lower rates of reoperation and recurrent AI. This confirms the notion that the VAJ in patients with bicuspid AV disease may continue to dilate over time and may cause repair failure.

Trileaflet AV repair

Different techniques may be used to correct cusp prolapse in trileaflet aortic valves. Free margin plication and free margin resuspension are the most commonly used techniques. Studies comparing the two techniques demonstrate equivalent durability in terms of freedom from reoperation or recurrent AI.[16,28] Another important question in the repair of trileaflet aortic valves is the appropriate detection and localization of cusp prolapse. We examined echocardiographic and intraoperative features that could predict the need for cusp prolapse repair in trileaflet aortic valves with or without aortic root pathology. We found that the presence of a preoperative eccentric AI jet, regardless of severity, and the presence of a transverse fibrous band (Figure 4.4) were most useful in the detection and correct localization of cusp prolapse.[7]

Valve-related complications

A consistent finding across all longitudinal studies of aortic valve repair outcome is the low incidence of valve-related events. For prosthetic aortic valve replacements, the rate of thromboembolic events is typically between 1% and 2% per year.[29,30] For patients with mechanical aortic valves, the rate of anticoagulant-related hemorrhage is also 1–2% per year. Furthermore, valve thrombosis and prosthetic valve endocarditis are infrequent but devastating complications. In contrast, the combined rate of thromboembolism, bleeding events, and endocarditis following aortic valve repair has been reported in several studies to be less than 0.5% per year.[6,17,31] This is particularly attractive for young patients who continue to accrue the risk of valve-related events over time.

Conclusions

Over the past two decades, important advances have been made in the field of aortic valve repair. These include a better understanding of the functional anatomy of the aortic valve, the development of a repair-oriented classification system for aortic insufficiency, the application of valve-sparing techniques to the preservation and repair of regurgitant aortic valves, and the development of cusp repair techniques. Increasing data is now available indicating the durability of aortic valve repair up to 10 years. Further long-term studies and those comparing aortic valve repair to replacement are needed to define the role of aortic valve repair in patients with aortic insufficiency.

References

1. **Anderson RH** (2000). Clinical anatomy of the aortic root. *Heart*, **84**(6), 670–3.

2. **Boodhwani M, El Khoury G** (2010). Principles of aortic valve repair. *J Thorac Cardiovasc Surg*, **140**(6 Suppl), S20–2; discussion S45–51.

3. **Underwood MJ, El Khoury G, Deronck D, Glineur D, Dion R** (2000). The aortic root: structure, function, and surgical reconstruction. *Heart*, **83**(4), 376–80.

4. **Boodhwani M, El Khoury G** (2009). Aortic valve repair. *Op Tech Thorac Cardiovasc* Surg, **14**(4), 266–80.

5. **Carpentier A** (1983). Cardiac valve surgery—the "French correction". *J Thorac Cardiovasc Surg*, **86**(3), 323–37.

6. **Boodhwani M, de Kerchove L, Glineur D,** *et al.* (2009). Repair-oriented classification of aortic insufficiency: impact on surgical techniques and clinical outcomes. *J Thorac Cardiovasc Surg*, **137**(2), 286–94.

7. **Boodhwani M, de Kerchove L, Watremez C,** *et al.* (2011). Assessment and repair of aortic valve cusp prolapse: implications for valve-sparing procedures. *J Thorac Cardiovasc Surg*, **141**(4), 917–25.

8. **David TE, Feindel CM** (1992). An aortic valve-sparing operation for patients with aortic incompetence and aneurysm of the ascending aorta. *J Thorac Cardiovasc Surg*, **103**(4), 617–21; discussion 622.

9. **Yacoub MH, Gehle P, Chandrasekaran V,** *et al.* (1998). Late results of a valve-preserving operation in patients with aneurysms of the ascending aorta and root. *J Thorac Cardiovasc Surg*, **115**(5), 1080–90.

10. **Lansac E, Di Centa I, Sleilaty G,** *et al.* (2010). An aortic ring: from physiologic reconstruction of the root to a standardized approach for aortic valve repair. *J Thorac Cardiovasc Surg*, **140**(6 Suppl), S28–35; discussion S45–51.

11. **Scharfschwerdt M, Pawlik M, Sievers HH, Charitos EI** (2011). *In vitro* investigation of aortic valve annuloplasty using prosthetic ring devices. *Eur J Cardiothorac Surg*, **40**(5), 1127–30.

12. **Boodhwani M, de Kerchove L, El Khoury G** (2009). Aortic root replacement using the reimplantation technique: tips and tricks. *Interact Cardiovasc Thorac Surg*, **8**(5), 584–6.

13. **de Kerchove L, Boodhwani M, Glineur D, Noirhomme P, El Khoury G** (2011). A new simple and objective method for graft sizing in valve-sparing root replacement using the reimplantation technique. *Ann Thorac Surg*, **92**(2), 749–51.

14. **Boodhwani M, de Kerchove L, Glineur D, El Khoury G** (2010). A simple method for the quantification and correction of aortic cusp prolapse by means of free margin plication. *J Thorac Cardiovasc Surg*, **139**(4), 1075–7.

15. **David TE, Armstrong S** (2010). Aortic cusp repair with Gore-Tex sutures during aortic valve-sparing operations. *J Thorac Cardiovasc Surg*, **139**(4), 1075–7.

16. **de Kerchove L, Boodhwani M, Glineur D,** *et al.* (2009). Cusp prolapse repair in trileaflet aortic valves: free margin plication and free margin resuspension techniques. *Ann Thorac Surg*, **88**(2), 455–61; discussion 461.

17. **Boodhwani M, de Kerchove L, Glineur D,** *et al.* (2010). Repair of regurgitant bicuspid aortic valves: a systematic approach. *J Thorac Cardiovasc Surg*, **140**(2), 276–84.e1.

18. **Sievers HH, Schmidtke C** (2007). A classification system for the bicuspid aortic valve from 304 surgical specimens. *J Thorac Cardiovasc Surg*, **133**(5), 1226–33.

19. **Van Dyck MJ, Watremez C, Boodhwani M, Vanoverschelde JL, El Khoury G** (2010). Transesophageal echocardiographic evaluation during aortic valve repair surgery. *Anesth Analg*, **111**(1), 59–70.

20. **le Polain de Waroux JB, Pouleur AC,** *et al.* (2009). Mechanisms of recurrent aortic regurgitation after aortic valve repair: predictive value of intraoperative transesophageal echocardiography. *JACC Cardiovasc Imaging*, **2**(8), 931–9.

21. **David TE, Feindel CM, Webb GD,** *et al.* (2007). Aortic valve preservation in patients with aortic root aneurysm: results of the reimplantation technique. *Ann Thorac Surg*, **83**(2), S732–5; discussion S785–90.

22. **David TE, Maganti M, Armstrong S** (2010). Aortic root aneurysm: principles of repair and long-term follow-up. *J Thorac Cardiovasc Surg*, **140**(6 Suppl), S14–9; discussion S45–51.

23. **Aicher D, Langer F, Lausberg H, Bierbach B, Schafers HJ** (2007). Aortic root remodeling: ten-year experience with 274 patients. *J Thorac Cardiovasc Surg*, **134**(4), 909–15.

24. **de Kerchove L, Boodhwani M, Glineur D,** *et al.* (2009). Effects of preoperative aortic insufficiency on outcome after aortic valve-sparing surgery. *Circulation*, **120**(11 Suppl), S120–6.

25. **Schafers HJ, Aicher D, Langer F, Lausberg HF** (2007). Preservation of the bicuspid aortic valve. *Ann Thorac Surg*, **83**(2), S740–5; discussion S785–90.

26. **Aicher D, Kunihara T, Abou Issa O,** *et al.* (2011). Valve configuration determines long-term results after repair of the bicuspid aortic valve. *Circulation*, **123**(2), 178–85.

27. **Alsoufi B, Borger MA, Armstrong S, Maganti M, David TE** (2005). Results of valve preservation and repair for bicuspid aortic valve insufficiency. *J Heart Valve Dis*, **14**(6), 752–8; discussion 758–9.

28. **de Kerchove L, Glineur D, Poncelet A,** *et al.* (2008). Repair of aortic leaflet prolapse: a ten-year experience. *Eur J Cardiothorac Surg*, **34**(4), 785–91.

29. **Peterseim DS, Cen YY, Cheruvu S,** *et al.* (1999). Long-term outcome after biologic versus mechanical aortic valve replacement in 841 patients. *J Thorac Cardiovasc Surg*, **117**(5), 890–7.

30. **Ruel M, Masters RG, Rubens FD,** *et al.* (2004). Late incidence and determinants of stroke after aortic and mitral valve replacement. *Ann Thorac Surg*, **78**(1), 77–83; discussion 83–74.

31. **Aicher D, Fries R, Rodionycheva S,** *et al.* (2010). Aortic valve repair leads to a low incidence of valve-related complications. *Eur J Cardiothorac Surg*, **37**(1), 127–32.

Chapter 5

Aortic valve: Conventional valve replacement and transcatheter valve implantation

Jörg Kempfert and Thomas Walther

Introduction

The natural history of untreated severe aortic valve stenosis (AS), with an average survival of 3 years after the onset of angina or syncope and only 1½ years after onset of heart failure,[1] strongly suggests early surgical therapy which represents the only curative option. Since the first pioneering work in the early 1960s, conventional aortic valve replacement (AVR) has become a routine procedure performed more than 200,000 times annually worldwide.

General considerations and literature: Current issues in conventional aortic valve replacement (AVR)

Current outcome in "low-risk" patients

Over the past decades the surgical technique of AVR has evolved to a highly standardized procedure resulting in excellent outcome and patient safety. According to the Society of Thoracic Surgeons (STS) National Database, 30-day mortality decreased over the last decade by 24% despite increased patient age and risk profile.[2] Today, most centers report a 30-day mortality rate of 2–3% in elective "low-risk" patients.

Tissue *vs.* mechanical valves

According to the STS National Database, a dramatic shift toward the use of bioprosthetic valves occurred over the last decade.[2] Generally, the selection of a tissue valve is supported by the recently updated American Heart Association (AHA) guidelines in patients over 65 years of age.[3] However, the avoidance of a second operation due to potential tissue valve degeneration should be balanced against the cumulative risk for bleeding or thromboembolism of mechanical valves in each individual patient. For quality of life and lifestyle reasons, even younger patients might opt for a tissue valve. Given the lack of evidence proving the superiority of mechanical over tissue valves in younger patients regarding long-term mortality,[4] this recent trend seems to be justified. According to a recent analysis the merits and drawbacks of tissue and mechanical valves outbalance at an age crossing point of 60 years.[5] In addition, the operative risk for a second surgical AVR has been demonstrated to be not significantly increased in younger patients compared to the primary procedure.[6] Although still evolving, the transcatheter "valve-in-a-valve" option might have further impact on the decision to choose bioprosthetic valves in younger patients in the near future.[7]

Patient-prosthesis mismatch

Since the introduction of the theoretical concept of patient–prosthesis mismatch (PPM) following AVR this phenomenon has been of much debate in the literature over the last decade. PPM is generally accepted to be severe if the indexed effective orifice area (IEOA) is less than 0.65 cm^2/m^2 and moderate in patients with an IEOA less than 0.85 cm^2/m^2.[8] The published data on the topic of PPM is very conflicting. According to a recent analysis,[9] severe PPM seems to be associated with impaired short-, mid-, and long-term outcome, and should be always avoided. The potential impact of moderate PPM is more complex. It seems to be well tolerated in elderly patients with preserved left ventricular function, who represent most patients undergoing AVR for AS. On the other hand, moderate PPM should be avoided in patients with impaired left ventricular function or marked hypertrophy and in young and/or physically active patients. To avoid severe PPM in the small aortic annulus both, annular enlargement techniques[10] or full root replacement using a stentless valve[11] results in good hemodynamical outcome without a significant increase in the operative risk.

Stentless valves

At time of introduction into clinical practice, the concept of stentless valves was seen as revolutionary. The hope was that these new valves would show hemodynamic performance similar to a native aortic valve and that this benefit regarding low gradients and large effective orifice area would transduce into improved patient outcome and quality of life. In addition, better flow kinetics would result in less stress on the artificial valve leaflets. Thus, improved long-term durability was anticipated.

Now, almost 15 years later some long-term data regarding the durability of the valves became available and are somehow conflicting. Whereas the Medtronic Freestyle valve demonstrated extremely low rates of valvular degeneration at 10-year follow-up,[12] data for the St. Jude Toronto valve were disappointing at 12-year follow-up,[13] despite good 8-year results.[14]

The drawback of all stentless valves is that the implantation itself is technically more demanding. In case of subcoronary implantation, the coronary ostia do not have to be reimplanted, but this technique is prone to increased transvalvular gradients especially in small aortic roots.[15] The other option, a full root replacement seems to be the treatment of choice in case of a small aortic annulus to avoid PPM but the necessity to reimplant the coronary arteries adds complexity. Nevertheless, several randomized trials have proven that stentless valve implantation does not increase the operative mortality in specialized centers but results in beneficial hemodynamic performance associated with accelerated regression of ventricular hypertrophy.[16,17]

Regarding survival, several studies claimed a benefit due to the implantation of stentless valves. Unfortunately, the evidence is not very valid as most studies were non-randomized and there was a clear bias present toward using stentless valves in younger patients, which certainly affected the reported long-term data. On the other hand, the literature data strongly suggest a significant benefit for stentless valves in case of a small aortic root or impaired left ventricular function.[18]

For most patients presenting for AVR due to degenerative AS in their late seventies, the easiness and safety of a quick procedure using a stented valve probably outbalance the potential benefits of a more complex stentless valve. In younger patients, where hemo-dynamic performance, especially during exercise, is a more relevant issue, the potential risks of a reoperation associated with stentless valves[19] should be taken into consideration. In summary, stentless valves are an excellent option in carefully selected patients but more data regarding the long-term durability and valve designs allowing for an easier implant-ation technique are required to further increase the acceptance of the "stentless" concept.

Minimally invasive access aortic valve replacement

Minimally invasive access aortic valve replacement (MA-AVR) was introduced more than 10 years ago.[20] It facilitates standard AVR using either an upper partial sternotomy or a right lateral mini-thoracotomy. Both approaches have been proven to be safe and feasible, are less invasive regarding cosmetics and surgical trauma and spare sternal stability com-pared to full-sternotomy AVR. The upper sternotomy access is probably more "straight-forward" and does not require any special instruments.[21] On the other hand, the lateral approach provides the benefit of not dividing the sternum at all, but usually requires a set of special minimally invasive instruments and is associated with prolonged cross-clamp times reflecting the technical challenges.[22]

Several studies have shown that MA-AVR can be performed as safely as with a full sternotomy without affecting the quality of the valve procedure itself. Furthermore, a recent meta-analysis[23] demonstrated a significant benefit for the MA-AVR technique regarding length of hospital stay, length of intensive care stay, and length of ventilation. Tabata et al.[21] reported remarkably good results in elderly patients (>80 years, n = 179) with the MA-AVR technique resulting in a 30-day mortality rate of 1.7% only despite the age of this particular patient group. In another recent study, MA-AVR was even identified as an independent factor for decreased 30-day mortality in a subgroup of high-risk elderly patients.[24]

Although safety of the minimally invasive approach is clearly proven and significant benefit regarding outcome is most likely, MA-AVR is still not standard of care more than 10 years after its introduction. For example, in 2008 only 8.3% of all isolated AVR proced-ures were performed using a minimally invasive access in Germany.[25]

MA-AVR is well suited for younger patients as it facilitates the use of "classic" valve prosthesis with known long-term durability while at the same time offering a less inva-sive option is certainly appreciated by the patients. Regarding elderly high-risk patients, MA-AVR in combination with a new sutureless valve prosthesis[26] may become an inter-mediate step between conventional AVR and transcatheter techniques.

Older patients

The prevalence of AS increases with age, it reaches 8.1% at 85 years.[27] Combined with the phenomenon of the aging population, AS is expected to become a major factor in cardiovascular practice in the near future.[28] After the onset of symptoms, the prognosis of AS is grave and it is even worse in presence of advanced age.[29] Given the poor natural history of AS in older people, surgical valve replacement seems to be justified even in octogenarians to improve survival.

Over the past few years several groups have demonstrated that today, conventional surgical aortic valve replacement is feasible in octogenarians with an acceptable outcome. Consistent with the good outcomes observed in older people, age alone has been shown not to be an independent risk factor for conventional AVR.[30] In addition to the known improvement of short-term outcome by surgical intervention, it has been demonstrated recently that surgical AVR in elderly patients is also associated with an excellent long-term outcome.[31]

Today, conventional AVR clearly leads to a significant survival benefit even in octogenerians. On the other hand, survival alone should probably not be the preliminary endpoint in these patients. Therefore, several groups have investigated quality of life (QoL) after conventional AVR over the past years reporting significant benefit.[32,33] However, some studies have demonstrated that QoL may not to be significantly different after AVR compared to an age-matched "healthy" population.[34]

Current issues in transcatheter aortic valve implantation (TAVI)

The concept of transcatheter valves

Given the good outcome of conventional AVR, the question is: Do we really need anything new? According to the data of the European Heart Survey one-third of all elderly patients suffering from severe symptomatic AS were never referred to a cardiac surgeon because the referring cardiologists believed the surgical risk to be unacceptably high.[35] A similar "non-referral" pattern has been demonstrated in a study from California where even 61% of patients with severe AS never underwent aortic valve replacement.[36] Although the observed "non-referral" pattern can be partially explained by the fact that the referring physicians are often not aware of the true outcome of conventional AVR in elderly patients at present, it still clearly demonstrates the need for a less invasive option in carefully selected elderly high-risk patients.

The idea itself is not new and aortic valve balloon valvuloplasty was advocated in the 1980s for selected patients, but it became quickly evident that this technique is associated with modest and short-lived clinical improvement only.[37,38] After the development of a valve stent[39] the concept regained interest and finally resulted in its first human implantation in 2002 using an antegrade transfemoral transseptal approach.[40]

After initial pioneering, TAVI has evolved to an almost routine procedure in specialized centers. Valve delivery is either performed using a retrograde transvascular approach (transfemoral, transsubclavian, transaortal) or the surgical antegrade transapical access. Theoretically, the transcatheter concept offers several advantages:

1. The technique facilitates valve implantation with minimal surgical trauma only (transapical) or even with a purely percutaneous approach (transfemoral) and avoids sternotomy.

2. General anesthesia is not required for the transfemoral approach and even when using the apical technique, it can be avoided in selected patients.[41]

3. The technique allows for valve implantation off-pump, thus avoiding the potentially harmful effects of cardiopulmonary bypass. However, potential drawbacks such as procedure-related complications (vascular injury, ventricular tear, paravalvular leak, valve dislocation, and so on) must be kept in mind.

Which patients should undergo TAVI instead of conventional AVR?

Although the concept itself offers some obvious advantages, the benefit of TAVI compared to conventional AVR is unproven yet. Given the excellent results of conventional AVR and the unknown long-term durability of the TAVI valves, the technique should stay restricted to "true" elderly high-risk patients until convincing scientific data is available justifying a broadening of the indication. Otherwise, a development similar to the inglorious story of coronary artery bypass graft (CABG) versus PCI might repeat itself. Clinical practice must stay supported by best scientific evidence available. At present most groups accept the recommendations recently published by the European Association for Cardio-Thoracic Surgery (EACTS) and ESC.[42] Accordingly, patients are eligible for TAVI if they present with advanced age (>75) AND additional risk factors (STS-score >10%, logistic EuroSCORE (ES) >20%) such as severe respiratory dysfunction, chest radiation, mediastinitis, previous CABG with patent left internal mammary artery (LIMA), and other risk factors not represented by the STS or EuroSCORE (i.e., porcelain aorta, liver failure, immobility, or severe hematological disorders).

The true risk of this special subgroup of patients is hard to estimate. In addition to scoring systems issues as biological age and frailty are not routinely measurable. On the other hand, scoring systems are needed to compare the outcome of different techniques. It is well accepted that the logistic EuroSCORE generally overestimates the true risk[43] and the STS-score should be probably favored as it is more accurate in these patients.[44]

Transfemoral versus transapical access

TAVI is feasible using either the retrograde transfemoral, or the antegrade transapical approach with good outcomes.[45,46] There is currently no scientific evidence proving the superiority of the one or the other approach. The strengths of the transfemoral access are certainly that it can be performed under local anesthesia. On the other hand, the transapical approach is clinically advantageous due to the direct and antegrade access to the aortic valve, hence very precise device manipulation and positioning is feasible. In addition, sheath size and quality of the femoral vessels are not an issue with the apical access. Another advantage of the antegrade transapical approach might be the fact that this technique is associated with limited manipulations around the aortic arch only. This might result in a lower stroke rate compared to the transfemoral approach especially in "high-risk" patients with a calcified aortic arch. In patients with severe lung dysfunction, the awake transfemoral approach might be advantageous whereas the apical approach should be favored in case of stenotic or calcified femoral vessels. In addition, there are other approaches that include transaortic and trans-subclavian routes which are appropriate in selected patients.

In conclusion, for most patients both options will lead to good results. A "transfemoral first strategy" is not supported by any scientific evidence although advocated by some groups. When comparing the results in regard to the access site, the overall risk profile (logistic EuroSCORE and most importantly STS-score) must be taken into account for a "fair" comparison.

Current outcome of TAVI

After an initial pioneering phase, the results have now stabilized. Unfortunately, most groups seem to favor a "transfemoral first strategy" which results in two groups of patients hardly comparable. In the transfemoral group a 30 d-mortality rate of 7% with a logistic EuroSCORE less than 25% has to be expected. In the transapical group, patients usually have a higher risk profile (logEuroSCORE >30%) that translates to a higher 30 d-mortality rate of approximately 10%.

Over recent years, TAVI emerged to become the treatment of choice for inoperable patients and the preferred alternative for high-risk patients with severe, symptomatic aortic stenosis. The randomized PARTNER trial reported the benefit of TAVI in patients with inoperable aortic stenosis.[47] Evidence continues to emerge rapidly as ongoing trials are conducted. The PARTNER trial reported no structural valve deterioration requiring surgical aortic valve replacement (SAVR) was detected after 5 years and the valve area as well as the mean transvalvular gradient remained stable. The reported durability of TAVI devices appears sufficient for high high-risk patients, but long-term studies are necessary to prove comparable durability to SAVR valves. As regards Vascular complication rates, this has significantly declined as the size of TF-TAVI delivery sheaths has decreased significantly compared with the first-generation systems.

The results of randomized trials of TAVI in intermediate-risk patients are eagerly awaited.

Technical key steps

Conventional AVR

The technique of conventional full-sternotomy AVR today is a highly standardized procedure. Therefore, we would just like to share our approach for the small aortic root. In case of younger patients, we believe that the full root replacement is the best solution to avoid any PPM. A mechanical conduit is a good choice to avoid a potential risky redo root replacement in the future in younger patients. If the patient decides to have a tissue valve, the long-term durability of the Freestyle valve seems to be excellent and comparable to a homograft. In case of elderly "active" patients we would favor a posterior root enlargement in combination with a modern supraannular stented tissue valve to keep the procedure relatively straightforward. In case of elderly rather "inactive" patients we believe that with the use of a modern supraannular biological stented valve, acceptable hemodynamic performance can be anticipated in most patients and a moderate PPM is acceptable obviating the need for more complex procedures in this patient group.

Minimally invasive access AVR

We believe that minimally invasive access AVR should be increasingly used in isolated aortic valve procedures. The lateral parasternal access offers the advantage of completely sparing the sternum and several groups have reported excellent outcome with this approach. However, reported cross-clamp duration is rather long with this technique. In comparison we favor the upper partial mini-sternotomy, as this technique is technically straightforward translating into shorter procedure and cross-clamp times and does not require special instruments.

In most cases, we use a 6–8 cm long skin incision and a J-shaped mini-sternotomy into the fourth or fifth right intercostal space. Usually a conventional chest X-ray is sufficient to plan the procedure avoiding the radiation and the contrast load of a CT-scan. The access allows for standard cannulation of the ascending aorta and the right atrial appendage in most patients (Figure 5.1). Alternatively, the venous cannula can be placed through an

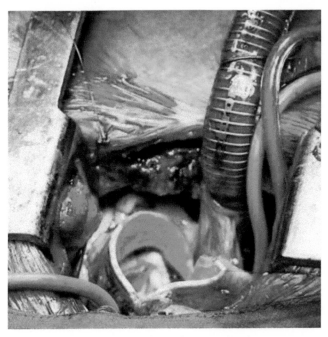

Figure 5.1 Minimally invasive access aortic valve replacement (AVR).

additional epigastric incision or a percutaneous venous cannula can be used with vacuum assisted drainage. Placement of the vent into the upper right pulmonary vein is almost always possible; in rare cases, venting of the pulmonary artery is an option. Once access is established, the procedure can be performed similar to a full sternotomy procedure using antegrade cardioplegia.

A few pitfalls were identified over time:

1. A typical site of bleeding is the right internal thoracic artery (RITA) due to the J-shaped sternotomy.

2. Placement of the epicardial pacing lead and the chest drain is a lot easier and safer to achieve once the heart is still unloaded on-pump.

3. The limited access does not allow for full visualization of the right and left ventricle—transesophageal echo (TEE) is mandatory to identify potential ventricular distension. Deairing is relatively difficult—therefore CO_2 field flush should be routinely used.

TAVI (focusing on the surgical transapical approach):

Specific issues observed during the learning-curve, in addition to useful tips and tricks with the transapical technique using the Edwards SAPIEN prosthesis are highlighted here.[48]

The setup

The optimal environment for TAVI procedures is a fully equipped hybrid operative room (OR). If such a room is not available, an "upgraded" cath-lab should be favored over a regular OR with a mobile C-arm as imaging quality is key. In addition, a TEE and a regular cardiopulmonary bypass system (CPB) should be available. The procedures should be performed by a specialized team—made up of surgeons, cardiologists, and anesthetists—to ensure optimal patient safety. The setup should be designed with potential "bail-out" scenarios in mind, ranging from simple procedures like surgical femoral cut-down to complex worst-case settings like redo aortic arch replacement in type A dissection.

In order to provide immediate CPB support if necessary, a femoral "safety-net" (percutaneous venous wire in addition to the arterial sheath) should be placed prior to skin incision.[49]

Apical access

Although transapical valve implantation has been proven feasible in awake patients,[42] general anesthesia is used in most cases. When trying to identify the optimal access site, echocardiography might be helpful to locate the ape. Alternatively, the sixth intercostal space with an incision of 5–6 cm beginning at the mid-clavicular line to the lateral aspect usually provides good exposure (Figure 5.2). In patients with enlarged ventricles, a more lateral approach is chosen. Once an intercostal space is slightly opened the apex can be easily palpated and, accordingly, an intercostal space higher or lower can be selected prior to insertion of the rib spreader without significantly increasing the overall trauma. With

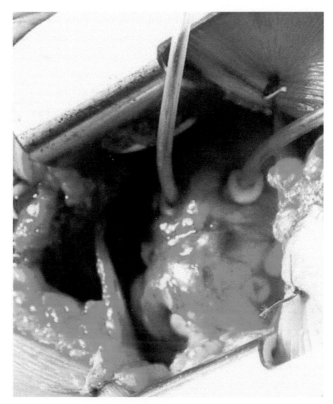

Figure 5.2 Apical access for transcatheter aortic valve implantation (TAVI).

the help of four to six pericardial stay-sutures, the exposure of the apex is then optimized. The stay-sutures allow for regular bilateral lung ventilation.

Although different techniques have been suggested with good results, we always use two separate 2-0 Prolene purse strings (large medium half (MH) needle) with five small Teflon pledget-supported interruptions to secure the apex. Sufficiently deep bites should be taken to avoid tearing of the epicardium. The optimal target site is the muscular spot cranial to the anatomical left ventricular apex lateral of the left anterior descending artery (LAD) to avoid the fatty tissue at the true apex.

After the valve is implanted both purse strings are tied. In case of high systolic blood pressure, a brief episode of rapid ventricular pacing might be used. If residual bleeding is present, deep felt strip supported 2-0 Prolene U-stiches provide adequate haemostasis. "Uncontrollable" apical bleeding or tearing requires temporary CPB support to unload the ventricle. In case of persistent arterial bleeding without a clear source at the apex the rare event of annular rupture is suspected and ruled out by repeat root angiography.

Imaging: Optimal angulation of the C-arm

As already mentioned, we believe that good imaging quality is one of the key steps for a successful TAVI program. A new imaging modality (DynaCT) was developed and might be of utmost help to achieve a perfectly perpendicular angulation of the C-arm.[50] If not available, however, the optimal angulation (hint: start at LAO/cranial 10°/10°) must be identified by repeat root angiography. The importance of a truly perpendicular angulation of the C-arm cannot be emphasized enough and is often underestimated at the beginning of each team's learning-curve. Figure 5.3 demonstrates a non-perpendicular (A) versus an optimal angulation (B). This ensures precise and controlled positioning of the prosthesis.

Valve positioning and implantation

Ideally, the valve should be positioned one-third to one-half above the aortic annulus but strictly subcoronary. In our experience, too low a position is associated with a higher rate of paravalvular leak. On the other hand, a high position might result in coronary obstruction—a rare but devastating complication. The distance between the aortic annulus

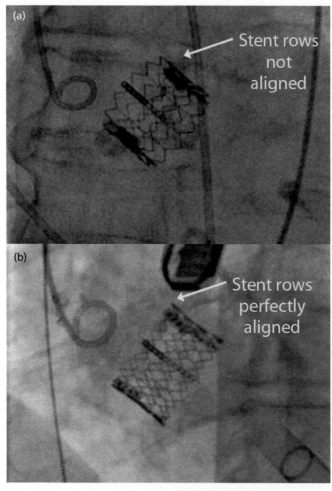

Figure 5.3 Optimal C-arm angulation: (a) non-perpendicular, (b) perpendicular.

and the coronary ostia can be usually assessed on the preoperative coronary angiogram. If in doubt, an additional CT-scan is indicated. A rather wide aortic root configuration (pronounced aortic sinus) allows for a more "aggressive" positioning close to the ostia, whereas in a small more tubular shaped root, a position on the "lower side" is more advisable.

In contrast to the femoral access, the transapical approach allows adjusting the tilting of the valve within the aortic annulus by either tightening the guidewire or giving some extra slack (Figure 5.4). Furthermore, some minor positional adjustments are feasible even during valve implantation by stepwise balloon inflation. The implantation sequence is as follows:

1. The valve is positioned including adjustment of the wire tension and all team members agree after the final angiographic control.

2. Ventilation is stopped to minimize side motion.

3. Rapid pacing is initiated (180–220 bpm, in case of "non-capture" try a *slower* rate to avoid 2:1 conduction).

4. The anesthetist confirms: "No output."

5. A final contrast injection into the root is given during the rapid pacing. This allows for implantation into the contrasted aortic root and thus for optimal visualization of all key target structures, including the aortic annulus and the coronary ostia.

6. The balloon is gradually inflated to 50%.

7. If required final adjustments are made (to avoid uncontrolled jumping due to initial friction between the sheath and the catheter it is best to manipulate the whole system only).

8. Once the team is satisfied, full inflation is performed.

Potential complications and "bail-out" suggestions

Given the high-risk nature of the patients treated with the TAVI technique, a variety of complications might occur. We would like to share the more frequent complications and how we would react according to the specific situation:

• **Valve deployed too low:** The delivery system should be retrieved immediately to be prepared for a second valve-in-a-valve implantation with a slightly higher position.

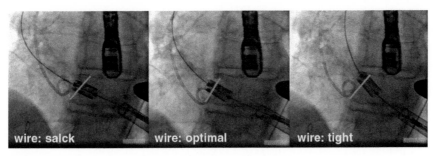

Figure 5.4 Adjustment of the valve tilting by wire manipulation.

- **Valve deployed too high, leading to coronary occlusion or impingement:** If a guidewire can be placed, consider stent-implantation. If not, sternotomy and surgical bypass grafts beating-heart on-pump should be performed. To decrease the time until myocardial reperfusion retrograde continuous coronary sinus perfusion can be established immediately after start of CPB especially in case of left main occlusion.

- **Paravalvular leak (>grade 1+):** Reballooning adding 1 mL of extra volume should be attempted.

- **Central leak (>grade 1+):** If one leaflet is not moving mobilization by pigtail manipulation might be feasible. Valve function often dramatically improves once the arterial pressure has fully recovered. In case the maneuver is not successful consider second valve-in-valve implantation eventually slightly higher to avoid interference of the native aortic valve cusps.

- **Hemodynamical instability:** Low-dose epinephrine (2–10 mL of 1 mg diluted to 100 mL saline) into the aortic root over the pigtail is often helpful. In case of persistent low-output convert to CPB using the "Safety-Net" for reperfusion. Bridge with chest compressions until full CBP flow is established. To prevent left ventricular distension (especially in case of higher degree of aortic regurgitation) consider apical venting.

References

1. Ross J Jr, Braunwald E (1968). Aortic stenosis. *Circulation*, **38**, 61–7.
2. Brown JM, O'Brien SM, Wu C, *et al.* (2009). Isolated aortic valve replacement in North America comprising 108,687 patients in 10 years: changes in risks, valve types, and outcomes in the Society of Thoracic Surgeons National Database. *J Thorac Cardiovasc Surg*, **137**, 82–90.
3. Bonow RO, Carabello BA, Chatterjee K, *et al.* (2008). Focused update incorporated into the ACC/AHA 2006 guidelines for the management of patients with valvular heart disease. *Circulation*, **118**, e523–661.
4. Ruel M, Kulik A, Lam BK, *et al.* (2005). Long-term outcomes of valve replacement with modern prostheses in young adults. *Eur J Cardiothorac Surg*, **27**, 425–33; discussion 433.
5. Puvimanasinghe JP, Takkenberg JJ, Edwards MB, *et al.* (2004). Comparison of outcomes after aortic valve replacement with a mechanical valve or a bioprosthesis using microsimulation. *Heart*, **90**, 1172–8.
6. Potter DD, Sundt TM, 3rd, Zehr KJ, *et al.* (2005). Operative risk of reoperative aortic valve replacement. *J Thorac Cardiovasc Surg*, **129**, 94–103.
7. Walther T, Kempfert J, Borger MA, *et al.* (2008). Human minimally invasive off-pump valve-in-a-valve implantation. *Ann Thorac Surg*, **85**, 1072–3.
8. Pibarot P, Dumesnil JG (2006). Prosthesis-patient mismatch: definition, clinical impact, and prevention. *Heart*, **92**, 1022–9.
9. Urso S, Sadaba R, Aldamiz-Echevarria G (2009). Is patient-prosthesis mismatch an independent risk factor for early and mid-term overall mortality in adult patients undergoing aortic valve replacement? *Interact Cardiovasc Thorac Surg*, **9**, 510–8.
10. Dhareshwar J, Sundt TM, 3rd, Dearani JA, *et al.* (2007). Aortic root enlargement: what are the operative risks? *J Thorac Cardiovasc Surg*, **134**, 916–24.
11. Ennker JA, Ennker IC, Albert AA, *et al.* (2009). The Freestyle stentless bioprosthesis in more than 1000 patients: a single-center experience over 10 years. *J Card Surg*, **24**, 41–8.

12. **Bach DS, Kon ND, Dumesnil JG**, *et al*. (2005). Ten-year outcome after aortic valve replacement with the freestyle stentless bioprosthesis. *Ann Thorac Surg*, **80**, 480–6; discussion 486–7.

13. **David TE, Feindel CM, Bos J**, *et al*. (2008). Aortic valve replacement with Toronto SPV bioprosthesis: optimal patient survival but suboptimal valve durability. *J Thorac Cardiovasc Surg*, **135**, 19–24.

14. **Yadav S, Hodge AJ, Hilless AD**, *et al*. (2006). Outcomes with Toronto stentless porcine aortic valve: the Australian experience. *Interact Cardiovasc Thorac Surg*, **5**, 709–15.

15. **Albert A, Florath I, Rosendahl U**, *et al*. (2007). Effect of surgeon on transprosthetic gradients after aortic valve replacement with Freestyle stentless bioprosthesis and its consequences: a follow-up study in 587 patients. *J Cardiothorac Surg*, **2**, 40.

16. **Ali A, Halstead JC, Cafferty F**, *et al*. (2006). Are stentless valves superior to modern stented valves? A prospective randomized trial. *Circulation*, **114**, I535–40.

17. **Walther T, Falk V, Langebartels G**, *et al*. (1999). Prospectively randomized evaluation of stentless versus conventional biological aortic valves: impact on early regression of left ventricular hypertrophy. *Circulation*, **100**, II6–10.

18. **Gulbins H, Reichenspurner H** (2009). Which patients benefit from stentless aortic valve replacement? *Ann Thorac Surg*, **88**, 2061–8.

19. **Borger MA, Prasongsukarn K, Armstrong S**, *et al*. (2007). Stentless aortic valve reoperations: a surgical challenge. *Ann Thorac Surg*, **84**, 737–43; discussion 743–34.

20. **Cosgrove DM, 3rd, Sabik JF** (1996). Minimally invasive approach for aortic valve operations. *Ann Thorac Surg*, **62**, 596–7.

21. **Tabata M, Umakanthan R, Cohn LH**, *et al*. (2008). Early and late outcomes of 1000 minimally invasive aortic valve operations. *Eur J Cardiothorac Surg*, **33**, 537–41.

22. **Plass A, Scheffel H, Alkadhi H**, *et al*. (2009). Aortic valve replacement through a minimally invasive approach: preoperative planning, surgical technique, and outcome. *Ann Thorac Surg*, **88**, 1851–6.

23. **Murtuza B, Pepper JR, Stanbridge RD**, *et al*. (2008). Minimal access aortic valve replacement: is it worth it? *Ann Thorac Surg*, **85**, 1121–31.

24. **Grossi EA, Schwartz CF, Yu PJ**, *et al*. (2008). High-risk aortic valve replacement: are the outcomes as bad as predicted? *Ann Thorac Surg*, **85**, 102–6; discussion 107.

25. **Gummert JF, Funkat A, Beckmann A**, *et al*. (2009). Cardiac surgery in Germany during 2008. A report on behalf of the German Society for Thoracic and Cardiovascular Surgery. *Thorac Cardiovasc Surg*, **57**, 315–23.

26. **Shrestha M, Folliguet T, Meuris B**, *et al*. (2009). Sutureless perceval S aortic valve replacement: a multicenter, prospective pilot trial. *J Heart Valve Dis*, **18**, 698–702.

27. **Iung B, Baron G, Butchart EG**, *et al*. (2003). A prospective survey of patients with valvular heart disease in Europe: the Euro Heart Survey on Valvular Heart Disease. *Eur Heart J*, **24**, 1231–43.

28. **Nkomo VT, Gardin JM, Skelton TN**, *et al*. (2006). Burden of valvular heart diseases: a population-based study. *Lancet*, **368**, 1005–11.

29. **Varadarajan P, Kapoor N, Bansal RC**, *et al*. (2006). Clinical profile and natural history of 453 nonsurgically managed patients with severe aortic stenosis. *Ann Thorac Surg*, **82**, 2111–5.

30. **Melby SJ, Zierer A, Kaiser SP**, *et al*. (2007). Aortic valve replacement in octogenarians: risk factors for early and late mortality. *Ann Thorac Surg*, **83**, 1651–6; discussion 1656–7.

31. **Likosky DS, Sorensen MJ, Dacey LJ**, *et al*. (2009). Long-term survival of the very elderly undergoing aortic valve surgery. *Circulation*, **120**, S127–33.

32. **Kolh P, Lahaye L, Gerard P**, *et al*. (1999). Aortic valve replacement in the octogenarians: perioperative outcome and clinical follow-up. *Eur J Cardiothorac Surg*, **16**, 68–73.

33. **Huber CH, Goeber V, Berdat P,** *et al.* (2007). Benefits of cardiac surgery in octogenarians--a postoperative quality of life assessment. *Eur J Cardiothorac Surg,* **31,** 1099–105.

34. **Maillet JM, Somme D, Hennel E,** *et al.* (2009). Frailty after aortic valve replacement (AVR) in octogenarians. *Arch Gerontol Geriatr,* **48,** 391–6.

35. **Sundt TM, Bailey MS, Moon MR,** *et al.* (2000). Quality of life after aortic valve replacement at the age of >80 years. *Circulation,* **102,** III70–4.

36. **Iung B, Cachier A, Baron G,** *et al.* (2005). Decision-making in elderly patients with severe aortic stenosis: why are so many denied surgery? *Eur Heart J,* **26,** 2714–20.

37. **Pai RG, Kapoor N, Bansal RC,** *et al.* (2006). Malignant natural history of asymptomatic severe aortic stenosis: benefit of aortic valve replacement. *Ann Thorac Surg,* **82,** 2116–22.

38. **Bashore TM, Davidson CJ** (1991). Follow-up recatheterization after balloon aortic valvuloplasty. Mansfield Scientific Aortic Valvuloplasty Registry Investigators. *J Am Coll Cardiol,* **17,** 1188–95.

39. **Cribier A, Savin T, Saoudi N,** *et al.* (1986). Percutaneous transluminal valvuloplasty of acquired aortic stenosis in elderly patients: an alternative to valve replacement? *Lancet,* **1,** 63–7.

40. **Knudsen LL, Andersen HR, Hasenkam JM** (1993). Catheter-implanted prosthetic heart valves. Transluminal catheter implantation of a new expandable artificial heart valve in the descending thoracic aorta in isolated vessels and closed chest pigs. *Int J Artif Organs,* **16,** 253–62.

41. **Cribier A, Eltchaninoff H, Bash A,** *et al.* (2002). Percutaneous transcatheter implantation of an aortic valve prosthesis for calcific aortic stenosis: first human case description. *Circulation,* **106,** 3006–8.

42. **Mukherjee C, Walther T, Borger MA,** *et al.* (2009). Awake transapical aortic valve implantation using thoracic epidural anesthesia. *Ann Thorac Surg,* **88,** 992–4.

43. **Vahanian A, Alfieri O, Al-Attar N,** *et al.* (2008). Transcatheter valve implantation for patients with aortic stenosis: a position statement from EACTS and ESC, in collaboration with EAPCI. *Eur Heart J,* **29,** 1463–70.

44. **Dewey TM, Brown D, Ryan WH,** *et al.* (2008). Reliability of risk algorithms in predicting early and late operative outcomes in high-risk patients undergoing aortic valve replacement. *J Thorac Cardiovasc Surg,* **135,** 180–7.

45. **Wendt D, Osswald BR, Kayser K,** *et al.* (2009). Society of Thoracic Surgeons score is superior to the EuroSCORE determining mortality in high-risk patients undergoing isolated aortic valve replacement. *Ann Thorac Surg,* **88,** 468–74; discussion 474–65.

46. **Piazza N, Grube E, Gerckens U,** *et al.* (2008). Procedural and 30-day outcomes following transcatheter aortic valve implantation using the third generation Corevalve revalving system. *EuroIntervention,* **4,** 242–9.

47. **Kapadia SR, Leon MB, Makkar RR,** *et al.* (2015). 5-year outcomes of transcatheter aortic valve replacement compared with standard treatment for patients with inoperable aortic stenosis (PARTNER 1): a randomised controlled trial. *Lancet,* **385,** 2485–91.

48. **Walther T, Dewey T, Borger MA,** *et al.* (2009). Transapical aortic valve implantation: step by step. *Ann Thorac Surg,* **87,** 276–83.

49. **Kempfert J, Walther T, Borger MA,** *et al.* (2008). Minimally invasive off-pump aortic valve implantation: the surgical safety net. *Ann Thorac Surg,* **86,** 1665–8.

50. **Kempfert J, Falk V, Schuler G,** *et al.* (2009). Dyna-CT during minimally invasive off-pump transapical aortic valve implantation. *Ann Thorac Surg,* **88,** 2041.

Chapter 6

Open and endovascular treatment options in thoracic aortic surgery

Ourania Preventza and Joseph S. Coselli

Introduction

The thoracic aorta is divided into the proximal aorta, the transverse arch, and the descending and thoracoabdominal aorta. Each segment is addressed differently with regard to pathology. Open endovascular and hybrid repairs have emerged for treating these different segments. A full median sternotomy is the standard approach for proximal aortic disease and proximal and transverse arch repairs. Other minimally invasive approaches such as upper mini-sternotomy and right mini-thoracotomy have emerged for treating proximal aortic and arch disease. Until recently, a left thoracotomy and thoracoabdominal approach has been the sole approach for treating lesions of the descending and thoracoabdominal thoracic aorta. In the mid-1980s, Volodos and associates[1] reported the first aortic repair with a self-fixing endoprosthesis. In 1991, Parodi and colleagues[2] popularized the technique by using a stent graft to treat an abdominal aortic aneurysm, and 3 years later, Dake and colleagues[3] described the use of a homemade stent graft to treat thoracic aortic aneurysms. These initial attempts to treat aortic aneurysms with a minimally invasive procedure led to robust research and development of this technology. As a result, the United States Food and Drug Administration (FDA) approved two devices for treating abdominal aortic aneurysms in 1999 and the first device for the endovascular treatment of thoracic aortic aneurysms in 2005.

Diagnostic modalities in thoracic aortic surgery

Different imaging modalities can provide critical information to guide treatment options in the thoracic aorta. The availability of imaging equipment and experienced operators varies among institutions, and this variability results in differences in current thoracic aortic practices among different centers. Nevertheless, recent guidelines attempt to standardize image acquisition and reporting with regard to basic key points: location of aortic pathology (including calcification and extension of abnormalities into branch vessels); maximum external aortic diameters; evidence of rupture or internal filling defects; and comparison with previous imaging studies.[4]

Although plain radiography of the chest and abdomen can aid the initial suspicion or even diagnosis of a thoracic aortic aneurysm (characterized by a convex shadow to the right of the cardiac silhouette, widening of the descending thoracic aortic shadow with a rim of calcification, and a convexity in the right superior mediastinum), the results may also appear completely normal. Aneurysms of the mid and lower descending thoracic aorta can reside undetected within the cardiac silhouette. Computed tomography (CT)—with or without intravenous contrast agents—of the chest, abdomen, and pelvis can image the entire thoracic and abdominal aorta with multiplanar and three-dimensional aortic reconstructions. Measurements should be taken in standard anatomic locations and should be obtained perpendicular to the direction of blood flow.[4] By detecting aortic dissections (acute and chronic), aneurysms, mural thrombi, inflammatory reactions around saccular aneurysms, contained aortic ruptures, and mediastinal and retroperitoneal hematomas, CT scanning permits accurate diagnosis of thoracic aortic pathology. In patients with previous thoracic aortic surgery, a CT scan can provide valuable information with regard to the results of that surgery (i.e., the integrity of previously placed Dacron grafts or the position of previously placed endovascular stent grafts), as well as the fate of the remaining native aorta. This modality is also a useful tool for follow-up evaluation and comparison. Moreover, in patients with proximal and arch aneurysms and previous sternotomies for whom a debranching hybrid or a traditional open procedure is being considered, CT scanning provides valuable information regarding the proximity of the sternum to the thoracic aorta or the relationship of a previous left internal thoracic mammary artery bypass to the back of the sternum. The frequent use of CT scanning for a multitude of indications has led the discovery of numerous asymptomatic thoracic and abdominal aortic aneurysms that a few decades ago would have gone undetected until rupture or death.

Although radiation exposure is not inconsequential, in these patients the impact on renal function is of more concern. Contrast-induced nephropathy, defined as an increase of 25% or more in the serum creatinine level compared to the baseline level within 1 to 4 days after contrast administration, is responsible for 10% of hospital-acquired cases of renal failure and is the major adverse effect of CT scanning with an intravenous contrast agent.[5,6] This complication is associated with patient-related risk factors such as congestive heart failure, advanced age, anemia, chronic renal disease, reduced effective circulating volume, and the type and volume of contrast agent.[5,6] Non-ionic, low-osmolar contrast medium is used in most studies.[5,6] Preoperative hydration with sodium chloride and sodium bicarbonate has proven quite helpful.[5,6] Use of oral N-acetylcysteine has no consistent efficacy.[6-8] For long-term follow-up, since in the asymptomatic patient the primary diagnostic feature is the outer diameter of the aorta, CT scanning without the use of intravenous contrast is adequate for routine surveillance in most cases.

Magnetic resonance angiography (MRA) can be another useful tool for imaging the entire aorta, because this approach requires no exposure to ionizing radiation and offers excellent visualization and detection of branch-vessel stenosis.[9] However, gadolinium, the contrast material used for MRA, has been implicated in nephrogenic systemic fibrosis in patients with advanced renal insufficiency.[10] For patients who require long-term follow-up observation, MRA can be an excellent imaging tool.

Other diagnostic modalities for visualizing the thoracic aorta include two-dimensional (2D) echocardiography (transthoracic and transesophageal), which provides excellent visualization of the aortic root and the ascending aorta.[11,12] In addition, this approach can assess wall-motion abnormalities, detect and grade aortic insufficiency, and identify other valvular abnormalities and intracardiac defects.[11] Echocardiography is considered the diagnostic imaging procedure of choice in patients with unstable proximal aortic dissection and is cost-effective in following up most aortic diseases.[13,14] Invasive aortic angiography, once considered the gold standard, has been replaced by CT scanning and MRA except for intraoperative use during in endovascular aortic procedures. A 3D image fusion of a preoperative CT with live fluoroscopy and carbon dioxide digital subtraction angiography (DSA) instead of iodine DSA has been used in patients with renal insufficiency.[15] Cardiac catheterization still plays an important role in preoperative planning and diagnosis, especially in patients with aortic root pathology, known coronary artery disease, and prior coronary artery bypass.

Preoperative assessment before thoracic aortic surgery

Before any elective thoracic aortic procedure, every patient should undergo a detailed evaluation, with an emphasis on the assessment and optimization of pulmonary, cardiac, and renal status. With regard to pulmonary assessment, every patient should undergo arterial blood gas measurement and spirometry. Patients with a forced expiratory volume of more than 1.0 L in 1 second (FEV_1) and a partial pressure of carbon dioxide ($PaCO_2$) of less than 45 mmHg are considered surgical candidates. Poor preoperative pulmonary function does not preclude repair of an aneurysm or dissection, but special consideration must be given to preserving the left recurrent laryngeal nerve, the phrenic nerve, and diaphragmatic function. Smoking cessation, exercise, weight loss, and treatment of bronchitis a few months before the repair procedure can be beneficial in patients with borderline pulmonary function.

Preoperative cardiac evaluation consists of transthoracic echocardiography to evaluate cardiac and valvular function. A dipyridamole-thallium myocardial perfusion scan to identify reversible ischemia in the myocardium can be beneficial, especially in older and less mobile patients with peripheral vascular disease. If any of these tests suggests coronary artery disease, or if the left ventricular ejection fraction is less than 30%, cardiac catheterization and coronary angiography should be performed. Any significant coronary artery or valvular disease can be addressed in the same procedure as the proximal aortic surgery. If the repair involves the distal aorta, coronary revascularization should be performed before the thoracic aortic procedure.

Baseline renal function is extremely important, because in up to 25–30% of patients requiring thoracoabdominal aortic replacement, significant renal artery stenosis may be encountered. Renal artery endarterectomy, stenting, or bypass may be necessary in selected patients. In the event of precipitous decline in renal function, temporary hemodialysis may be necessary after surgery.

Surgical indications for replacement of the proximal aorta and/or aortic root

Ascending aortic dissection and variants

Acute ascending aortic dissection (Stanford A or DeBakey type I or II), defined as occurring within 2 weeks after the onset of pain, and spontaneous aortic rupture are the two main emergency indications for intervention and replacement of the ascending aorta. The timing of intervention is critical because of two potential severe cardiac complications related to disruption of normal anatomic relationships: (1) acute aortic regurgitation (AR), manifesting as an insignificant diastolic murmur or even as congestive heart failure and cardiogenic shock[16]; and (2) myocardial infarction due to extension of the dissection into the coronary ostia or compression of the coronary arteries. Because the latter condition is an infrequent complication of acute type I aortic dissection, it is likely to be misdiagnosed as primary myocardial infarction and treated inappropriately.[17] Another complication of proximal aortic dissection is heart failure, which can have an atypical presentation and possibly a delayed diagnosis.[16] Pericardial tamponade, a frequent complication of acute ascending aortic dissection, necessitates immediate repair. Syncope due to cardiac, neurologic, vascular, and volume-related causes is another manifestation of acute type A (or type I) aortic dissection. It requires special attention and prompt intervention because affected patients have a significantly greater risk of death than patients without a history of syncope.[18]

Malperfusion (cerebral, visceral and lower extremity) associated with acute Type I aortic dissection predicts poor outcomes and deserves special consideration.[19] A significant dilemma with regard to the method and timing of intervention exists in the case of patients who present with stroke. According to recent data from the International Registry of Acute Aortic Dissection (IRAD), stroke was the presenting symptom in 6% of patients with acute proximal aortic dissection.[20] These patients tended to be older, to be hypertensive, and to have aortic-arch-vessel involvement. They had less surgical treatment and significantly higher in-hospital mortality and morbidity but not long-term mortality. In these patients, aggressive surgical intervention and its effect on in-hospital morbidity need to be examined and tailored to each patient's circumstances, including age, comorbidities, and potential for meaningful recovery.

Intramural hematoma (IMH) is a variant of aortic dissection and a dynamic process.[21] Ten to twenty percent of patients with a clinical picture of aortic dissection have IMH without an intimal tear on diagnostic imaging.[22] According to some reports,[23,24] a microscopic tear in the intima, versus hemorrhage of the vasa vasorum within the media, can also result in an intramural hematoma. Intramural hematoma has the same indication for surgical intervention as acute type A (type I) aortic dissection, except in very elderly individuals or patients with multiple comorbidities, in whom medical management with blood pressure control and serial imaging is essential.

Chronic dissection of the ascending aorta, defined as dissection that occurs more than 6 weeks after the onset of initial symptoms,[25] is not an emergency, but the threshold for intervention is low. In these patients, the thoracic aorta tends to dilate, and the dissection should be managed like an enlarging aneurysm.

Penetrating atherosclerotic ulcer (PAU), or ulceration of the internal elastic lamina that allows hematoma formation within the media of the aortic wall, can occur anywhere in the aorta but is most commonly located in the descending thoracic aorta and can result in IMH or aortic dissection.[26] It can be treated more or less aggressively.[21] Its presence in the ascending aorta is another surgical indication for non-urgent replacement. Patients with connective tissue disorders and acute type A (type I) aortic dissection require replacement not only of the ascending aorta, but also of the aortic root.

Ascending aortic aneurysm

The most common indication for ascending aortic replacement is a degenerative aneurysm. All symptomatic patients are referred for urgent or emergent repair. According to the current recommendations,[27] surgical repair is recommended in suitable candidates when the ascending aorta or sinus reaches a diameter of 5.5 cm in asymptomatic patients, or when the growth rate exceeds 0.5 cm per year regardless of the size. In patients with genetic disease, an aortic or sinus diameter of 5 cm is an indication for repair unless the patient has a family history of aortic dissection, which could lower the threshold for repair. For patients who undergo any cardiac operation, the recommended size for ascending aortic replacement is 4.5 cm. In patients with a connective tissue disorder, aortic root repair or replacement is required in addition to ascending aortic replacement.

Bicuspid aortic valve

A bicuspid aortic valve is the most common cardiovascular defect, having a prevalence of 1–2% and affecting four times as many males as females. Bicuspid aortic valve (BAV) may be associated with thoracic aortic aneurysm formation, aortic dissection, and coarctation. A normally functioning BAV and an ascending aorta exceeding 5 cm in diameter is an indication for ascending aortic replacement.[27] Because as many as 15% of patients with proximal aortic dissection have BAV, and 12.5% of patients with an ascending aortic diameter of less than 5 cm could have aortic dissection,[28,29] an abnormally functioning BAV alone may be an indication for ascending aortic repair. Even though current guidelines[4] suggest replacing the ascending aorta during aortic valve replacement in patients with BAV when the diameter of the ascending aorta is greater than 4.5 cm, this recommendation is not supported by all.[30] The mortality rate associated with elective repair with or without ascending aortic replacement should be less than 1%.[27] Bicuspid aortic valve is more likely to cause AR in younger patients and aortic stenosis (AS) in older ones. Aortic regurgitation and a dilated sinotubular junction in patients with BAV indicate the need for root repair or replacement.

Infection

Infection of a previously placed Dacron graft is an indication for proximal aortic replacement. Fungal or bacterial endocarditis is another indication for aortic root replacement with additional proximal ascending aortic replacement.

Porcelain aorta

A porcelain aorta with an eggshell appearance due to extensive calcification, as seen on a CT scan or a simple chest radiogram,[31] can be found during operations for valvular heart disease or coronary artery disease. Aortic cross-clamping and direct ascending aortic cannulation for arterial inflow is prohibited in these patients because these maneuvers pose an extreme risk of embolic stroke. Replacing the ascending aorta with a tube graft has been recommended, in addition to other suggested techniques for dealing with the porcelain aorta.[32,33]

Special considerations: Pregnancy

Increases in blood pressure, maternal blood flow, and stroke volume can lead to greater aortic wall tension and shear forces, especially during the third trimester of pregnancy and the peripartum period, resulting in a higher incidence of dissection during that period.[27,34] In cases of acute proximal dissection during the first and second trimester of pregnancy, emergent repair is indicated, with additional aggressive fetal monitoring and the involvement of an experienced high risk maternal-fetal team.[27] Cardiopulmonary bypass and hypothermia can be detrimental, potentially even resulting in fetal loss. If the proximal aortic dissection occurs during the third semester of pregnancy, a cesarean section followed by aortic repair provides the best chance for survival of both the unborn child and the mother.[27]

Surgical indications for repair/replacement of the aortic arch

Rarely is aortic pathology confined to the aortic arch, sparing the remainder of the aorta. As a result, the indications for surgical intervention in the aortic arch are quite similar to those for treating the ascending or descending aorta. Acute type A (type I) aortic dissection with a tear inside the arch and marked dilation of the arch (to >5 cm) is an indication for aortic arch replacement in addition to ascending aortic replacement.[27] Proximal aortic dissection alone, without arch dilatation, is not considered an indication for aortic arch replacement. In an attempt to decrease the rate of late reoperations on the distal aorta, a few surgeons[35,36] have advocated extensive total arch replacement at the time of the initial ascending repair. Others have advocated antegrade stent delivery into the descending thoracic aorta to promote distal aortic remodeling and, possibly, to help patients with malperfusion.[37,38] In patients with a previous ascending aortic repair and remaining distal dissection, we replace the aortic arch if there is evidence of continuous enlargement (0.5 cm/year) during the follow-up period or if the diameter of the aortic arch is 5.5 cm or greater. In patients with connective tissue disorders and a remaining dissecting aortic arch, we proceed with arch replacement when the aortic diameter is ≥5 cm.

Fusiform or saccular aneurysms are another indication for replacement of the aortic arch. Saccular aneurysms of the aortic arch are rarely encountered and are usually secondary to an infection (mycotic aneurysm), degeneration of a heavily atherosclerotic penetrating ulcer, trauma, previous surgery, or focal dissection.[37,39] In all of these circumstances, it is our practice to intervene surgically to replace or exclude the aneurysm.

Surgical indications for repair/replacement of the descending and the thoracoabdominal aorta

Descending thoracic and thoracoabdominal aneurysms

According to Elefteriades,[40] who reported the natural history of 1,600 patients with thoracic aortic aneurysms and dissections, aneurysms greater than 6.0 cm in diameter are associated with a yearly rupture rate of 3.6%, a dissection rate of 3.7%, a death rate of 10.8%, and a rupture, dissection, or death rate of 14.1%. The growth rate of thoracic aortic aneurysms varies; descending and thoracoabdominal aneurysms grow at a rate of 0.19 cm/year. Fast-growing aneurysms are more likely to rupture.[40] No level A or B scientific evidence from prospective, randomized studies is available regarding the timing of operative intervention according to aneurysm size. Practice guidelines recommend that an asymptomatic descending thoracic aneurysm be repaired at an aortic diameter of 5.5 cm.[4] Our practice is to proceed with surgical intervention in patients with a family history of Marfan syndrome and aneurysms 5.0 cm or greater in diameter; patients without a family history of Marfan syndrome and aneurysms of 5.5 cm or larger; and patients with aneurysms that have a documented growth rate of more than 1 cm/year. We also intervene for rapidly expanding aneurysms, those more than twice the diameter of the normal contiguous aorta, and those that produce symptoms.

Type B or DeBakey type III aortic dissection and its variants

In the acute phase of the dissection, the following conditions are considered specific indications for immediate intervention: a contained rupture; a rapidly expanding aortic diameter; increasing periaortic or pleural fluid; uncontrollable pain; persistent hypertension not responding to medical therapy; evidence of malperfusion manifesting as lower-extremity ischemia; and renal or mesenteric ischemia. Acute dissection superimposed on a chronic dissection or an existing aneurysm needs special consideration and is another indication for surgery. In uncomplicated cases of acute type B (type IIIa, type IIIb) aortic dissection, medical therapy alone is satisfactory even though it does not improve long-term survival.[41,42] Remodeling of the distal aorta and thrombosis of the false lumen induced by the stent graft after endovascular intervention has been reported, but long-term results are not yet available.[43] In chronic distal aortic dissection, late complications occur in 20–50% of patients.[44–46] Crawford[44] found that in 23% of patients who presented with rupture of a chronically dissected aorta, the descending aorta was between 5 and 6 cm in diameter. We intervene when the diameter of a chronic dissecting aneurysm reaches 5.5 cm in patients with no genetically triggered thoracic aortic disease and 5 cm in patients with genetic thoracic aortic disease.

With IMH of the descending or thoracoabdominal aorta, the indications for intervention are similar to those in acute type B (type IIIa, type IIIb) lesions. Recurrent pain, increasing hematoma size, and aortic leak are indications for urgent repair.[41] With regard to PAU, there is controversy about the indications for intervention. Eighty percent (80%) of these patients may have an associated IMH.[26] Although it is usually our practice to intervene in patients with PAU who are acceptable surgical candidates, it is unclear whether any surgical intervention affects long-term survival in these patients, who usually have multiple comorbidities.[42]

Treatment options for aortic root and ascending aortic pathology

Surgical treatment of thoracic aortic pathologies involving the proximal aorta is traditionally performed via a median sternotomy with the aid of cardiopulmonary bypass. A variety of different procedures, with or without circulatory arrest, are used, ranging from a straightforward ascending aortic replacement with a Dacron tube graft to replacement of the entire proximal aorta and the hemiarch, with additional aortic root replacement and reimplantation of the coronary arteries. In all cases, intraoperative transesophageal echocardiography is performed, and near-infrared spectroscopy (NIRS) probes are placed over the cranium to monitor cerebral perfusion pressure and regional cerebral oxygen saturation (rSO_2). For arterial inflow, different cannulation strategies have been implemented: since 2008, innominate artery cannulation has been our preferred strategy for proximal aortic aneurysms and aortic dissections unless the patient's condition (i.e., in extremis or hemodynamically unstable) indicates using an alternative site.[47-48] Our previous preferred approach, right axillary artery cannulation, is currently our second choice, followed by femoral and/or direct aortic cannulation if the patient is hemodynamically unstable. An 8-mm graft is sewn to the right axillary or innominate artery as previously described elsewhere.[47-48] Antegrade and retrograde cardioplegia is administered for myocardial protection throughout the procedure.

Regardless of whether we are treating an ascending aortic aneurysm involving the proximal arch or a proximal dissection, we perform an open distal anastomosis.[37,47-48] Only in the rare case in which the distal ascending aorta and arch are absolutely normal, not at risk, and without dissection do we use a cross-clamp. In cases of open distal anastomosis, hypothermia to 24°C is targeted. Moderate hypothermia (24–28°C) is our usual practice for elective total arch and hemiarch replacements.[49] Ice is placed around the patient's head, and mannitol and hydrocortisone are administered to prevent cerebral edema. Systemic circulatory arrest is initiated once the target temperature is reached. Once the proximal innominate artery is secured, the pump flows are decreased to 10–15 mL/kg/min. This provides unilateral antegrade perfusion via the right common carotid artery. Additional or bilateral perfusion can be achieved by adding a 9F Pruitt® perfusion catheter (LeMaitre Vascular, Inc.; Burlington, Massachusetts, USA), which is inserted into the left common carotid artery by direct access once the arch is open. After completion of the distal anastomosis, pump flow is re-established via the innominate artery to its full level, and the period of circulatory arrest is ended. The newly placed Dacron graft is clamped, and the proximal aortic pathology (involving the aortic valve [AV]) is addressed.

The following options cover the entire spectrum of treatment for AV pathology. The repair can be as simple as (1) AV commissural plication for patients with mild-to-moderate regurgitation and a normal sinus of Valsalva segment, or (2) AV resuspension with or without commissural plication in patients with proximal dissection with or without regurgitation in whom the false and true lumens extend through the aortic annulus. The following conditions are indications for aortic root replacement: aortic root aneurysm (annuloaortic ectasia); Marfan syndrome or other connective tissue disorder; endocarditis of the AV with extensive involvement of the root; endocarditis of a prosthetic AV; recurrent perivalvular leak; and a small aortic root requiring a new AV prosthesis. In cases of complex proximal dissection with or without a dilated sinus of Valsalva, aortic root replacement can be considered. The coronary artery reattachments are performed by using either free buttons or an inclusion technique. Patients with type A (DeBakey Type I) aortic dissection undergo aortic root replacement with a composite Valsalva valved graft (Terumo, VASCUTEK, Inchinnan, Scotland) or, less commonly, a valve-sparing procedure if the aortic valve leaflets are normal. In our practice, in cases of acute proximal dissection in which the aortic root is involved and requires replacement, we either place a composite Valsalva valved graft with an attachment of free coronary buttons or place a bioroot (Medtronic Freestyle Bioroot). We very rarely perform AV-sparing procedures in patients with aortic dissection.

We consider AV repair with AV-sparing techniques in cases of non-dissection in young patients with BAV, mild-to-moderate dilation of the sinus of Valsalva, and mild-to-moderate AR; in all young individuals with AR and dilated sinuses of Valsalva; and in patients with connective tissue disorders in whom the AV leaflets are of suitable quality for repair. We prefer the David I reimplantation technique of valve-sparing aortic root replacement over the remodeling procedure (Yacoub or David II technique). In the remodeling procedure, the sinuses and the ascending aorta are replaced with three "tongues" to simulate the normal sinuses. These tongues are sewn to the scalloped contour of the aortic annulus. In the reimplantation procedure (David I), the Dacron graft (we use a Valsalva non-valved graft) is placed around the skeletonized AV and is secured below the annulus. The remnant of sinus tissue and the annulus are sewn to the inside of the graft. This technique stabilizes the annulus and prevents future dilation, especially in patients with connective tissue disorders. The remodeling technique can lead to aortic annular dilation. The surgeon's experience and degree of confidence play a critical role in successful and durable valve-sparing procedures.[50–52]

Treatment options for aortic arch pathology

The treatment armamentarium for repair/replacement of the aortic arch includes open surgical repair, hybrid repair, and endovascular replacement of the aortic arch. The choice of repair technique for the various thoracic arch lesions is influenced by the patient's comorbidities and age.

Open aortic arch repair

The first open aortic arch repair was reported by Cooley and DeBakey in 1955.[53] This was for its time an extremely challenging operation that involved a considerable risk of stroke and death. Because of advances in cardiopulmonary bypass techniques, simplification of surgical technique, and the development of protective adjuncts—such as selective antegrade cerebral protection and moderate hypothermia—for better brain protection, recent outcomes are a substantial improvement over those obtained in the past.[54-56] As previously mentioned, our preferred route for arterial inflow in treating ascending aortic lesions and performing arch reconstruction is via an 8-mm Dacron graft anastomosed end-to-side to the innominate artery.[47-48] Although the first arch reconstructions were enabled by deep hypothermic circulatory arrest (DHCA), this technique has adverse effects on the coagulation system and is limited to 30 minutes at 18°C.[57] Retrograde cerebral perfusion, introduced by Ueda[57] in 1990 as an adjunct to DHCA, yields better results by routing oxygenated blood through the superior vena cava and flushing air and debris out of the cerebral circulation. Despite initial adoption by our surgical group,[58] retrograde cerebral perfusion failed to improve neurologic and metabolic outcomes,[59] and antegrade cerebral perfusion has become the preferred means of brain protection for our group, as well as for others.[60] In addition, moderate or even mild hypothermia (26–30°C) may be safe and effective for brain protection, although the upper safe temperature limit has not yet been determined.[49,61,62] The open arch repair technique varies from the traditional "island-and-en bloc" supra-aortic-arch-vessel anastomosis to the four-branched arch graft and the Y-graft technique.[63,64] In cases of extensive aneurysmal disease also involving the descending thoracic or thoracoabdominal aorta, the elephant trunk procedure as described by Hans Borst is used.[65]

Here is how we conduct the operation: After cardiopulmonary bypass has been established, cooling of the patient is initiated. For open arch reconstruction, we prefer the Y-graft technique,[55,71] although we use the island technique as needed, depending on the patient's anatomy. During cooling, the arch vessels are dissected, and the left subclavian and left common carotid arteries are bypassed with an off-the-shelf trifurcated graft (Terumo, Vascutek). Once the targeted temperature has been achieved (24°C), the innominate artery is snared or clamped, and blood flows are decreased to 10–15 mL/kg/min. Antegrade cerebral perfusion is initially established unilaterally via the innominate artery, and then bilaterally by adding a balloon-tipped catheter at the proximal end of the Y-graft. In the event of a significant decline in the left-sided NIRS, or a known large dominate left vertebral artery, an additional perfusion cannula can be added to the origin of the left subclavian artery. The arch is opened, and the main body of the Y-graft is anastomosed to the innominate artery. After de-airing has been performed, the Y-graft is clamped, and the distal anastomosis is performed, usually between the left subclavian and left common carotid artery. For the elephant trunk, we use Terumo's (Terumo, VASCUTEK, Inchinnan, Scotland) skirted elephant-trunk graft. If a dissecting arch has extensive aneurysmal disease in the descending aorta, the elephant trunk technique is required. The graft is placed inside the true lumen of the dissecting descending thoracic aorta, or a fenestration is created and the graft is placed inside a common lumen.

For patients in whom the descending thoracic aorta is amenable to future endovascular therapy, we perform the frozen elephant trunk procedure with our custom-made frozen elephant trunk graft.[66] After the distal anastomosis has been completed, the graft is clamped, and the proximal part of the operation takes place. At that point, pump flows are restored to normal, and systemic perfusion is re-established. After completion of the proximal reconstruction, the main body of the Y-graft is anastomosed to the main aortic graft at an angle that will minimize kinking of the Y-graft. We rewarm patients to a nasopharyngeal temperature of 36.5°C. Throughout the procedure, we monitor the NIRS and use retrograde and antegrade cardioplegia for myocardial protection.

Hybrid arch repair

"Hybrid" arch repair is a combination of open supra-aortic vessel debranching and the endovascular exclusion of pathologic conditions that affect the aortic arch. The first hybrid arch repair was described by Volodos and colleagues in 1991.[67] It has been advocated as an effective alternative that produces acceptable mortality and morbidity rates in patients at high risk from traditional open procedures.[68,69] Our technique for aortic arch debranching has previously been reported.[69,70] Via a median sternotomy, we reroute the supra-aortic arch vessels by using commercially available branched grafts (Terumo, Vascutek). First, we create the proximal anastomosis between the main trunk of the bifurcated or trifurcated Y-graft and the ascending aorta by applying a partial occluding clamp to the ascending aorta. We then create the individual distal anastomoses: first to the left subclavian artery, then to the left common carotid artery, and last to the innominate artery. The endovascular portion of the procedure is then carried out by performing antegrade or retrograde stent graft delivery to exclude the aortic arch pathology. The complexity of the hybrid procedure depends on the extent of the aortic disease.[70] In an attempt to avoid a median sternotomy, extra-anatomic bypass for full rerouting of the arch vessels has been also reported.[69] Cardiopulmonary bypass is not required unless the ascending aorta is aneurysmal and needs to be replaced. Off-pump coronary artery bypass can be added as necessary.

Direct comparison of the hybrid procedure and open arch surgery may be unfair because of a lack of homogeneity in the patient populations.[71] Newer endovascular stent grafts are currently on trial for hybrid procedures of the aortic arch.

Endovascular repair of the aortic arch

Custom-made branched grafts have been used for patients' specific anatomy and pathology. Various endovascular techniques have been described in an attempt to overcome the lack of available technology.[72] Because reports are limited, it is difficult to compare this approach to hybrid or open arch repair.

Treatment options for descending and thoracoabdominal aortic pathologies

Open and endovascular treatment options are available for various aortic pathologies involving the descending and thoracoabdominal aorta (Figure 6.1).

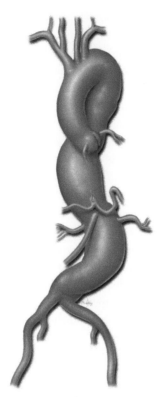

Figure 6.1 Aneurysm extending into the descending and thoracoabdominal aorta.
Printed with permission from Baylor College of Medicine

Descending thoracic aorta

Descending thoracic aneurysms: Open surgical repair

No level A or B scientific evidence from prospective, randomized studies exists regarding the timing of operative intervention according to aneurysm size. The following conditions justify operative intervention[41]: aneurysms with a diameter of 5.0 or larger in patients with a family history of Marfan syndrome; aneurysms with a diameter of 5.5 cm in patients without a family history of Marfan syndrome; aneurysms with a documented growth rate of more than 1 cm/year; and aneurysms that are rapidly expanding, are more than twice the diameter of the normal contiguous aorta, or are producing symptoms.

Open surgical repair is performed via a left posterolateral thoracotomy. The following techniques are appropriate for the open surgical treatment of descending thoracic aneurysms.

Clamp-and-sew technique—Before cross-clamp application, heparin is given (1.5 U/kg). The cross-clamp is applied whenever possible distal to the left subclavian artery. In patients with aortic dissection, the clamp is most commonly applied just distal to the left common

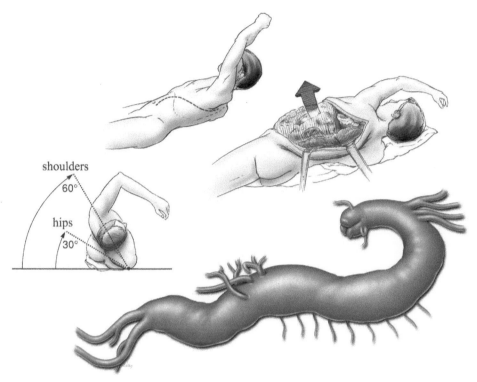

shoulders

60°

hips

30°

Figure 6.2 Right lateral decubitus position for a left posterolateral thoracotomy, which extends from the left scapula to the left, toward the umbilicus.
Printed with permission from Baylor College of Medicine

carotid artery. In cases involving an enlarging thoracic aneurysm secondary to chronic dissection, the thrombus is removed from the false lumen; then the septum is divided, and the true lumen is opened. Small proximal intercostal vessels that give rise to active back-bleeding are oversewn. Large distal intercostal vessels with slow back-bleeding are usually considered for reattachment. After completing the proximal anastomosis and applying the intercostal patch, we perform an open distal anastomosis. In chronic dissection, the septum is fenestrated during reconstruction of the distal anastomosis to allow inflow into both the true and false lumens distally.

Clamp-and-sew technique with left-sided heart bypass—Partial left-sided heart bypass (LHB) is used as an adjunct to provide distal aortic perfusion and maintain blood flow to visceral vessels and the spinal cord during the repair. This technique is used most for extent I and II TAAA repairs (Figures 6.2 and 6.3). The LHB circuit is established through an outflow cannula inserted into the left atrium via the left inferior pulmonary vein, and through an inflow cannula in the lower descending thoracic aorta or, less frequently, in a femoral artery. Left-sided heart bypass is preferred if the repair is prolonged and complicated, because LHB lowers the risk of paraplegia and paraparesis after thoracoabdominal aortic aneurysm repair, especially extent II repair.[73]

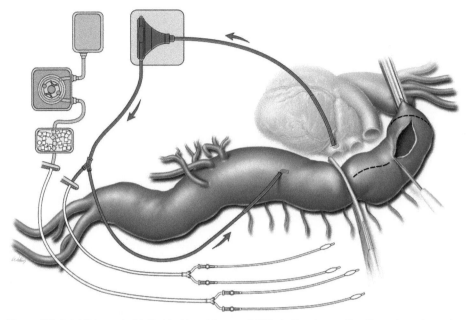

Figure 6.3 Establishment of left-sided heart bypass (LHB) via the descending thoracic aorta and left pulmonary vein.
Printed with permission from Baylor College of Medicine

Deep hypothermic circulatory arrest (DHCA)—If the aneurysm extends proximally into the distal arch and cross-clamping is not possible, DHCA may be necessary to construct an open proximal anastomosis. Cardiopulmonary bypass is usually initiated via the femoral artery and vein, or via the junction of the inferior vena cava with the right atrium. The patient is cooled to a target temperature of 18°C. When the targeted temperature is achieved, the proximal aorta is opened with a distal clamp in the mid-descending aorta or lower to allow flow of 2–3 L/min. Once the proximal anastomosis is completed, the pump is restarted, usually via a pre-attached 8-mm side graft just below the distal arch anastomosis. The graft is cross-clamped, and the open distal anastomosis is performed during rewarming with the patient on cardiopulmonary bypass.

Descending thoracic aneurysms: Endovascular repair (TEVAR)

In March 2005, the FDA approved for commercial use the Gore TAG thoracic endograft (W.L. Gore and Associates, Flagstaff, AZ, USA) for treatment of descending thoracic aneurysms. Since then, more devices have gained approval. Despite the sole indication approved by the FDA in 2005, thoracic aortic endografting is rapidly emerging as the treatment of choice for a variety of thoracic pathologies.[41,74–76] Recently, the FDA has approved endovascular therapy for both traumatic injury and aortic dissection of the descending thoracic aorta. During the evaluation for endografting in the descending thoracic aorta, the following points should be addressed: the proximal landing zone and its relationship to the origin of the great vessels (left subclavian and left common carotid artery); the distal landing zone and its relationship to the celiac axis; the iliofemoral artery's diameter; the presence of calcification, thrombus, or dissection; the tortuosity of the thoracic aorta; and the potential for compromise of critical branch flow. Depending on the size of the access vessels, the native iliofemoral vessels or iliac-conduit or aorto-conduit access is used. Left subclavian artery revascularization with left carotid–to–subclavian artery bypass or transposition is an absolute indication in patients with a patent left internal mammary artery and prior coronary artery bypass, a functioning arteriovenous fistula in the left upper extremity, or a dominant left vertebral artery. Coverage of a long segment of the descending thoracic aorta is a relative indication for left subclavian revascularization for spinal cord protection.

The following are the basic procedural steps: the femoral artery is accessed (percutaneously or open), and heparin (5,000 U) is administered. Under fluoroscopic guidance, a soft wire is advanced into the ascending aorta. In cases of acute or chronic aortic dissection, using intravascular ultrasound (IVUS) to confirm the placement of the guidewire inside the true lumen of the thoracic aorta is recommended. Occasionally, accessing the true lumen can be challenging, in which case inserting the soft wire via the right brachial artery and snaring this wire via the femoral artery can be very helpful. The soft wire is exchanged for a stiff Lunderquist guidewire, and the sheath, stent endograft, or both are advanced under fluoroscopy. Before the endograft is placed, preoperative arch and descending thoracic angiography, IVUS, or both are necessary to confirm the origin of the left subclavian artery, the left common carotid artery, and the celiac axis. During deployment of the endograft, the systolic pressure is kept below 100 mmHg; immediately after deployment, we raise the mean pressure to at least 90 mmHg and/or the systolic blood pressure to 150–170 mmHg for spinal cord protection. The sheath is removed, and the femoral artery is repaired under direct vision or percutaneously. Protamine is given to reverse heparin. Preferably, the patient is extubated in the operating room. A cerebrospinal fluid drain is used for spinal cord protection during the TEVAR when we cover more than 15 cm of the descending thoracic aorta and when the patient has previously undergone open or endovascular abdominal aortic aneurysm replacement.

Descending thoracic aortic dissection: Acute Stanford type B, or DeBakey type IIIA, and/or DeBakey type IIIB aortic dissection

Special considerations

The initial treatment for all patients with suspected or confirmed acute aortic dissection is aggressive blood pressure control or anti-impulse therapy to stabilize the dissection and to prevent rupture. Intravenous beta-adrenergic blockers, direct vasodilators, calcium channel blockers, and angiotensin-converting enzyme inhibitors are used. Beta antagonists are administered to all patients unless there are strong contraindications. Medical therapy provides better outcomes in non-complicated acute descending thoracic dissection than open surgical therapy.[77] Serial CT scanning of the chest and abdomen during the patient's hospitalization is recommended, and meticulous follow-up after hospital discharge and aggressive blood pressure control are imperative. Surgical intervention is indicated in cases of complicated acute type B, IIIA, or IIIB aortic dissection, which are characterized by contained rupture, malperfusion, continuous pain, uncontrollable hypertension, and periaortic hematoma. Three goals should be achieved during any open or endovascular repair for acute type B aortic dissection: exclude the primary tear, eliminate all aneurysmal disease, and permit perfusion to all distal organs and major aortic branches. Endovascular therapy is becoming the preferred approach for complicated acute descending thoracic aortic dissection. According to the IRAD registry, TEVAR is associated with lower 5-year mortality than medical therapy.[78] For patients with a connective tissue disorder, endografting is not recommended, and endovascular stent grafting, if needed, may be used as a bridge to later definitive repair.[79]

Chronic Stanford type B (type IIIA and/or type IIIB) aortic dissection

The presence of symptoms, evidence of an enlarging dissecting thoracic aneurysm, and acute dissection superimposed on a chronic aneurysm with imminent rupture or malperfusion are the indications for surgical intervention in chronic descending thoracic aortic dissection. The same open technique used to treat open thoracoabdominal aortic aneurysms (described next) can be used with these patients. Special attention is given to the septum, which should be divided to identify the true and false lumens and all the important branch vessels.

With regard to endovascular therapy, recent 5-year results of the INSTEAD-XL trial (Investigation of Stent-grafts in Aortic Dissection) revealed that TEVAR improved 5-year aorta-specific survival and delayed disease progression when used in addition to optimal medical treatment.[80] In stable type B dissection with suitable anatomy, the conclusion was that pre-emptive TEVAR should be considered to improve late outcome.

We consider treatment options tailored to each patient's anatomy, age, and comorbid conditions. The endovascular repair, with regard to technical considerations, can be challenging—even more so than in acute disease. The principles followed during TEVAR in patients with acute descending thoracic dissection are also followed during TEVAR in patients with chronic dissection.

Thoracoabdominal aorta

Thoracoabdominal aortic aneurysms (TAAA): Open repair

Surgical repair of TAAA is categorized by the extent of aortic replacement according to the Crawford classification. Extent I thoracoabdominal aortic aneurysm repair (TAAA ext I) involves the descending thoracic aorta, beginning near the left subclavian artery, and extends into visceral vessels (celiac, superior mesenteric, and both renal arteries). Extent II repair (TAAA ext II; Figure 6.1) also begins near the left subclavian artery but extends distally into the aortic bifurcation. Extent III repair (TAAA ext III) extends from the lower descending thoracic aorta (below the sixth rib) into the abdomen. Extent IV repair (TAAA ext IV) begins at the diaphragmatic hiatus at the level of the visceral vessels and often involves the entire abdominal aorta. Exposure is achieved by thoracoabdominal incision. In TAAA ext I and ext II repair, we routinely use LHB, permissive hypothermia, and cold (4°C) crystalloid solution (25 g of mannitol and 125 mg of methylprednisolone in 1 L of Ringer's lactate solution) for renal perfusion and protection.[73,81,82] Cerebrospinal fluid drainage, in addition to sequential cross-clamping and selective reimplantation of intercostal or lumbar arteries, is used for spinal cord protection,[83,84] especially in ext I and II repairs. The steps of the operation have been previously described (Figure 6.2). Left heart bypass is initiated (Figure 6.3), the cross-clamp is placed for performing the proximal anastomosis (Figure 6.4), and large intercostal arteries with slow back-bleeding are reimplanted (Figure 6.5). For extensive aneurysms ("mega aorta") involving the ascending aorta, transverse arch, and descending thoracic aorta, we proceed with staged operations. When the descending or thoracoabdominal component is symptomatic or is disproportionately large (compared with the ascending aorta), the distal segment is treated during the initial operation, and repair of the ascending aorta and transverse aortic arch is performed as a second procedure. A reversed elephant trunk repair can be performed during the first operation.[85] Frozen elephant trunk repair can be performed in patients with ascending and arch aneurysms that extend through the upper or the entire descending thoracic aorta.[86] Although spinal cord ischemia and renal failure warrant special consideration postoperatively, the most common complication after extensive repair is respiratory

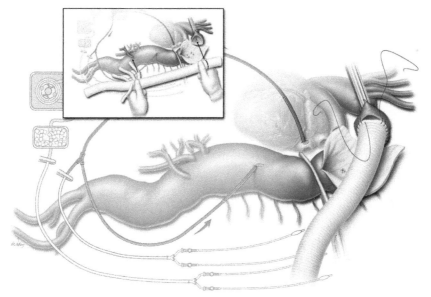

Figure 6.4 After LHB is established, placement of the cross-clamp and performance of the proximal anastomosis follow.
Printed with permission from Baylor College of Medicine

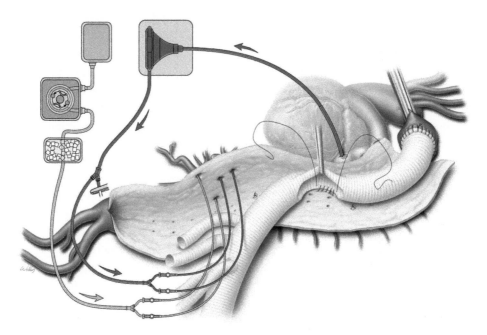

Figure 6.5 Intercostal patch placement.
Printed with permission from Baylor College of Medicine

failure. In addition, the vagus and left recurrent laryngeal nerves are susceptible to injury. Vocal cord paralysis can be treated by direct cord medialization. In patients with patent left internal thoracic artery grafts from prior coronary artery bypass in whom there is need to clamp proximal to the left subclavian artery, a left common carotid-to-subclavian bypass is performed before TAAA repair.

Completion elephant trunk repair

This repair can be performed with endovascular techniques in patients whose aneurysm ends at the diaphragm, whereas open repair is necessary in patients with more extensive pathology. Occasionally, advancing a stent graft in retrograde fashion from the femoral artery into the elephant trunk can be very challenging; advancing a wire antegrade via the right brachial artery may be useful in these cases. For the past few years, in cases in which the completion stage can be performed endovascularly, we have been placing a short (10-cm) stent inside the trunk of the elephant graft to facilitate the second/completion stage.[86,66]

Thoracoabdominal aortic aneurysms (TAAA): Hybrid and endovascular repair

A combination of open surgery to reroute the blood supply of the visceral vessels to avoid visceral ischemia, allowing their aortic origin to be covered by stent graft, is the mainstay of hybrid therapy for TAAA. The endovascular portion of the hybrid therapy procedure can be performed concomitantly with the open portion, or it can be done later as a separate procedure. The results of these procedures vary.[87,88] We do not favor the hybrid approach for TAAA. Although it requires a less extensive incision than does thoracoabdominal exposure for TAAA, debranching usually requires substantial retroperitoneal or transperitoneal exposure. Total endovascular repair for TAAA with the use of fenestrated and branched endografts has been used extensively with promising results.[89] However, mortality and spinal cord ischemia risks remain considerable.

Conclusion

Innovative and standard open surgical approaches are used to treat the various thoracic aortic pathologies. Having open, endovascular, and hybrid repair options creates an opportunity to maximize the benefit of repair for the individual patient.

References

1. Volodos NL, Shekhanin VE, Karpovich IP, Troian VI, Gur'ev Iu A (1986). [A self-fixing synthetic blood vessel endoprosthesis]. *Vestn Khir Im I I Grek*, **137**, 123–5.
2. Parodi JC, Palmaz JC, Barone HD (1991). Transfemoral intraluminal graft implantation for abdominal aortic aneurysms. *Ann Vasc Surg*, **5**, 491–9.
3. Dake MD, Miller DC, Semba CP, *et al.* (1994). Transluminal placement of endovascular stent-grafts for the treatment of descending thoracic aortic aneurysms. *N Engl J Med*, **331**, 1729–34.
4. Hiratzka LF, Creager MA, Isselbacher EM, *et al.* (2016). Surgery for aortic dilatation in patients with bicuspid aortic valves: a statement of clarification from the American College of Cardiology/American Heart Association Task Force on Clinical Practice Guidelines. *J Am Coll Cardiol*, **67**, 724–31.
5. Brar SS, Shen AY, Jorgensen MB, *et al.* (2008). Sodium bicarbonate vs sodium chloride for the prevention of contrast medium-induced nephropathy in patients undergoing coronary angiography: a randomized trial. *JAMA*, **300**, 1038–46.
6. Subramaniam RM, Suarez-Cuervo C, Wilson RF, *et al.* (2016). Effectiveness of prevention strategies for contrast-induced nephropathy: a systematic review and meta-analysis. *Ann Intern Med*, **164**, 406–16.
7. Duong MH, MacKenzie TA, Malenka DJ (2005). N-acetylcysteine prophylaxis significantly reduces the risk of radiocontrast-induced nephropathy: comprehensive meta-analysis. *Catheter Cardiovasc Interv*, **64**, 471–9.
8. Goldenberg I, Shechter M, Matetzky S, *et al.* (2004). Oral acetylcysteine as an adjunct to saline hydration for the prevention of contrast-induced nephropathy following coronary angiography. A randomized controlled trial and review of the current literature. *Eur Heart J*, **25**, 212–8.
9. Danias PG, Manning WJ (2000). Coronary MR angiography: current status. *Herz*, **25**, 431–9.
10. Ergun I, Keven K, Uruc I, *et al.* (2006). The safety of gadolinium in patients with stage 3 and 4 renal failure. *Nephrol Dial Transplant*, **21**, 697–700.
11. Erbel R (1993). Role of transesophageal echocardiography in dissection of the aorta and evaluation of degenerative aortic disease. *Cardiol Clin*, **11**, 461–73.
12. Rodríguez-Palomares JF, Teixidó-Tura G, Galuppo V, *et al.* (2016). Multimodality assessment of ascending aortic diameters: Comparison of different measurement methods. *J Am Soc Echocardiogr*, **29**, 819–26.

13. Evangelista A, Flachskampf FA, Erbel R, *et al.* (2010). Echocardiography in aortic diseases: EAE recommendations for clinical practice. *Eur J Echocardiogr*, **11**, 645–58.

14. Flachskampf FA (2006). Assessment of aortic dissection and hematoma. *Semin Cardiothorac Vasc Anesth*, **10**, 83–8.

15. Koutouzi G, Henrikson O, Roos H, Zachrisson K, Falkenberg M (2015). EVAR guided by 3D image fusion and CO_2 DSA: a new imaging combination for patients with renal insufficiency. *J Endovasc Ther*, **22**, 912–17.

16. Januzzi JL, Eagle KA, Cooper JV, *et al.* (2005). Acute aortic dissection presenting with congestive heart failure: results from the International Registry of Acute Aortic Dissection. *J Am Coll Cardiol*, **46**, 733–5.

17. Hansen MS, Nogareda GJ, Hutchison SJ (2007). Frequency of and inappropriate treatment of misdiagnosis of acute aortic dissection. *Am J Cardiol*, **99**, 852–6.

18. Nallamothu BK, Mehta RH, Saint S, *et al.* (2002). Syncope in acute aortic dissection: diagnostic, prognostic, and clinical implications. *Am J Med*, **113**, 468–71.

19. Berretta P, Trimarchi S, Patel HJ, *et al.* (2018). Malperfusion syndromes in type A aortic dissection: what we have learned from IRAD. *J Vis Surg*, **4**, 65.

20. Bossone E, Corteville DC, Harris KM, *et al.* (2013). Stroke and outcomes in patients with acute type A aortic dissection. *Circulation*, **128**, S175–9.

21. Lansman SL, Saunders PC, Malekan R, Spielvogel D (2010). Acute aortic syndrome. *J Thorac Cardiovasc Surg*, **140**(6 Suppl), S92–7; discussion S142–S146.

22. Evangelista A, Mukherjee D, Mehta RH, *et al.* (2005). Acute intramural hematoma of the aorta: a mystery in evolution. *Circulation*, **111**, 1063–70.

23. Nienaber CA, Sievers HH (2002). Intramural hematoma in acute aortic syndrome: more than one variant of dissection? *Circulation*, **106**, 284–5.

24. O'Gara PT, DeSanctis RW (1995). Acute aortic dissection and its variants. Toward a common diagnostic and therapeutic approach. *Circulation*, **92**, 1376–8.

25. VIRTUE Registry Investigators (2014). Mid-term outcomes and aortic remodelling after thoracic endovascular repair for acute, subacute, and chronic aortic dissection: the VIRTUE Registry. *Eur J Vasc Endovasc Surg*, **48**, 363–71.

26. Cho KR, Stanson AW, Potter DD, *et al.* (2004). Penetrating atherosclerotic ulcer of the descending thoracic aorta and arch. *J Thorac Cardiovasc Surg*, **127**, 1393–9; discussion 9–401.

27. Svensson LG, Adams DH, Bonow RO, *et al.* (2013). Aortic valve and ascending aorta guidelines for management and quality measures: executive summary. *Ann Thorac Surg*, **95**, 1491–505.

28. Larson EW, Edwards WD (1984). Risk factors for aortic dissection: a necropsy study of 161 cases. *Am J Cardiol*, **53**, 849–55.

29. Svensson LG, Kim KH, Lytle BW, Cosgrove DM (2003). Relationship of aortic cross-sectional area to height ratio and the risk of aortic dissection in patients with bicuspid aortic valves. *J Thorac Cardiovasc Surg*, **126**, 892–3.

30. Kaneko T, Shekar P, Ivkovic V, *et al.* (2018). Should the dilated ascending aorta be repaired at the time of bicuspid aortic valve replacement? *Eur J Cardiothorac Surg*, **53**(3), 560–8.

31. Chiu KM, Lin TY, Chen JS, *et al.* (2006). Images in cardiovascular medicine. Left ventricle apical conduit to bilateral subclavian artery in a patient with porcelain aorta and aortic stenosis. *Circulation*, **113**, e388–9.

32. Aranki SF, Nathan M, Shekar P, Couper G, Rizzo R, Cohn LH (2005). Hypothermic circulatory arrest enables aortic valve replacement in patients with unclampable aorta. *Ann Thorac Surg*, **80**, 1679–86; discussion 86–7.

33. Girardi LN, Krieger KH, Mack CA, Isom OW (2005). No-clamp technique for valve repair or replacement in patients with a porcelain aorta. *Ann Thorac Surg*, **80**, 1688–92.

34. **Pacini L, Digne F, Boumendil A**, *et al.* (2009). Maternal complication of pregnancy in Marfan syndrome. *Int J Cardiol*, **136**, 156–61.

35. **Kazui T, Washiyama N, Muhammad BA**, *et al.* (2000). Extended total arch replacement for acute type A aortic dissection: experience with seventy patients. *J Thorac Cardiovasc Surg*, **119**, 558–65.

36. **Uchida N, Shibamura H, Katayama A**, *et al.* (2009). Operative strategy for acute type A aortic dissection: ascending aortic or hemiarch versus total arch replacement with frozen elephant trunk. *Ann Thorac Surg*, **87**, 773–7.

37. **Preventza O, Cervera R, Cooley DA**, *et al.* (2014). Acute type I aortic dissection: traditional versus hybrid repair with antegrade stent delivery to the descending thoracic aorta. *J Thorac Cardiovasc Surg*, **148**, 119–25.

38. **Vallabhajosyula P, Szeto WY, Pulsipher A**, *et al.* (2014). Antegrade thoracic stent grafting during repair of acute Debakey type I dissection promotes distal aortic remodeling and reduces late open distal reoperation rate. *J Thorac Cardiovasc Surg*, **147**, 942–8.

39. **Preventza O, Coselli JS** (2015). Saccular aneurysms of the transverse aortic arch: treatment options available in the endovascular era. *Aorta (Stamford)*, **3**, 61–6.

40. **Elefteriades JA** (2002). Natural history of thoracic aortic aneurysms: indications for surgery, and surgical versus nonsurgical risks. *Ann Thorac Surg*, **74**, S1877–80; discussion S92–8.

41. **Svensson LG, Kouchoukos NT, Miller DC**, *et al.* (2008). Expert consensus document on the treatment of descending thoracic aortic disease using endovascular stent-grafts. *Ann Thorac Surg*, **85**, S1–41.

42. **Umana JP, Miller DC, Mitchell RS** (2002). What is the best treatment for patients with acute type B aortic dissections—medical, surgical, or endovascular stent-grafting? *Ann Thorac Surg*, **74**, S1840–3; discussion S57–63.

43. **Brunkwall J, Kasprzak P, Verhoeven E, Heijmen R, Taylor P, the Adsorb Trialists** (2014). Endovascular repair of acute uncomplicated aortic type B dissection promotes aortic remodelling: 1-year results of the ADSORB trial. *Eur J Vasc Endovasc Surg*, **48**, 285–91.

44. **Crawford ES** (1990). The diagnosis and management of aortic dissection. *JAMA*, **264**, 2537–41.

45. **Doroghazi RM, Slater EE, DeSanctis RW**, *et al.* (1984). Long-term survival of patients with treated aortic dissection. *J Am Coll Cardiol*, **3**, 1026–34.

46. **Fann JI, Smith JA, Miller DC**, *et al.* (1995). Surgical management of aortic dissection during a 30-year period. *Circulation*, **92**, II113–21.

47. **Preventza O, Garcia A, Tuluca A**, *et al.* (2015). Innominate artery cannulation for proximal aortic surgery: outcomes and neurological events in 263 patients. *Eur J Cardiothorac Surg*, **48**, 937–42; discussion 942.

48. **Preventza O, Price MD, Spiliotopoulos K**, *et al.* (2018). In elective arch surgery with circulatory arrest, does the arterial cannulation site really matter? A propensity score analysis of right axillary and innominate artery cannulation. *J Thorac Cardiovasc Surg*, **155**, 1953–60.

49. **Preventza O, Coselli JS, Garcia A**, *et al.* (2017). Moderate hypothermia at warmer temperatures is safe in elective proximal and total arch surgery: results in 665 patients. *J Thorac Cardiovasc Surg*, **153**, 1011–8.

50. **David TE, Armstrong S, Ivanov J**, *et al.* (2001). Results of aortic valve-sparing operations. *J Thorac Cardiovasc Surg*, **122**, 39–46.

51. **David TE, Feindel CM** (1992). An aortic valve-sparing operation for patients with aortic incompetence and aneurysm of the ascending aorta. *J Thorac Cardiovasc Surg*, **103**, 617–21; discussion 22.

52. **Yacoub MH, Gehle P, Chandrasekaran V**, *et al.* (1998). Late results of a valve-preserving operation in patients with aneurysms of the ascending aorta and root. *J Thorac Cardiovasc Surg*, **115**, 1080–90.

53. **Cooley DA, Mahaffey DE, De Bakey ME** (1955). Total excision of the aortic arch for aneurysm. *Surg Gynecol Obstet*, **101**, 667–72.

54. **Bachet J, Guilmet D** (2002). Brain protection during surgery of the aortic arch. *J Card Surg*, **17**, 115–24.

55. **LeMaire SA, Price MD, Parenti JL**, *et al.* (2011). Early outcomes after aortic arch replacement by using the Y-graft technique. *Ann Thorac Surg*, **91**, 700–7; discussion 7–8.

56. **Patel HJ, Nguyen C, Diener AC**, *et al.* (2011). Open arch reconstruction in the endovascular era: analysis of 721 patients over 17 years. *J Thorac Cardiovasc Surg*, **141**, 1417–23.

57. **Ueda Y, Miki S, Kusuhara K**, *et al.* (1990). Surgical treatment of aneurysm or dissection involving the ascending aorta and aortic arch, utilizing circulatory arrest and retrograde cerebral perfusion. *J Cardiovasc Surg (Torino)*, **31**, 553–8.

58. **Coselli JS** (1994). Retrograde cerebral perfusion via a superior vena caval cannula for aortic arch aneurysm operations. *Ann Thorac Surg*, **57**, 1668–9.

59. **Harrington DK, Bonser M, Moss A**, *et al.* (2003). Neuropsychometric outcome following aortic arch surgery: a prospective randomized trial of retrograde cerebral perfusion. *J Thorac Cardiovasc Surg*, **126**, 638–44.

60. **Spielvogel D, Kai M, Tang GH, Malekan R, Lansman SL** (2013). Selective cerebral perfusion: a review of the evidence. *J Thorac Cardiovasc Surg*, **145**, S59–62.

61. **Preventza O, Garcia A, Kashyap SA**, *et al.* (2016). Moderate hypothermia ≥24 and ≤28°C with hypothermic circulatory arrest for proximal aortic operations in patients with previous cardiac surgery. *Eur J Cardiothorac Surg*, **50**, 949–54.

62. **El-Sayed Ahmad A, Papadopoulos N**, *et al.* (2017). The standardized concept of moderate-to-mild (≥28°C) systemic hypothermia during selective antegrade cerebral perfusion for all-comers in aortic arch surgery: single-center experience in 587 consecutive patients over a 15-year period. *Ann Thorac Surg*, **104**, 49–55.

63. **Kazui T, Washiyama N, Muhammad BA**, *et al.* (2000). Total arch replacement using aortic arch branched grafts with the aid of antegrade selective cerebral perfusion. *Ann Thorac Surg*, **70**, 3–8; discussion 9.

64. **Spielvogel D, Strauch JT, Minanov OP, Lansman SL, Griepp RB** (2002). Aortic arch replacement using a trifurcated graft and selective cerebral antegrade perfusion. *Ann Thorac Surg*, **74**, S1810–4; discussion S25–32.

65. **Neri E, Massetti M, Sani G** (2004). The "elephant trunk" technique made easier. *Ann Thorac Surg*, **78**, e17–8.

66. **Preventza O, Coselli JS, Mayor J**, *et al.* (2017). The stent is not to blame: lessons learned with a simplified US version of the frozen elephant trunk. *Ann Thorac Surg*, **104**, 1456–63.

67. **Volodos NL, Karpovich IP, Troyan VI**, *et al.* (1991). Clinical experience of the use of self-fixing synthetic prostheses for remote endoprosthetics of the thoracic and the abdominal aorta and iliac arteries through the femoral artery and as intraoperative endoprosthesis for aorta reconstruction. *Vasa Suppl*, **33**, 93–5.

68. **Czerny M, Weigang E, Sodeck G**, *et al.* (2012). Targeting landing zone 0 by total arch rerouting and TEVAR: midterm results of a transcontinental registry. *Ann Thorac Surg*, **94**, 84–9.

69. **Preventza O, Bakaeen FG, Cervera RD, Coselli JS** (2013). Deployment of proximal thoracic endograft in zone 0 of the ascending aorta: treatment options and early outcomes for aortic arch aneurysms in a high-risk population. *Eur J Cardiothorac Surg*, **44**, 446–52; discussion 52–3.

70. **Preventza O, Aftab M, Coselli JS** (2013). Hybrid techniques for complex aortic arch surgery. *Tex Heart Inst J*, **40**, 568–71.

71. **Preventza O, Garcia A, Cooley DA**, *et al.* (2015). Total aortic arch replacement: a comparative study of zone 0 hybrid arch exclusion versus traditional open repair. *J Thorac Cardiovasc Surg*, **150**, 1591–8; discussion 8–600.

72. **Moulakakis KG, Mylonas SN, Dalainas I**, *et al.* (2013). The chimney-graft technique for preserving supra-aortic branches: a review. *Ann Cardiothorac Surg*, **2**, 339–46.

73. **Coselli JS** (2003). The use of left heart bypass in the repair of thoracoabdominal aortic aneurysms: current techniques and results. *Semin Thorac Cardiovasc Surg*, **15**, 326–32.

74. **Brinster DR, Wheatley GH, 3rd, Williams J**, *et al.* (2006). Are penetrating aortic ulcers best treated using an endovascular approach? *Ann Thorac Surg*, **82**, 1688–91.

75. **Preventza O, Wheatley GH, 3rd, Williams J**, *et al.* (2006). Endovascular approaches for complex forms of recurrent aortic coarctation. *J Endovasc Ther*, **13**, 400–5.

76. **Wheatley GH, 3rd, Nunez A, Preventza O**, *et al.* (2007). Have we gone too far? Endovascular stent-graft repair of aortobronchial fistulas. *J Thorac Cardiovasc Surg*, **133**, 1277–85.

77. **Hagan PG, Nienaber CA, Isselbacher EM**, *et al.* (2000). The International Registry of Acute Aortic Dissection (IRAD): new insights into an old disease. *JAMA*, **283**, 897–903.

78. **Fattori R, Montgomery D, Lovato L**, *et al.* (2013). Survival after endovascular therapy in patients with type B aortic dissection: a report from the International Registry of Acute Aortic Dissection (IRAD). *JACC Cardiovasc Interv*, **6**, 876–82.

79. **Preventza O, Mohammed S, Cheong BY**, *et al.* (2014). Endovascular therapy in patients with genetically triggered thoracic aortic disease: applications and short- and mid-term outcomes. *Eur J Cardiothorac Surg*, **46**, 248–53; discussion 253.

80. **Nienaber CA, Kische S, Rousseau H**, *et al.* (2013). Endovascular repair of type B aortic dissection: long-term results of the randomized investigation of stent grafts in aortic dissection trial. *Circ Cardiovasc Interv*, **6**, 407–16.

81. **Coselli JS, LeMaire SA, Preventza O**, *et al.* (2016). Outcomes of 3309 thoracoabdominal aortic aneurysm repairs. *J Thorac Cardiovasc Surg*, **151**, 1323–37.

82. **Koksoy C, LeMaire SA, Curling PE**, *et al.* (2002). Renal perfusion during thoracoabdominal aortic operations: cold crystalloid is superior to normothermic blood. *Ann Thorac Surg*, **73**, 730–8.

83. **Coselli JS, LeMaire SA, Koksoy C, Schmittling ZC, Curling PE** (2002). Cerebrospinal fluid drainage reduces paraplegia after thoracoabdominal aortic aneurysm repair: results of a randomized clinical trial. *J Vasc Surg*, **35**, 631–9.

84. **Coselli JS, de la Cruz KI, Preventza O, LeMaire SA, Weldon SA** (2016). Extent II thoracoabdominal aortic aneurysm repair: how I do it. *Semin Thorac Cardiovasc Surg*, **28**, 221–37.

85. **Coselli JS, Oberwalder P** (1998). Successful repair of mega aorta using reversed elephant trunk procedure. *J Vasc Surg*, **27**, 183–8.

86. **Preventza O, Al-Najjar R, Lemaire SA, Weldon S, Coselli JS** (2013). Total arch replacement with frozen elephant trunk technique. *Ann Cardiothorac Surg*, **2**, 649–52.

87. **Hughes GC, Andersen ND, Hanna JM, McCann RL** (2012). Thoracoabdominal aortic aneurysm: hybrid repair outcomes. *Ann Cardiothorac Surg*, **1**, 311–9.

88. **Patel R, Conrad MF, Paruchuri V**, *et al.* (2009). Thoracoabdominal aneurysm repair: hybrid versus open repair. *J Vasc Surg*, **50**, 15–22.

89. **Greenberg R, Eagleton M, Mastracci T** (2010). Branched endografts for thoracoabdominal aneurysms. *J Thorac Cardiovasc Surg*, **140**, S171–8.

Chapter 7

Mitral valve repair: Conventional open techniques

A. Marc Gillinov and Tomislav Mihaljevic

Mitral valve repair: Indications and results

Mitral valve repair *vs.* mitral valve replacement

Mitral valve repair is the preferred surgical option for nearly all patients with mitral re-gurgitation (MR). Advantages of mitral valve repair over mitral valve replacement include better preservation of left ventricular function, greater freedoms from endocarditis and anticoagulant-related hemorrhage, and, in some cases, improved survival.[1-4] Mitral valve repair has particular advantages in younger patients, who require lifelong anticoagulation if they receive mechanical prostheses. Mitral valve repair can be achieved in more than 90% of patients with MR caused by prolapse.[1-5]

Durability of mitral valve repair

The durability of mitral valve repair is widely recognized to be excellent.[1-7] However, it is clear that not all mitral valve repairs last a lifetime. In fact, a recent single center series reports an alarmingly high incidence of recurrent MR in patients who had repair for prolapse.[8] Other experienced centers report better durability.[1-7] Among patients having repair for posterior leaflet prolapse, the most common finding for 10-year freedom from reoperation is 97%, and 10-year freedom from moderately severe or severe MR is 80% to 90%.[7-9] Durability of repair for anterior leaflet prolapse has been somewhat lower in most series.[7-10] However, changes in surgical technique have improved results in patients with anterior prolapse. With the elimination of chordal shortening, standardized correc-tion of anterior prolapse with artificial chordae or chordal transfer, and routine use of an annuloplasty, durability of repair of anterior (or bileaflet) prolapse is similar to that for repair of posterior prolapse.[7]

Indications for mitral valve repair (*vs.* replacement)

There are no specific anatomic contraindications to mitral valve repair in patients with mitral valve prolapse. However, clinical judgment must be applied on a case-by-case basis. If an elderly patient with multiple comorbidities has complex valvar pathology (bileaflet prolapse, annular calcification), bioprosthetic mitral valve replacement should be considered. Conversely, mitral valve repair is preferred in a younger, healthier patient who has a similarly complex mitral valve.

Approaches to the mitral valve

Most mitral valve surgery is performed via median sternotomy. Advantages to median sternotomy include central cannulation, good surgical exposure, excellent access for de-airing the heart, and ability to perform concomitant procedures. Nevertheless, in a patient with isolated mitral valve disease, minimally invasive approaches should be considered. Currently applied less invasive approaches to the mitral valve include partial sternotomy (upper or lower), right mini-thoracotomy, and robotically assisted right chest approaches. In our practice, standard median sternotomy is indicated when concomitant procedures (e.g. coronary artery bypass grafting, aortic valve replacement) are necessary. Most other patients requiring mitral operation, including those with atrial fibrillation (AF), are approached minimally invasively.

Median sternotomy and mitral valve repair: Technical considerations

Before incision, the transesophageal echocardiogram is carefully studied. This is necessary to identify the precise mechanism(s) of MR and to formulate the final operative plan. The heart is exposed through a standard median sternotomy. In selected patients, a limited skin incision (10–12 cm) is employed for improved cosmesis. Cannulation is achieved via the ascending aorta, superior vena cava (right angle cannula), and inferior vena cava. Cardiopulmonary bypass is established, and antegrade and retrograde cardioplegia catheters are placed. The aorta is cross-clamped, and the heart arrested with antegrade and retrograde cardioplegia. Thereafter, retrograde cardioplegia is administered every 15 minutes. The operative field is flooded with CO_2 at 6 l/min. If the left atrium is small or the operation is a reoperation, the mitral valve is accessed via a transseptal incision that is carried onto the dome of the left atrium. In most other cases, the mitral valve is approached by a standard incision in the left atrium; this incision is constructed anterior to the right pulmonary veins and is taken beneath the superior and inferior vena cavae to enhance exposure. A self-retaining retractor with three blades is positioned in the left atrium, exposing the mitral valve. Next, systematic valve examination is undertaken, assessing each segment of the anterior and posterior leaflets, and clearly identifying site(s) of prolapse.

Repair techniques

Recent increased interest in minimally invasive approaches to mitral valve surgery has been complemented by introduction (or reintroduction) of surgical techniques that simplify mitral valve repair. These mitral valve repair techniques help to reduce operative time and can be applied through both minimally invasive and standard sternotomy approaches (Table 7.1). The specific repair technique applied depends primarily upon the site of prolapse. All leaflet and chordal repair techniques are accompanied by an annuloplasty. In

Table 7.1 Repair techniques: Evolution

Site of prolapse	Classic technique	Simplified technique	Alternate technique(s)
Posterior-low risk of systolic anterior motion (SAM)	Quadrangular resection	Triangular resection	Edge-to-edge
Posterior-high risk of SAM	Sliding repair	Folding repair	Edge-to-edge
Posterior-extensive resection	Sliding repair	Artificial chordae	
Anterior	Chordal transfer	Artificial chordae	Edge-to-edge
Commissure	Leaflet resection or chordal transfer	Commissuroplasty	
Bileaflet-posterior predominant	Sliding repair ± anterior leaflet procedure	Triangular resection, large annuloplasty	Edge-to-edge
Bileaflet-balanced, no flail	Sliding repair ± anterior leaflet procedure	Large annuloplasty alone	Edge-to-edge

patients with degenerative disease, durability does not appear to be strongly influenced by type of prosthetic annuloplasty.[5] Therefore, in such patients, we generally favor a posterior flexible band placed from trigone to trigone. It is technically simpler to use a flexible band than it is to employ a rigid ring. The band is sized according to the surface area of the anterior leaflet.

Posterior prolapse

Approximately 75% of patients with MR caused by degenerative disease have isolated prolapse of the posterior leaflet, most commonly the P2 segment (middle scallop).[5] The classic technique for managing this is quadrangular resection, with or without sliding repair.[1] The sliding repair was developed to reduce the risk of post-repair systolic anterior motion (SAM) in the setting of excessive leaflet tissue and/or a small, hyperdynamic left ventricle.[11] In our clinical practice, we have generally replaced standard quadrangular resection and sliding repair with triangular resection and folding plasty, respectively; these two simplified techniques for correction of posterior leaflet prolapse reduce the number of surgical maneuvers and thereby decrease operative time. When posterior prolapse is extensive or diffuse, we apply artificial chordae without leaflet resection.

Triangular resection

In the patient with segmental posterior leaflet prolapse, MR is caused by lack of coaptation at the site of chordal rupture or elongation. Therefore, it is logical to target the prolapsing free edge of the leaflet when addressing this problem.[12,13] A triangular resection entails resection of the portion of the free edge that prolapses, with incisions in the leaflet

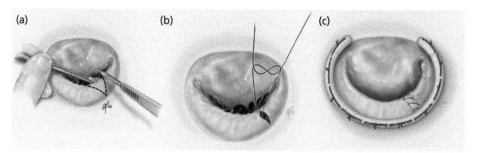

Figure 7.1 Triangular resection. (a) The prolapsing portion of the posterior leaflet is identified and excised as a triangle. (b) The leaflet edges are reapproximated. (c) Annuloplasty completes the repair.
Reprinted with permission, Cleveland Clinic Center for Medical Art & Photography © 2006–2016. All Rights Reserved

angled toward one another as the incision approaches the annular level (Figure 7.1).[12,13] No annular plication sutures are necessary; this simplifies the procedure and reduces the risk of circumflex artery distortion or kinking. After triangular resection, care should be exercised not to use too small an annuloplasty, as this may increase the risk of SAM.[14] We most frequently employ a posterior flexible band of labeled size 34–38 mm.

Folding plasty

The folding plasty is used to treat posterior leaflet prolapse when there is a high risk of SAM, replacing the sliding repair in most of these cases.[15] The prolapsing portion of the posterior leaflet is resected as for a quadrangular resection, leaving tall posterior leaflet remnants on either side (Figure 7.2). A suture is passed through the mid-portion of the cut leaflet edge on each side, and this suture is then passed through the annulus at the mid-portion of the area of resection; this maneuver reduces the posterior leaflet height. If necessary, suture placement is modified to ensure that the leaflet remnants are of similar height. Leaflet tissue is then approximated to the annulus, closing the gap at the annular level, and uniformly reducing the height of the posterior leaflet in this region. The leaflet edges are reapproximated in the middle and an annuloplasty completes the repair.

Artificial chordae

There has been considerable recent interest in the application of artificial expanded poly-tetrafluoroethylene (ePTFE) chordae (Gore-Tex, W.L. Gore and Assoc, Flagstaff, AZ) for correction of posterior leaflet prolapse. We use artificial chordae when there is diffuse posterior leaflet prolapse. If the prolapsing segment is very large, its resection may leave inadequate tissue for restoration of valve competence. In such cases, we create artificial chordae. The needle of an ePTFE suture is passed twice through the tip of a papillary muscle, creating a figure-of-eight stitch. Each of the needles is then passed twice through the free edge of the posterior leaflet, traversing from the ventricular to the atrial aspect each time. In most cases of diffuse prolapse, two sets of chordae are necessary. The ePTFE sutures are left untied, and the annuloplasty is placed. The ventricle is then filled with saline, and the sutures tied at a length that prevents leakage. In general, chordae to the

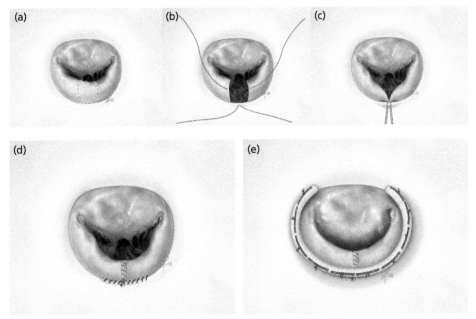

Figure 7.2 Folding plasty. (a) The posterior leaflet is tall. Quadrangular resection of the prolapsing portion is performed. (b) Sutures are passed through the mid-points of the cut leaflet edges and then through the annulus in the region of the defect. (c) Traction on these sutures folds the posterior leaflet toward the annulus, reducing its height. (d) The leaflet edges are sutured to the annulus, each bite reducing the height of the posterior leaflet and the leaflet edges are reapproximated in the middle. (e) Annuloplasty completes the repair.

Reprinted with permission, Cleveland Clinic Center for Medical Art & Photography © 2006–2016. All Rights Reserved

posterior leaflet are quite short, distracting the tip of the leaflet into the ventricle. The posterior leaflet then provides an excellent surface of coaptation for the more mobile anterior leaflet.

Anterior prolapse

Correction of anterior leaflet prolapse is traditionally more challenging than is correction of posterior leaflet prolapse. Classic techniques for management of anterior leaflet prolapse include chordal transfer, which usually requires manipulation of the posterior leaflet; chordal shortening, which is associated with reduced durability; and triangular resection.[16] Management of anterior prolapse by creation of artificial chordae or the edge-to-edge repair simplifies the procedure.

Artificial chordae

As for posterior prolapse, artificial chordae used to treat anterior prolapse are constructed of ePTFE. The key challenge with application of artificial chordae for anterior prolapse is determination of chordal length, and there are many techniques for estimating chordal length.[17,18] We generally create artificial chordae to the anterior leaflet using the same technique

(a) (b)

(c) (d)

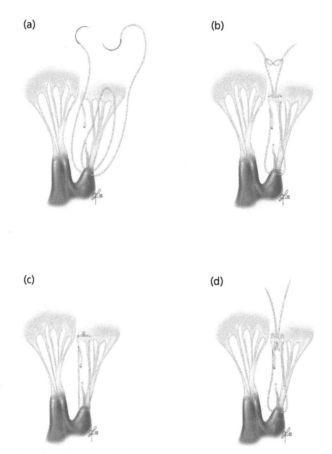

Figure 7.3 Creation of artificial chordae. (a) A figure-of-eight suture is passed through the tip of the papillary muscle. (b) Each needle is passed twice through the free edge of the unsupported leaflet. (c) After placing the annuloplasty and insufflating the ventricle, the ePTFE sutures are adjusted until the valve does not leak. The sutures are then tied at this length on the atrial aspect of the leaflet. (d) Completed chordae; each suture creates two chordae. In most instances, one or two sets of chordae are used to support the anterior leaflet.

described earlier for posterior leaflet prolapse (Figure 7.3). The ePTFE suture is affixed to a papillary muscle as a figure-of-eight stitch. Care is taken not to entrap other, normal chordae in this suture. Each needle is passed twice through the free edge of the prolapsing anterior leaflet. The annuloplasty is placed and then the ventricle insufflated with saline. The chordae are tied at a length that ensures valve competence. Great care must be exercised to ensure that chordae to the anterior leaflet are not too short; this is the most common error.

Alternatively, a caliper may be used for direct measurement and construction of chordal loops, as described by Von Uppell and Mohr.[17] With this technique, the caliper is used to measure the length of a normal chord or, if there is no reference chord, the distance from the papillary muscle head to the annulus. Chordal loops of this length are constructed

(a)

(b)

(c)

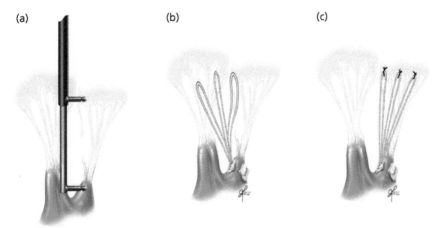

Figure 7.4 Creation of pre-measured artificial chordae. (a) A caliper is used to measure a normal chord to the anterior leaflet. The caliper is then locked. (b) A group of chordal loops is fashioned from a single stitch by tying the loops around the caliper, locking each loop to ensure that its length is constant. (c) The set of chordal loops is affixed to a papillary muscle using pledgets, and the loops are attached to the unsupported free edge of the anterior leaflet.

and affixed to a papillary muscle; for repair of anterior prolapse, the length is most commonly 22–24 mm. Finally, the loops are affixed to the free edge of the prolapsing leaflet with a Gore-Tex suture (Figure 7.4). This technique may also be applied for correction of posterior leaflet prolapse, in which case the chordae are generally 12–14 mm in length.[19]

Edge-to-edge repair

Described by Alfieri and coworkers, the edge-to-edge repair is the simplest maneuver for correction of prolapse.[20] With this technique, the prolapsing segment of the anterior leaflet is sutured to normal posterior leaflet directly opposite, ensuring coaptation and preventing prolapse. Sutures are taken several millimeters deep into the leaflet and span the entire region of prolapse. The stitch should normally not exceed 1 cm in length. Of note, the edge-to-edge technique can also be employed to manage posterior prolapse and bileaflet prolapse; however, it is rarely our primary repair technique.

Commissural prolapse

Commissuroplasty is a simple and reproducible solution for management of commissural prolapse involving the anterior leaflet, posterior leaflet, or both leaflets.[21] The edge of the prolapsing segment is sutured to the free edge of the opposite leaflet. A relatively large annuloplasty device is employed to avoid mitral stenosis.

Bileaflet prolapse

Bileaflet prolapse is often a consequence of Barlow's disease. Management of this entity depends upon valve pathology. Nearly all of these patients have excessive leaflet tissue and annular dilatation. In selected patients with symmetric bileaflet prolapse, a central jet of MR, and no flail, repair can frequently be accomplished by insertion of a large annuloplasty device alone (typically labeled size 36 or greater); this reduces annular diameter and increases leaflet coaptation. In many patients with bileaflet prolapse, prolapse is asymmetric, and the predominant lesion is prolapse of the middle scallop of the posterior leaflet, producing an anteriorly directed jet of MR. In such cases, mitral valve repair is most often achieved by resection of the middle scallop of the posterior leaflet (folding repair, sliding repair, or triangular resection, depending upon leaflet height and extent of resection). A relatively large annuloplasty is applied in order to reduce the risk of SAM. In patients with severe bileaflet prolapse and obvious pathology of chordae to both leaflets, it is necessary to perform repair of both the anterior and posterior leaflets. This generally necessitates a combination of repair techniques, frequently incorporating resection and sliding repair for the posterior leaflet, artificial chordae for the anterior leaflet, and annuloplasty to increase leaflet coaptation.

Special situations

Annular calcium

Mitral annular calcification complicates mitral valve repair.[22] The calcium tends to be along the posterior annulus. If the valve is to be repaired, it is nearly always necessary to remove the calcium. In most cases, the primary problem is posterior leaflet prolapse. The posterior leaflet is detached from the annulus as for a sliding repair, and the prolapsing segment is resected. The annular calcium is then removed. Although the calcium occasionally comes out as a single bar, the more common situation is that the calcium is resected piecemeal. Great care must be taken not to allow calcium to fall into the ventricle or atrium. If the resection has been particularly deep or extensive, an autologous pericardial patch is sewn to the ventricle and the atrium, excluding the area of resection and preventing rupture of the atrioventricular groove. The posterior leaflet tissue is then reattached to the annulus (or pericardial patch) and an annuloplasty is placed.

Atrial fibrillation

In patients with AF, surgical ablation is performed before the mitral valve procedure. We favor a biatrial lesion set in most patients, replicating the lesions of the classic Maze III procedure with alternate energy sources. In the left atrium, this includes a pulmonary vein encircling lesion and connecting lesions to the mitral annulus and to the left atrial appendage. A cryolesion is created on the epicardial aspect of the coronary sinus, corresponding to the endocardial connection to the mitral annulus. The left atrial appendage is excised, or, in a reoperative setting, oversewn from inside the left atrium. Right atrial lesions include incisions in the body of the right atrium and the right atrial appendage, with connecting lesions to the tricuspid annulus and a lesion from the superior vena cava to the inferior vena cava.

The only instance in which we would perform pulmonary vein isolation alone is in the patient with recent onset paroxysmal AF and normal left atrial size.

Recommendations

When faced with the need for mitral valve surgery, patients tend to focus on (1) valve repair (*vs*. replacement) and (2) minimally invasive approaches. It is the surgeon's responsibility to deliver the highest probability of repair with the safest approach. While minimally invasive procedures are certainly desirable, patient characteristics, as already outlined, may dictate a sternotomy as the approach of choice. Less invasive approaches should be considered only after the surgeon has mastered standard repair techniques via sternotomy.

References

1. Braunberger E, Deloche A, Berrebi A, *et al*. (2001). Very long-term results (more than 20 years) of valve repair with Carpentier's techniques in nonrheumatic mitral valve insufficiency. *Circulation*, **104**, I8–11.
2. Mohty D, Orszulak TA, Schaff HV, *et al*. (2001). Very long-term survival and durability of mitral valve repair for mitral valve prolapse. *Circulation*, **104**, I1–7.
3. Shuhaiber J, Anderson RJ (2007). Meta-analysis of clinical outcomes following surgical mitral valve repair or replacement. *Eur J Cardio-Thorac Surg*, **31**, 267–75.
4. Gillinov AM, Blackstone EH, Nowicki ER, *et al*. (2008). Valve repair versus valve replacement for degenerative mitral valve disease. *J Thorac Cardiovasc Surg*, **135**, 885–93.
5. Gillinov AM, Cosgrove DM, Blackstone EH, *et al*. (1998). Durability of mitral valve repair for degenerative disease. *J Thorac Cardiovasc Surg*, **116**, 734–43.
6. David TE, Ivanov J, Armstrong S, Rakowski H (2003). Late outcomes of mitral valve repair for floppy valves: implications for asymptomatic patients. *J Thorac Cardiovasc Surg*, **125**, 1143–52.
7. David TE, Ivanov J, Armstrong S, Christie D, Rakowski H (2005). A comparison of outcomes of mitral valve repair for degenerative disease with posterior, anterior, and bileaflet prolapse. *J Thorac Cardiovasc Surg*, **130**, 1242–9.
8. Flameng W, Herijgers P, Bogaers K (2003). Recurrence of mitral valve regurgitation after mitral valve repair in degenerative valve disease. *Circulation*, **107**, 1609–13.
9. Johnston DR, Gillinov AM, Blackston EH, *et al*. (2010). Surgical repair of posterior mitral valve prolapse: implications for guidelines and percutaneous repair. *Ann Thorac Surg*, **89**, 1385–94.
10. Gillinov AM, Blackstone EH, Abdulrahman A, *et al*. (2008). Outcomes after repair of the anterior mitral leaflet for degenerative disease. *Ann Thorac Surg*, **86**, 708–17.
11. Gillinov AM (1999). Cosgrove DM III. Modified sliding leaflet technique for repair of the mitral valve. *Ann Thorac Surg*, **68**, 2356–7.
12. Suri RM, Orszulak TA (2005). Triangular resection for repair of mitral regurgitation due to degenerative disease. *Oper Techniq Thorac Cardiovasc Surg*, **10**, 194–9.
13. Gazoni LM, Fedoruk LM, Kern JA, *et al*. (2007). A simplified approach to degenerative disease: triangular resections of the mitral valve. *Ann Thorac Surg*, **83**, 1658–65.
14. Brown ML, Abel MD, Click RL, *et al*. (2007). Systolic anterior motion after mitral valve repair: is surgical intervention necessary? *J Thorac Cardiovasc Surg*, **133**, 136–43.
15. Calafiore AM, Di Mauro M, Iaco AL, *et al*. (2006). Overreduction of the posterior annulus in surgical treatment of degenerative mitral regurgitation. *Ann Thorac Surg*, **81**, 1310–6.

16. **Gillinov AM, Cosgrove DM III** (2004). Chordal transfer for repair of anterior leaflet prolapse. *Semin Thorac Cardiovasc Surg*, **16**, 169–73.

17. **Von Oppel UO, Mohr FW** (2000). Chordal replacement for both minimally invasive and conventional mitral valve surgery using premeasured Gore-Tex loops. *Ann Thorac Surg*, **70**, 2166–8.

18. **Gillinov AM, Banbury MK** (2007). Pre-measured artificial chordae for mitral valve repair. *Ann Thorac Surg*, **84**, 2127–9.

19. **Falk V, Seeburger J, Czesla M,** *et al.* (2008). How does the use of polytetrafluoroethylene neochordae for posterior mitral valve prolapse (loop technique) compare with leaflet resection? A prospective randomized trial. *J Thorac Cardiovasc Surg*, **136**, 1200–6.

20. **Lapenna E, Torracca L, De Bonis M, La Canna G, Crescenzi G, Alferi O** (2005). Minimally invasive mitral valve repair in the context of Barlow's disease. *Ann Thorac Surg*, **79**, 1496–9.

21. **Gillinov AM, Shortt KG, Cosgrove DM III** (2005). Commissural closure for repair of mitral commissural prolapse. *Ann Thorac Surg*, **80**, 1135–6.

22. **Bichell DP, Adams DH, Aranki SF, Rizzo RJ, Cohn LH** (1995). Repair of mitral regurgitation from Myxomatous degeneration in the patient with a severely calcified posterior annulus. *J Card Surg*, **10**, 281–4.

Chapter 8

Minimally invasive mitral valve repair

Evelio Rodriguez and W. Randolph Chitwood, Jr

History

In 1996 Cosgrove and Cohn demonstrated that either a parasternal incision or a partial sternotomy could be used to perform MV operations safely.[1-3] Carpentier first used videoscopic assistance and cold ventricular fibrillation to repair a mitral valve (MV) via a right mini-thoracotomy.[4] Shortly thereafter, Mohr and Chitwood reported independently their experiences with minimally invasive mitral valve surgery (MIMVS) at their respective institutions.[5-7] Since then, the logical trend has moved toward less invasive techniques using robotic assistance. Initially, the main robotic component was the AESOP 3000 voice-activated camera manipulator[8] and more recently the da Vinci™ Surgical System (Intuitive Surgical, Sunnyvale, CA). The use of the Zeus robotic system was short lived with only a few MV cases performed.[9,10]

In 1999 Carpentier reported the first MV operation using true robotic assistance.[11] In May 2000, our center performed the first da Vinci™ robotic-assisted MV repair in the United States, which consisted of a leaflet resection with a repair and a band annuloplasty. Since then many international centers have establish different levels of MIMVS program sophistication but few have used the da Vinci™ robotic-assisted approach consistently. Recently, Gammie *et al.* reviewed less invasive MV operative trends in the United States.[12] They identified 28,143 patients, archived in the Society of Thoracic Surgeons (STS) Adult Surgical Database that had undergone an isolated MV operation between 2004 and 2008. During that period, adoption of MIMVS increased from 12% to 20%, with 35% of the latter having been performed using robotic techniques. These data demonstrate that cardiac surgeons are increasingly embracing MIMVS techniques, and this trend has been mirrored in many international centers. Nevertheless, adoption of a MIMVS strategy has been much slower than that in other surgical disciplines. It is not surprising that robotic cardiac surgery, and especially MIMVS, would have a significant penetration phase lag, as the complexity is much greater than in extirpative operations.

Outcomes

Cardiac surgeons have moved toward less invasive MV surgery as these operations result in less morbidity than traditional sternotomy operations. Less invasive approaches often result in faster recovery, shorter hospitalizations, and more rapid return to normal activities and productivity, compared to patients undergoing a full sternotomy. Although several reports have addressed these issues, sufficient statistical power has not been present to accurately compare MIMVS to sternotomy-based MV surgery in a prospective randomized manner. Thus, definitive evidence has not arisen to support many surgeons' belief that MIMVS is superior, or at least equivalent to traditional MV surgery. Despite our desire to prove superiority, patients and referring physicians now consider MIMVS very beneficial and, therefore, prefer not to participate in randomized trials. To this end, we are forced to rely on large published series for direction, knowing that many have limitations. Moreover, it is important for surgeons adopting MIMVS to keep detailed databases so that they can provide accurate information to their patients.

Different reports have demonstrated that MIMVS is associated with decreased bleeding, transfusions, and re-explorations for bleeding when compared to traditional approaches.[5,13–15] Moreover, these studies suggest that patients have less wound infections,[13,16] better pain control,[17] improved quality of life,[18,19] shorter hospitalizations,[20] and faster return to normal activities.[5] In addition, most patients are very satisfied with the cosmetic results associated with a right mini-thoracotomy incision.[21] At the same time, however, MIMVS has been associated with longer cardiopulmonary and cross-clamp times, as well a slight increase in perioperative strokes.

Recently, Modi *et al.* published a meta-analysis of many MIMVS publications.[22] They identified 43 reports, of which two were from randomized trials, 17 were from case control studies, and 24 from were cohort studies. Of 2,827 cohort patients, 1,358 were in the MIMVS group and 1,469 were in the sternotomy group. The operative mortality was equivalent. The MIMVS cohort had less bleeding, and there was a trend toward shorter hospitalizations. These benefits were demonstrated despite longer cardiopulmonary perfusion and cardiac arrest times. Moreover, these studies consistently showed that after both primary MIMVS and reoperations, patients had less pain and had a more rapid recovery.

Cohn *et al.* published a comprehensive review that analyzed the recent MIMVS literature.[23] He concluded that in both approaches mortality and valve quality were similar. However, in MIMVS, femoral perfusion may potentially cause complications. Moreover, cardiopulmonary and cross-clamp times are longer, despite the learning curve improvements even in high volume centers. Interestingly, when compared to patients having a full sternotomy, MIMVS was shown to be safer for obese patients[24] and equal in safety for patients over 70 years old.[25] Prior publications also showed beneficial MIMVS outcomes for older patients (>70 years) when compared to traditional mitral operations.[26,27]

Today, the da Vinci™ robotic system facilitates the least invasive MV operations with the best visualization and instrument ergonomics. Surgeon adoption is increasing steadily and several centers in the United States now have reported excellent results. To date, at the *East Carolina Heart Institute*, we have performed over 650 robotic MV repairs, either singularly or in combination with other cardiac procedures. Between May of 2000 and January of 2010, 530 patients with either moderately severe or severe preoperative mitral insufficiency had an isolated robotic MV repair. Specific repair techniques included: (1) leaflet resection with an annuloplasty (LRA); (2) a LRA plus a sliding-plasty and/or chordal procedure (CP); (3) a CP with an annuloplasty; (4) a LRA with CP; and (5) an annuloplasty alone (N = 99, 18.4%; N = 130, 24.5%; N = 64, 12.1%; N = 144, 27.0%, N = 58, 11.2%, respectively). Other techniques were used in 34 (6.6%) patients. Every patient had an annuloplasty band implanted. The mean age was 57.2 ± 0.9 years (mean ± SEM) and 329 (62.1%) were men. Cardiopulmonary bypass, cross-clamp, and total robot repair times were 162.0 ± 2.3, 126.0 ± 3.0 and 90.0 ± 2.0 minutes, respectively. For the group, the mean operating room time was 285.5 ± 3.0 minutes. The overall mortality was 1.5% (N = 8) and average length of hospitalization was 4.8 ± 0.2 days. Complex repairs were done in 82% of patients, and 96.5% had either mild or less MR by follow-up transesophageal echocardiography.[28]

Other recent publications also have suggested that robotic MV surgery is safe and efficacious. Murphy et al. reported 127 robotic mitral operations, in which five patients were converted to a median sternotomy and one had a thoracotomy. Seven patients had prosthetic replacements and 114 had a repair [29]. There was one in-hospital death, one late death, two strokes, and 22 patients developed new postoperative atrial fibrillation. Blood product transfusions were required in 31% with re-explorations for bleeding in two patients (1.7%). Post-discharge echocardiograms were available in 98 patients with no more than mild residual MR in 96.2% at a mean follow-up of 8.4 months.

Chitwood et al. reported results from their first 300 robotic MV repairs that were operated upon between May 2000 and November 2006. This series was strengthened by 100% patient follow-up and interval echocardiographic studies in 93%.[30] Overall there were two (0.7%) early deaths (30 days), six (2.0%) late mortalities, and no conversions to a sternotomy. Immediate post-repair transesophageal echo studies revealed the following levels of mitral regurgitation: none/trivial, 294 (98%); mild, three (1.0%); moderate, three (1.0%); and severe, 0 (0.0%). Operative complications included two (0.7%) strokes, two transient ischemic attacks, three (1.0%) myocardial infarctions, and seven (2.3%) reoperations for bleeding. The mean hospital length of stay was 5.2 +/- 4.2 (+/-SD) days. Sixteen (5.3%) patients required a reoperation for recurrent MV regurgitation. Interval follow-up transthoracic echocardiograms showed the following amounts of mitral insufficiency: none/trivial, 192 (68.8%); mild, 66 (23.6%); moderate, 15 (5.4%); and severe, six (2.2%).

Mihaljevic et al. reported outcomes from 759 patients who had a posterior leaflet mitral repair at the Cleveland Clinic between 2006 and 2009.[31] They compared patients having a complete sternotomy (n = 114), a partial sternotomy (n = 270), a right mini-thoracotomy (n = 114), or a right mini-thoracotomy with robot assistance (n = 261). There were no in-hospital deaths and both cardiopulmonary bypass and cardiac arrest times were longest in the robotic group and shortest in the sternotomy group. There were no group differences in quality of the mitral repairs. The robotic group had the lowest occurrence of postoperative atrial fibrillation and the shortest hospitalization (median 4.2 days). Neurological, pulmonary, and renal complications were similar between groups. Folliguet et al. compared robot-assisted MV repair patients to a matched sternotomy cohort (N = 25 each group). The robotic group had a shorter hospital stay (7 days *vs.* 9 days, $P = 0.05$) with no other differences between groups.[32] Lastly, Woo et al. showed in a non-randomized single surgeon experience that robotic surgery patients had a significant reduction in blood transfusions and hospitalization compared to their sternotomy patients.[15]

In summary, the outcomes reported for MIMVS have been excellent and in many ways appear to be better that those for conventional sternotomy surgery. Our series and those of others suggest that results from robot-assisted mitral repairs are as good as those performed via sternotomy and are associated with less transfusions, rapid recovery, and better cosmetic effects. We believe that patient selection and preoperative vascular screening will decrease the number of perioperative strokes, as peripheral cannulation with retrograde perfusion may be responsible for some of these events. We believe that both central and axillary cannulation continue to be the best perfusion routes for higher-risk patients (older, previous strokes, and significant peripheral and/or aortic vascular disease). Lastly, completed learning curves for operating surgeons and surgical teams, as well as higher patient volumes, will foist robotic programs toward excellent outcomes in these patients. At the same time, other MIMVS methods provide patients with most of the modern benefits of a less invasive operation. No doubt evolving technology in preoperative planning, echocardiographic modeling, instrumentation, and perfusion will bring surgeons asymptotic to "non-invasive" mitral repairs having structural perfection.

Operative approach: MIMVS

Patient selection

For our early mini-thoracotomy video-assisted (1996) and da Vinci™ robot-assisted (2000) mitral valve operations, patient selection criteria were very stringent. However, after subsequent experience, the exclusion criteria for isolated MV and/or atrial fibrillation operations have been modified to include: (1) a previous right thoracotomy; (2) significant pulmonary dysfunction and/or severe pulmonary hypertension; and (3) a highly calcified mitral annulus. Some of our earlier contraindications, such as older patients and reoperations, have been abandoned as we have determined that MIMVS often provides better outcomes in the circumstances than a conventional sternotomy.

Preoperative planning

Today, patient evaluations are similar to standard ones for those undergoing sternotomy MV surgery. However, a major evaluation criterion is related to cannulation and perfusion strategies for individual patients. Computed tomography (CT) scanning and/or MRI studies best evaluate the descending aorta and peripheral vasculature. As endoballoon aortic occlusion with retrograde perfusion may be dangerous in the presence of mobile aortic atheroma and/or diseased ileo-femoral arteries, preoperative imaging is essential in suspect patients.[33]

Intraoperative transesophageal echocardiography (TEE) now has become standard for planning of any MV repair. Over the past few years we have relied on intraoperative 3D-TEE to determine detailed valve and annular structure and pathology. This modality has enhanced our planning of all MV repairs. By TEE we always measure P_1, P_2, and P_3 leaflet scallop lengths as well as that of the anterior leaflet. We also define the location and direction of all regurgitant jets to determine which MV segments needs a repair. Also, ideal post-repair leaflet lengths that will provide optimal coaptation can be predicted. In addition, preoperative topographic MV models can be synthesized and help us define leaflet regions that need reconstruction. Recently, we have paired this precise imaging with simple repair techniques. By defining precisely abnormal leaflet coaptation sites from dynamic echo studies, surgeons have been able to abandon many complex repair techniques of the past. Simplified techniques now include limited triangular and posterior leaflet "haircut" resections,[34] the "American Correction,"[35] folding plasties, and chordal replacements with polytetrafluoroethylene (PTFE) neochords.[36]

Anesthesia and patient position

After positioning the patient supine, intubation is performed using a double lumen endotracheal tube. Alternatively, a single lumen tube with a bronchial blocker can be used to deflate the right lung. Thereafter, the TEE probe is passed to the level of the left atrium. For superior vena caval drainage a 15 or 17 Fr thin-walled Bio-Medicus cannula (Medtronic, Minneapolis, MN) is passed into the right internal jugular vein via the Seldinger technique and under TEE guidance. Thereafter, a Swan-Ganz pulmonary artery catheter is inserted either into the subclavian or internal jugular vein (using a "double-puncture" method) (Figure 8.1). To monitor adequate limb perfusion during cardiopulmonary perfusion, oxygen saturation sensors are placed on each leg and levels measured using the

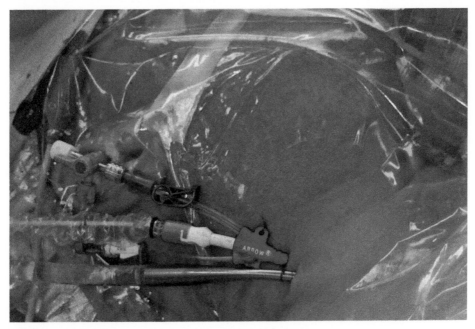

Figure 8.1 Neck cannulation using double-puncture technique.
SGC, Swan-Ganz catheter.

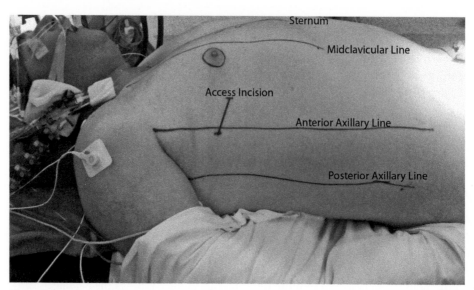

Figure 8.2 Patient positioning.

Invos® System (Somanetics Inc., Troy, MI). When arterial oxygen saturations fall significantly in the cannulated leg, we pass either a 5 Fr catheter or 14-gauge angiocatheter over a guidewire into the distal femoral artery. Thereafter, it is attached to an arterial shunt that originates from the perfusion circuit. For the remainder of the operation, patients are rotated into a semi-left lateral decubitus position (30°) as shown in Figure 8.2.

Cardiopulmonary perfusion and myocardial protection

Typically, the right femoral artery and vein are used for peripheral cannulation. To facilitate arterial cannulation, diagnostic catheterizations should be performed via the left femoral artery. A 2-cm oblique incision is made over the femoral vessels. To minimize lymphocele formation, only the anterior vessel surface is exposed after minimal dissection. Adventitial purse-string sutures (4-0 Prolene, Johnson & Johnson, Piscataway, NJ) are placed in each vessel near the inguinal ligament. After adequate heparinization, 17–19 Fr arterial and 21 Fr venous Bio-Medicus cannulas (Medtronic, Minneapolis, MN) are positioned using the guidewire technique under TEE guidance. In corpulent patients, cannulas can be tunneled through the subcutaneous tissue to allow vessel entrance at a 45° angle. If the angle is too acute, entry is difficult and the potential for vessel disruption or dissection of the posterior wall is increased. After appropriate positioning of the cannulas, cardiopulmonary perfusion can be instituted. For patients with severe peripheral vascular disease, either axillary arterial or direct ascending aortic cannulation (second intercostal space) should be used to maintain antegrade perfusion. For axillary cannulation, a 10-mm woven graft is anastomosed to the artery using a 5-0 Prolene suture (Figure 8.3). For cardiac protection, cold blood cardioplegia is infused into the ascending aorta every 15 minutes through a long dual-lumen cardioplegia/root vent catheter. This is

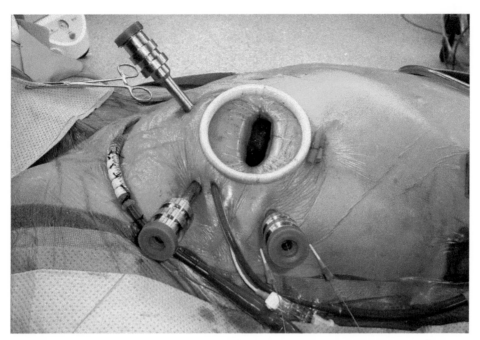

Figure 8.3 Axillary artery cannulation set-up and port placement.

positioned in the proximal ascending aorta through the access incision and secured with a pledgeted 4-0 PTFE suture.

For cardiac arrest, we most often use the Chitwood transthoracic aortic cross-clamp (Scanlan International, Minneapolis, MN). This clamp is passed into the thorax through a small second intercostal space incision placed near the posterior axillary line. The posterior tine of the clamp is passed through the transverse sinus and behind the aorta. Care must be taken to avoid injury to the right pulmonary artery, the left atrial appendage, or left main coronary artery. Alternatively, the balloon Endoclamp™ system can be used (Edwards Lifesciences, Irvine, CA). This device obviates the need for placement of an aortic cardioplegia catheter and avoids conflicts between a transverse sinus cross-clamp and robot left instrument arms. This method is a very good option for reoperations. It avoids the need for aortic exposure and possible injury to pre-existing bypass grafts. However, it is an expensive technology and requires detailed vascular CT/MRI imaging prior to surgery. For retrograde administration of cardioplegia, a percutaneous EndoPlege™ coronary sinus catheter (Edwards Lifesciences, Irvine, CA) can be inserted via the internal jugular vein.

Incision and port placement

Our standard MIMVS access is via a 4-cm right mini-incision, placed in the inframammary fold with the chest entered most often through the fourth intercostal space. The right superior pulmonary vein is the landmark for the best intra-atrial access. Thus, chest entrance may need to be higher or lower than the fourth interspace. If in doubt pre-operative imaging will help to establish the best entry point. The pericardium should be opened 3–4 cm anterior to the phrenic nerve after beginning cardiopulmonary bypass (CPB). Transthoracic traction sutures are placed through the pericardial edges under tension to distract the heart toward the incision. Care must be taken not to stretch the phrenic nerve with this maneuver. The interatrial groove does not have to be developed as much as in conventional sternotomy mitral surgery. However, fat surrounding both pulmonary veins should be displaced medially to reveal the left atrial margin. To displace intercardiac air, 14-gauge transthoracic angiocath is inserted for continuous CO_2 thoracic insufflation.

The planning of non-robot-assisted MIMVS is very similar to our robotic operation. However, for da Vinci™ robotic operations, the instrument arms are deployed through ports placed in the second and fifth interspaces most frequently. The HD-3D endoscope can be placed either through the access incision, or through a separate port placed in the same interspace as the access incision. For left atrial retractor deployment, a fourth port should be introduced at a point over the right pulmonary veins in the third intercostal space (Figure 8.4).

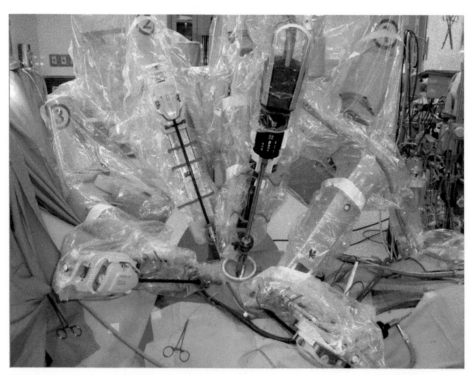

Figure 8.4 Da Vinci™ robotic surgical system deployed.

Mitral operation

Using either long-shafted or da Vinci™ robotic instruments, mitral operations are performed using similar techniques as traditional operations. However, suture placement and management are different and new skills to manage these issues must be acquired. Repair techniques have been simplified as already described here. The use of PTFE neochords and limited leaflet resections has both facilitated and made MIMVS more reproducible. After incomplete left atriotomy closure, limiting pump venous return while ventilating both lungs expels air. The atrial closure is completed as the last air is removed. With aortic root vent maintained on suction and the right coronary origin compressed, the cross-clamp is removed. Some prefer to leave a left ventricular vent across the MV until all cardiac air absence is confirmed by TEE. Before weaning from CPB, a temporary bipolar right ventricular pacing wire should be placed on the diaphragmatic surface of the heart. After separation from CPB, a complete TEE study should be done to evaluate prosthetic implantation and/or repair integrity. We routinely return to CPB to remove the aortic root vent and secure the purse-string suture. Once satisfied both with the operative result and hemodynamic stability, protamine is given and is followed by cannula removal. Two small chest tubes are placed through port incisions, and the access incision closed.

References

1. Gillinov AM, Cosgrove DM (1999). Minimally invasive mitral valve surgery: mini-sternotomy with extended transseptal approach. *Semin Thorac Cardiovasc Surg*, **11**, 206–11.

2. Cohn LH, Adams DH, Couper GS, *et al.* (1997). Minimally invasive cardiac valve surgery improves patient satisfaction while reducing costs of cardiac valve replacement and repair. *Ann Surg*, **226**, 421–6; discussion 7–8.

3. Navia JL, Cosgrove DM 3rd (1996). Minimally invasive mitral valve operations. *Ann Thorac Surg*, **62**, 1542–4.

4. Carpentier A, Loulmet D, Le Bret E, *et al.* (1996). [Open heart operation under videosurgery and minithoracotomy. First case (mitral valvuloplasty) operated with success]. *C R Acad Sci III*, **319**, 219–23.

5. Chitwood WR Jr, Elbeery JR, Chapman WH, *et al.* (1997). Video-assisted minimally invasive mitral valve surgery: the "micro-mitral" operation. *J Thorac Cardiovasc Surg*, **113**, 413–4.

6. Chitwood WR Jr, Elbeery JR, Moran JF (1997). Minimally invasive mitral valve repair using transthoracic aortic occlusion. *Ann Thorac Surg*, **63**, 1477–9.

7. Mohr FW, Falk V, Diegeler A, *et al.* (1998). Minimally invasive port-access mitral valve surgery. *J Thorac Cardiovasc Surg*, **115**, 567–74; discussion 74–6.

8. Mohr FW, Falk V, Diegeler A, *et al.* (2001). Computer-enhanced "robotic" cardiac surgery: experience in 148 patients. *J Thorac Cardiovasc Surg*, **121**, 842–53.

9. Boehm DH, Detter C, Arnold MB, Deuse T, Reichenspurner H (2003). Robotically assisted coronary artery bypass surgery with the ZEUS telemanipulator system. *Semin Thorac Cardiovasc Surg*, **15**, 112–20.

10. Sawa Y, Monta O, Matsuda H (2004). [Use of the Zeus robotic surgical system for cardiac surgery]. *Nippon Geka Gakkai Zasshi*, **105**, 726–31.

11. **Carpentier A, Loulmet D, Aupecle B,** *et al.* (1998). [Computer-assisted open heart surgery. First case operated on with success]. *C R Acad Sci III*, **321**, 437–42.

12. **Gammie JS, Zhao Y, Peterson ED,** *et al.* (2010). J. Maxwell Chamberlain Memorial Paper for adult cardiac surgery. Less-invasive mitral valve operations: trends and outcomes from the Society of Thoracic Surgeons Adult Cardiac Surgery Database. *Ann Thorac Surg*, **90**, 1401–8, 10.e1; discussion 8–10.

13. **Grossi EA, Galloway AC, Ribakove GH,** *et al.* (2001). Impact of minimally invasive valvular heart surgery: a case-control study. *Ann Thorac Surg*, **71**, 807–10.

14. **Dogan S, Aybek T, Risteski PS,** *et al.* (2005). Minimally invasive port access versus conventional mitral valve surgery: prospective randomized study. *Ann Thorac Surg*, **79**, 492–8.

15. **Woo YJ, Nacke EA** (2006). Robotic minimally invasive mitral valve reconstruction yields less blood product transfusion and shorter length of stay. *Surgery*, **140**, 263–7.

16. **Grossi EA, LaPietra A, Ribakove GH,** *et al.* (2001). Minimally invasive versus sternotomy approaches for mitral reconstruction: comparison of intermediate-term results. *J Thorac Cardiovasc Surg*, **121**, 708–13.

17. **Felger JE, Nifong LW, Chitwood WR Jr** (2002). The evolution of and early experience with robot-assisted mitral valve surgery. *Surg Laparosc Endosc Percutan Tech*, **12**, 58–63.

18. **Yamada T, Ochiai R, Takeda J, Shin H, Yozu R** (2003). Comparison of early postoperative quality of life in minimally invasive versus conventional valve surgery. *J Anesth*, **17**, 171–6.

19. **Walther T, Falk V, Metz S,** *et al.* (1999). Pain and quality of life after minimally invasive versus conventional cardiac surgery. *Ann Thorac Surg*, **67**, 1643–7.

20. **Mihaljevic T, Cohn LH, Unic D,** *et al.* (2004). One thousand minimally invasive valve operations: early and late results. *Ann Surg*, **240**, 529–34; discussion 34.

21. **Casselman FP, Van Slycke S, Wellens F,** *et al.* (2003). Mitral valve surgery can now routinely be performed endoscopically. *Circulation*, **108**(Suppl 1), II48–54.

22. **Modi P, Hassan A, Chitwood WR Jr** (2008). Minimally invasive mitral valve surgery: a systematic review and meta-analysis. *Eur J Cardiothorac Surg*, **34**, 943–52.

23. **Schmitto JD, Mokashi SA, Cohn LH** (2010). Minimally-invasive valve surgery. *J Am Coll Cardiol*, **56**, 455–62.

24. **Santana O, Reyna J, Grana R,** *et al.* (2011). Outcomes of minimally invasive valve surgery versus standard sternotomy in obese patients undergoing isolated valve surgery. *Ann Thorac Surg*, **91**, 406–10.

25. **Holzhey DM, Shi W, Borger MA,** *et al.* (2011). Minimally invasive versus sternotomy approach for mitral valve surgery in patients greater than 70 years old: a propensity-matched comparison. *Ann Thorac Surg*, **91**, 401–5.

26. **Grossi EA, Galloway AC, Ribakove GH,** *et al.* (1999). Minimally invasive port access surgery reduces operative morbidity for valve replacement in the elderly. *Heart Surg Forum*, **2**, 212–5.

27. **Tabata M, Cohn LH** (2006). Minimally invasive mitral valve repair with and without robotic technology in the elderly. *Am J Geriatr Cardiol*, **15**, 306–10.

28. **Nifong LW, Rodriguez E, Chitwood WR** (2012). 540 consecutive robotic mitral valve repairs including concomitant atrial fibrillation cryoablation. *Ann Thorac Surg*, **94**(1), 38–42; discussion 43.

29. **Murphy DA, Miller JS, Langford DA, Snyder AB** (2006). Endoscopic robotic mitral valve surgery. *J Thorac Cardiovasc Surg*, **132**, 776–81.

30. **Chitwood WR, Jr., Rodriguez E, Chu MW,** *et al.* (2008). Robotic mitral valve repairs in 300 patients: a single-center experience. *J Thorac Cardiovasc Surg*, **136**, 436–41.

31. **Mihaljevic T, Jarrett CM, Gillinov AM,** *et al.* (2011). Robotic repair of posterior mitral valve prolapse versus conventional approaches: potential realized. *J Thorac Cardiovasc Surg*, **141**, 72–80. e1–4.

32. **Folliguet T, Vanhuyse F, Constantino X, Realli M, Laborde** F (2006). Mitral valve repair robotic versus sternotomy. *Eur J Cardiothorac Surg*, **29**, 362–6.

33. **Jeanmart H, Casselman FP, De Grieck Y,** *et al.* (2007). Avoiding vascular complications during minimally invasive, totally endoscopic intracardiac surgery. *J Thorac Cardiovasc Surg*, **133**, 1066–70.

34. **Chu MW, Gersch KA, Rodriguez E, Nifong LW, Chitwood WR Jr** (2008). Robotic "haircut" mitral valve repair: posterior leaflet-plasty. *Ann Thorac Surg*, **85**, 1460–2.

35. **Lawrie GM, Earle EA, Earle N** (2011). Intermediate-term results of a nonresectional dynamic repair technique in 662 patients with mitral valve prolapse and mitral regurgitation. *J Thorac Cardiovasc Surg*, **141**, 368–76.

36. **Seeburger J, Kuntze T, Mohr FW** (2007). Gore-tex chordoplasty in degenerative mitral valve repair. *Semin Thorac Cardiovasc Surg*, **19**, 111–5.

Chapter 9

Surgical therapy for heart failure

Stephen Westaby

Introduction

The clinical syndrome of congestive heart failure affects 23 million people worldwide, 5 million in North America and 7 million in Europe. Heart failure is the final pathway for many diseases that affect the myocardium. Successful intervention in acute coronary syndromes, together with improved management of idiopathic dilated cardiomyopathy and dysrhythmia provide an ever-increasing number of advanced heart failure patients spread over a wide age range. Young adults with surgically palliated congenital heart disease enter the lower end of the spectrum. In Western countries coronary artery disease is responsible for about 70% of patients with idiopathic dilated cardiomyopathy and valvular heart disease accounting for 15%.[1] The remainder have hypertension-related restrictive cardiomyopathy. Since 10% of patients older than 65 years suffer systolic left ventricular dysfunction, the numbers with heart failure will double within the next 25 years. The major component of healthcare costs is generated by repeated hospital admissions to escalate medical treatment and palliate intolerable levels of breathlessness and fatigue. This amounts to 2% of the healthcare budget in Western countries.

Ten percent (10%) of heart failure patients are categorized as Stage D (New York Heart Association (NYHA) Class IV) with advanced structural heart disease and marked symptoms at rest despite detailed medical or cardiac resynchronization therapy. The symptoms result from two pathological processes: raised left ventricular end diastolic pressure (LVEDP) results in pulmonary congestion and breathlessness, while decreased systemic blood flow triggers numerous cytokine and humoral responses causing salt and water retention and fatigue. The patients become progressively more dependent on hospital admissions for symptomatic stabilization and outpatient nursing for palliative care. Currently there are more than 300,000 Stage D patients in the USA, 60,000 in the UK, and 2.2 million worldwide. Twenty percent are under 65 years of age. Stage D heart failure carries a grim prognosis. In the CONSENSUS Trial, half of the patients in the control arm had died within 6 months.[2] In the REMATCH study, only 8% of patients in the medically treated group were alive at 2 years.[3]

For end-stage patients, cardiac transplantation provides the benchmark for increased longevity and symptomatic relief. However, the vast majority of Stage D patients are over 65 years of age or are referred with established comorbidity which precludes transplantation. For those patients less than 65 years of age (60,000 in the USA and 12,000 in the UK) there are only around 2,500 and 190 donor hearts per year, respectively. In his paper "The Evolving Challenge of Heart Failure Management" Adamson describes heart transplantation as an "epidemiologically insignificant intervention."[4] Thus in the global context, transplantation is recognized as irrelevant. Accordingly, the development of non-transplant surgical options is a clear priority.

Pathology-based heart failure surgery

Non-transplant surgery is a specialty in itself. The goal of both medical and surgical treatment is to arrest or reverse progression of the adverse cardiac remodeling process. Left ventricular shape and volume are important predictors of survival. In both ischemic and idiopathic-dilated cardiomyopathy, increased chamber sphericity and the onset of mitral regurgitation are markers of worse prognosis (one-year mortality 54–70%).[5] Mitral regurgitation occurs secondary to altered left ventricular geometry, papillary muscle dysfunction, and annular dilatation. Volume overload causes progressive left ventricular dilatation, worsening mitral regurgitation, and decreased survival. Patients with a left ventricular ejection fraction (LVEF) of less than 30% have a 5-year survival of only 54% when left ventricular end systolic volume index (LVESVI) exceeds 150 mL/m². An evidence-based approach to treatment is achieved using detailed investigation to identify the cause of heart failure and the extent of structural and functional abnormalities.[6] The team must then establish whether there is a lesion amenable for surgical repair, whether dysfunctional myocardium is recoverable, or in the event of neither of these, whether complete cardiac replacement or mechanical left ventricular assist are feasible.

It is always preferable to repair rather than replace the diseased heart. All Stage C and D patients should be jointly assessed by a multidisciplinary heart failure team including the surgeon. Significant comorbidity, particularly renal and hepatic status, must be taken into consideration before embarking on a particular procedure. The surgeon's role is to determine which operation or combination of surgical procedures best suits an individual and whether the operation can be undertaken with acceptable risk.

Ischemic cardiomyopathy

The ischemic cardiomyopathy ventricle contains microenvironments of necrosis or scar tissue together with viable myocardial cells in varying proportions.[7] When dyskinetic myocardial scar occupies more than 20% of the total left ventricular mass (as occurs in 40% of transmural myocardial infarctions), the left ventricle progressively enlarges with the onset of symptomatic heart failure. When more than 50% of the myocardium is impaired, increased wall tension causes subendocardial ischemia, which precipitates left ventricular failure. The relationship between the extent of myocardial infarction, degree of left ventricular dysfunction, and late mortality was defined by Yoshida and Gould.[8] They showed that a myocardial infarction more than 23% of left ventricular circumference reduced LVEF less than 45% with a 3-year mortality rate exceeding 40%. This contrasted with less extensive myocardial infarction where 3-year mortality was only 5%. Patients with an LVEF of more than 40% have modest annual mortality rate (<10%) whereas those with an LVEF of more than 30% have annual mortality rates more than 25%. In patients with an LVEF of 15–40%, there is an almost linear relationship between LVEF and annual mortality. However, LVEF alone is a poor predictor of mortality in patients with hibernating myocardium. The presence of viable myocardium is an independent predictor of survival and a marker for those with impaired LVEF who are most likely to benefit from coronary revascularization (CABG). The 3-year mortality rate in patients with an LVEF less than 45% and no viable myocardium was 63%, in contrast to 13% for those revascularized with viable myocardium.

Exercise capacity has a poor relationship with LVEF measured by echocardiography at rest. Stress- or exercise-related myocardial ischemia and stunning often result in left ventricular systolic and diastolic dysfunction, elevated LVEDP, and dyspnea with or without angina. If stunning occurs frequently with incomplete recovery of contractile function, this triggers the development of hibernation. Eventually the myocardium may progress from structurally normal recoverable hibernation to the development of abnormal contractile proteins, where recovery is unlikely after CABG. Some patients have moderately increased LVEDP at rest with considerably reduced exercise capacity but only mildly increased heart size on chest X-ray. These patients often have marked ischemic dysfunction in non-scarred parts of the ventricles, which can be helped by revascularization. Others have moderate or severe cardiomegaly, reduced cardiac index, and substantial elevation of right atrial pressure with hepatomegaly and fluid retention. This latter group usually has extensive myocardial scarring, which will not improve with CABG alone.

Coronary bypass or transplantation?

The vast majority of patients with ischemic cardiomyopathy are older than 65 years, are smokers with chronic obstructive airways disease, and have peripheral vasculopathy. They often have renal impairment and will never be considered for transplantation. In turn, less than 10% of potential heart transplant candidates (referred as opposed to selected for the waiting list) will eventually receive a donor organ. So which patients benefit from CABG as an alternative?

Studies suggest that as many as 50% of ischemic cardiomyopathy patients referred for cardiac transplantation have hibernating myocardium.[9] It is impossible on the basis of echocardiography or coronary angiography alone to determine which areas of myocardium might benefit from improved perfusion. An indication that segmental and global LVEF will improve after CABG is obtained using imaging methods to provide evidence for myocardial viability. These include contrast enhanced MRI and single photon emission tomography (SPECT) with thallium-210 or technicium-99M perfusion tracers.[10] MRI has the benefit of providing very accurate information about left ventricular volume indices, myocardial wall thickness, and mitral valve function. Heart failure patients who benefit from viability testing include those with suspected coronary disease or dilated cardiomyopathy under consideration for cardiac transplantation, and those with coronary disease and left ventricular (LV) dysfunction (LVEF <35%) who are asymptomatic or have breathlessness with only mild angina. Viability testing is redundant in patients with unstable angina, post infarction angina, and severe chronic stable angina because CABG is indicated for symptomatic relief.

For ischemic heart failure patients without angina, the combination of good target vessels and more than 25% myocardial viability suggests the potential to benefit from CABG. For those with less than 25% viability, poor target vessels, or in reoperative candidates CABG is unlikely to produce improvement. Other unfavorable patient characteristics include advanced age, female gender, severity of coronary disease, presence of dysrhythmias, and renal impairment.

Useful information regarding patient selection for high-risk revascularization has emerged from transplant centers where many candidates have been diverted for CABG instead.[11] Transplant recipients tended to have longer duration of symptoms, concomitant right heart failure, and a greater incidence of previous CABG. Operative risk in CABG patients was significantly higher for those with LVEDP more than 24 mmHg, low preoperative cardiac output (<2.0 L/min/m²), and for NYHA IV patients. Hospital mortality was 7.1% for CABG patients versus 18.2% in the transplant cohort. Survival for CABG patients was 79% at 6 years versus 69% for the transplant group. Reinvestigation of CABG patients showed a significant decrease in mean pulmonary artery and left atrial pressures. LVEF improved from a mean of 24% to 39% (P <0.001). Others have reported similar findings.[9] Symptomatic relief, quality of life benefit, and improved survival have been reported in these patients.

The value of viability testing was confirmed by Haas in a series of patients with three vessel disease and LVEF less than 35%.[12] Half were operated on the basis of angiographic findings alone while the remainder underwent viability testing. Patients with hibernating myocardium had lower hospital mortality (0% vs. 11.4%), fewer postoperative complications (33% vs. 67%), and rarely experienced low cardiac output syndrome (3% vs. 17%). One-year survival was better (97 ± 8% vs. 79 ± 8%). The LVEF increased from 26% to 35% in those with myocardial viability but was unchanged in those without. Myocardial viability index was the only independent predictor of event free survival. Though CABG may provide better short-term outcome than transplantation, the benefits may be time limited. Luciani showed only 47% of patients with poor left ventricular function (LVEF <20%) to be free from heart failure symptoms 5 years after CABG despite 75% survival at this time.[13]

Despite symptomatic and survival benefit after CABG, the myocardial functional response is unpredictable. Using detailed studies of regional perfusion and contractility, Bax showed improvement in only 70% of stunned segments and 31% of hibernating segments by 3 months after CABG.[14] Haas used intraoperative myocardial biopsy to investigate the time course of functional recovery in ischemic segments. Positron emission tomography was used to distinguish stunned from hibernating myocardium. Hibernation was associated with more severe depression of contractility and incomplete recovery. Disappointingly by one year after CABG only 31% of stunned and 18% of hibernating segments showed complete functional recovery.[15] Failure to improve was associated with more severe ultra-structural degeneration in the myocyte. Stunning was present more frequently than hibernation and myocardial morphology determined the degree of functional improvement.

The role of mitral valve repair and surgical ventricular reconstruction

Functional ischemic mitral regurgitation follows myocardial infarction with degenerative changes in valve–ventricular interaction. Usually there is no structural disease in the valve leaflets or chordae. Mitral regurgitation affects survival. The Duke University Cardiovascular database reports 3-year post CABG survival rates of 78%, 57%, and 54% for patients with 1+, 2+ and 3 to 4+ mitral regurgitation, respectively.[16] Mitral valve repair is reserved for patients with grade III or IV mitral regurgitation which causes breathlessness on exertion, orthopnea, and fatigue. The principle indication for mitral repair in ischemic cardiomyopathy is a calculated regurgitant fraction of more than 50% of the forward LVEF. Those with a lesser degree usually respond to CABG alone. There are three main clinical problems which cause mitral regurgitation. First, exercise-induced ischemia may impair papillary muscle function causing mitral regurgitation, pulmonary congestion, and dyspnea. Second, acute myocardial infarction located inferobasally (right coronary or dominant circumflex distribution) can cause sudden posteromedial papillary muscle dysfunction and mitral regurgitation. Acute catastrophic pulmonary edema occur if the papillary muscle tears away from the LV wall. The third, and largest, group comprises those with progressive left ventricular dilatation, chronic mitral regurgitation, and pulmonary hypertension. Though valve surgery has been widely advocated for these patients, the long-term outcome is not as satisfactory as once thought.

Ventricular reconstructive surgery is the successor to left ventricular aneurysmectomy (for full-thickness scar), now that thrombolysis or primary coronary angioplasty limits myocardial infarction before the transmural stage. The scar is then limited to the endocardial surface while the epicardium appears normal through a rim of reperfused muscle. This contrasts with the leather-like appearance of an expanding full thickness scar in a dyskinetic left ventricular aneurysm. As LV size increases, the progressively elevated systolic wall stress accounts for worsening symptoms. Stroke volume and global LVEF gradually decline. When more than 40% of the LV circumference becomes dyskinetic the normal left ventricular end systolic diameter index of 25 mL/m^2 increases beyond 60 mL/m^2, a level predictive of cardiac mortality. Once decompensation begins, functional impairment progresses rapidly as does the risk of surgical mortality. For this reason, left ventricular reconstruction surgery should be considered for patients with LVEF less than 30%, mean pulmonary artery pressure more than 25 mmHg, left ventricular akinesia or dyskinesia more than 60%, and left ventricular end diastolic volume more than 250 mL. Most of these patients are already NYHA Class III or IV, despite cardiac resynchronization therapy and maximum drug treatment.

The aim is to reduce LV chamber size by around 30% below baseline, restore the natural elliptic LV shape, and decrease wall stress.[17] At surgery, the ischemic cardiomyopathy ventricle has a globular shape with a veneer of normal epicardium on the anterolateral surface. The surgeon incises through the akinetic muscle to access and excise the scar. The reconstruction is then begun using a continuous suture passed along the border between endocardial scar and healthy septal and lateral myocardium. The suture is tied in such a way as to restore the curvature of the anterolateral LV wall. A small patch of Dacron is used to close the residual defect. By excluding the scar, progressive (adverse) ventricular remodeling is stopped and LV ejection fraction improves by 10–15%. The procedure is supplemented by CABG and mitral valve repair where necessary.

In contrast to the slow and unpredictable improvement in contractility after CABG, left ventricular reconstruction (± mitral repair) produces an immediate result. In a large series by Dor, LVEF improved from 17% to 37%.[17] Hospital mortality saw a 19% improvement with LVEF, and this was maintained with a late mortality of only 10% at 5 years. Following Dor's lead, an international cooperative study investigated the outcomes following LV reconstruction on a multicenter basis. Again, the baseline LVEF of 28% ± 10% and mean LVESVI of 110 mL/m^2 improved to an LVEF of 39% ± 12% with a reduction in LVESVI to 68 mL/m^2.[18] In addition to reconstruction of the ventricle, 96% of the patients underwent CABG and 23% mitral valve repair.

Whether LV reconstruction ± mitral repair adds to CABG alone can only be answered by a large randomized trial in ischemic cardiomyopathy patients. The Surgical Treatment of Ischemic Heart Failure (STICH) was performed on a multicenter international basis but surprisingly did not demonstrate survival or quality of life benefit over and above that achieved by CABG alone.[19] Those already convinced of the benefits of LV reconstruction criticized the conduct of the trial and the efficacy of the operations performed by low volume surgical centers. The benchmark for LV volume reduction is 30%, whereas the mean for STICH was only 19%. Nevertheless, it is possible that even adequate LV volume reduction may not produce symptomatic or survival benefit because the operation disturbs the three-dimensional architecture of the LV. Loss of the heart's coordinated helical structure may disturb diastolic function (LV filling) and offset the improvement in systolic function.

Significant doubt has been cast about the efficacy of both mitral valve repair and left ventricular remodeling surgery in ischemic cardiomyopathy. A landmark paper from the Cleveland Clinic provides the best aid to decision-making using prognostic factors for the individual patient.[20] A 10-year cohort of 1,468 patients subject to the operations described earlier or listed for transplantation had the following outcomes. One-, five-, and nine-year survival rates were as follows: CABG alone 92%, 72%, and 53%; CABG with mitral repair 88%, 57%, and 34%; CABG with ventricular reconstruction 93%, 76%, and 55%; and listing for cardiac transplantation 79%, 66%, and 54%. Coronary bypass alone and listing for transplantation appeared to maximize 5-year survival.[20] This appears to support the skepticism surrounding other procedures.

Cardiac transplantation

Clinical cardiac transplantation began with Barnard's landmark operation in 1967 then almost disappeared through limitations in early immunosuppression. With persistence and refinement of antirejection therapy, this compelling procedure emerged as an effective solution for a few highly selected patients without significant comorbidity. Hospital survival has improved from around 75% in the early 1980s to 85% by 2000. Ten-year survival is around 50%.[21] Currently the number of donor hearts is around 2,500 per annum in the United States and 190 in the UK. This contrasts with approximately 100,000 and 12,000 end-stage heart failure patients, respectively, under the age of 65 in these countries. Clearly the scarce donor hearts should be reserved for those most likely to benefit in life expectancy and quality of life. Young patients with congenital heart disease or idiopathic dilated cardiomyopathy fit this category. While arteriopaths with ischemic heart disease comprise the largest cohort of potential candidates, most prove ineligible through heart failure comorbidity or advanced age.

Left ventricular assist devices

Ventricular assist devices were introduced by DeBakey in the late 1960s in an attempt to salvage surgical patients who could not be weaned from cardiopulmonary bypass (CPB). With increasingly sophisticated bioengineering, the original temporary external pneumatic blood pumps have evolved into miniaturized fully implantable electrical devices suitable for the long-term treatment of chronic heart failure. Experimental evidence showing that pulse pressure is not necessary in the systemic circulation of large mammals allowed the development of small continuous flow devices.[22] Mechanical blood pumps are now capable of sustaining full systemic or pulmonary blood flow against physiological and, in some cases, pathological levels of vascular resistance.[23] While left (LVAD), right (RVAD), and biventricular (BIVAD) assist devices are possible options, 85% of acute and 99% of chronic heart failure patients receive only an LVAD. Currently, total artificial hearts (biventricular) are still used in a small number of cardiac transplant candidates.

Temporary mechanical circulatory support

Temporary extracorporeal ventricular assist devices (VADs) are used for "bridge to recovery" and for bridge to transplantation when the blood type suggests that the waiting time will be short (days to weeks). Recovery is followed by weaning from, and removal of the device. Typically, the patient has acute cardiogenic shock after cardiac surgery, acute inflammatory cardiomyopathies, or myocardial infarction. Criteria for beginning temporary circulatory support include a cardiac index less than 2.0 L/min/m^2, systolic blood pressure less than 90 mmHg, and pulmonary capillary wedge pressure more than 20 mmHg together with biochemical evidence of poor tissue perfusion (increasing serum creatinine and liver transaminases). The patient is oliguric and acidotic with cool extremities and obtunded mental state. When receiving maximum medical treatment, these are indices of impending death.

Evidence-based patient selection is crucial and numerous ethical considerations influence the decision to implant the VAD.[24] The most important of these is the likelihood of a successful outcome in the face of device costs and need for prolonged intensive care. The presence of irremediable renal, hepatic, or respiratory failure is an absolute contraindication to initiating support. Established stroke and sepsis are relative contraindications. Patients older than 70 years have decreased survival, though the potential for weaning is not affected by age. Risk stratification models show preimplantation mechanical ventilation, urine output less than 30 mL/hour, preoperative central venous pressure more than 16 mmHg, hepatic dysfunction (prothrombin time >16 seconds) and increasing serum creatinine and bilirubin levels to be adverse prognostic risk factors. Experience shows extracorporeal pulsatile versus non-pulsatile VADs, and extracorporeal membrane oxygenation to provide similar outcomes.

In cardiac surgical patients the time of beginning VAD support has an important effect on outcome. Early deployment based on predictive models (derived from hemodynamic parameters and level of intraoperative inotropic support) provides improved likelihood of survival to hospital discharge.[25] When VAD insertion occurs within 3 hours of the first attempt to wean from CPB, then 60% of patients can be separated from VAD support with 45% hospital discharge rate. This contrasts with 27% VAD separation and 7% discharge rate when VAD deployment is delayed more than 3 hours after CPB. Delay also increases the need for biventricular support. An episode of cardiac arrest before VAD insertion decreases survival from around 45–7%. If the patient was weaned from CPB on two high dose inotropes, hospital mortality is 42% versus 80% when three high dose inotropes were required.

Long-term circulatory support

"Destination therapy" is an increasingly realistic alternative to cardiac transplantation and a lifeline for the vast majority of heart failure patients rendered ineligible for transplantation through common heart failure comorbidities. The aims of long-term mechanical support are clear. The first is to provide symptomatic relief for the severely debilitated heart failure patient. The second is to extend survival, aiming for at least 5 years of good-quality life. The third objective is cost-effectiveness, by reducing the need for recurrent hospital admissions. The clinical objectives have already been achieved by the new miniaturized rotary blood pumps, but economic considerations delay the final aim of making LVAD technology available to the target population. Three developments have set the scene for long-term support.

First, considerable knowledge and expertise was gained from prolonged bridging to transplantation because of limited donor heart availability. The LVAD gradually reverses the chronic heart failure syndrome, relieves breathlessness, and fatigue and in most cases restores the patient to NYHA Class I. Mechanical unloading improves native heart function, particularly in idiopathic dilated and inflammatory cardiomyopathies.

Second, the REMATCH trial demonstrated improved survival with LVAD use compared with medical management of advanced heart failure. The first-generation pulsatile

HeartMate I LVAD dramatically reduced mortality by 48% over 2 years in non-transplant eligible patients. LVADs were subsequently approved for destination therapy by the Food and Drug Administration in 2002. Nevertheless, survival remained suboptimal in LVAD patients due to deaths from mechanical failure or infection.

Third, the new axial flow and centrifugal pumps (providing continuous as opposed to pulsatile blood flow) have now been shown to be as effective but safer than the large first-generation devices which provide stroke volume and pulse pressure.[26] These miniaturized LVADs are silent, less obtrusive, easier to implant, and more user-friendly. Patients are discharged from hospital within a few weeks and pursue an active life in the community.

Improvement in native heart contractility

The failing heart beats more than 120,000 times a day pumping around 7,000 L of blood against an increasing afterload. As the heart dilates ventricular wall tension, myocardial energy, and oxygen consumption (MVO_2) increase, while subendocardial blood flow decreases. LVAD deployment has two principal benefits. First the failing ventricle is unloaded thereby promoting functional improvement or rarely recovery in dilated cardiomyopathy patients.[27] Second systemic blood flow is sustained at physiological levels to preserve vital organ perfusion.

Our own clinical experience suggests that rotary blood pump patients experience better survival when native heart contractility improves. There are several potential explanations for this. Cardiac output is boosted by the native heart and there is less propensity for intraventricular thrombus formation when contractility and segmental wall motion improves. Pulsatility generated by the native left ventricle improves coronary blood flow and there is less risk of coronary thrombosis in obstructed vessels.

For many years it has been recognized that ventricular unloading with a blood pump eliminates left ventricular wall stress triggering reversal of the heart failure remodeling process at cellular and molecular level.[28] Reverse remodeling encompasses regression of myocyte hypertrophy, improvement in left ventricle geometry, and resolution of many genetic and molecular mechanisms responsible for heart failure.[29] While complete functional recovery and LVAD removal are rare, early studies showed around 50% of patients with idiopathic dilated cardiomyopathy and 17% with ischemic cardiomyopathy to manifest substantial improvement in cardiac function.[30] The shorter the duration of heart failure, the greater the likelihood of improvement. Others have shown initial improvement in LVEF over 30 days but subsequent deterioration virtually to baseline by 120 days in both idiopathic dilated cardiomyopathy and ischemic cardiomyopathy patients.[31] Left ventricular dimensions followed the same pattern with evidence for mild ventricular redilatation during longer periods of support. In contrast to the changes in LV function, right ventricular function improves continuously presumably because the right ventricle is indirectly unloaded through reduction in pulmonary artery pressure and right ventricular recovery occurs over a longer time trajectory than LV recovery.

In ischemic cardiomyopathy the potential for functional improvement is limited by impaired myocardial perfusion and areas of scar, hibernation, and stunning.[32] Without substantial improvement in myocardial blood flow, functional recovery is unlikely. This is the group where an LVAD together with myocardial cell therapy holds the greatest promise. Mesenchymal stem cells appear to convey reparative processes by angiogenesis, extracellular matrix stabilization, and endogenous stem cell recruitment.[33,34] The objective is to improve capillary growth and vascularity in hibernating myocardium and thereby boost contractility.[35] Meanwhile LVAD unloading promotes the genetic and cellular mechanisms of reverse remodeling in the ventricle as a whole.

Current evidence suggests that intramyocardial injection of bone marrow stem cells is a more effective method of delivery than intracoronary infusion.[36] We have therefore undertaken a dual approach by implanting the LVAD to remove wall stress and injecting autologous bone marrow stem cells to areas of carefully delineated hibernating myocardium.[37]

In two innovative ongoing studies, the University of Minnesota and the University of Michigan are employing direct intramyocardial delivery of bone marrow derived mononuclear cells in patients undergoing bridge to cardiac transplantation. Tagged bone marrow stem cells or placebo are injected directly into the territory of the left anterior descending coronary artery and marked with titanium surgical clips. Myocardium from the core of the left ventricle obtained at the time of LVAD implantation will then be compared with myocardium marked with clips from the explanted heart after the transplant. Both ischemic and non-ischemic patients are included in this study.

Maximizing survival in high-risk cardiac surgery

The mean age and risk profile of patients referred for cardiac surgery is constantly increasing. Surgeons are now inclined to accept high-risk patients because interventional cardiology provides less invasive alternatives for an overlapping patient cohort. As risk profile increases, so does hospital mortality. A survey of 8,641 patients who underwent coronary artery bypass operations in New England showed an overall mortality of 4.48% of which 65% could be directly attributed to postcardiotomy myocardial failure.[38] In the PURSUIT trial which randomized coronary bypass patients with unstable angina to a glycoprotein IIb/IIIa inhibitor or placebo, the 7-day mortality or myocardial infarction rate was 22.3% in almost 700 patients in the control arm.[39] A collective review of 279 dialysis dependent coronary bypass patients reported a 12.2% hospital mortality.[40] Similarly, the Mayo Clinic Group reported a 14% perioperative mortality for aortic valve replacement patients with a LVEF less than 35% and a borderline transvalvular gradient. Intraoperative myocardial injury remains prevalent in the increasingly elderly surgical population because tolerance to ischemia is reduced in aged myocardium.

Patients who are difficult to wean from CPB and those who subsequently deteriorate into a low cardiac output state have mortality rates of between 50% and 80%.[41] In established cardiogenic shock, conventional treatment with inotropes, the intra-aortic balloon pump (IABP) or temporary circulatory support devices has not substantially improved survival. In an analysis of risk factors and outcomes for postcardiotomy mechanical support in 19,985 Cleveland Clinic patients, 0.5% received circulatory support with overall survival of 35%.[42] Included were patients who were converted to the HeartMate I implantable system and bridged to transplantation with 72% survival. In the absence of the transplant option, more innovative circulatory support strategies are required to improve survival in the postcardiotomy setting.

Prediction of postoperative low cardiac output syndrome

Coronary and valve patients with very poor ventricular function often have the most to gain from a successful operation. This is also the group at greatest risk from post-ischemic myocardial dysfunction. Because risk-scoring systems provide insufficient weight to very poor ventricular function, some patients may be declined surgery on the grounds of elevated risk.[43] Paradoxically, refined operative techniques and myocardial protection should widen the availability of surgical repair to high-risk groups. Improved processes are needed to identify very high-risk patients and improve their survival.

Poor LVEF is the most important index of mortality because these patients have less margin for recovery from postoperative stunning.

Management of patients at risk from low cardiac output syndrome

Three categories of patient are at substantial risk. First are those who present urgently for surgery, already in cardiogenic shock, often with a complication of myocardial infarction or infective endocarditis. Second is the group submitted for high-risk non-transplant heart failure surgery with LVEF less than 20% together with renal impairment or aorto-iliac disease, which precludes the use of an IABP. The third category includes patients who sustain an unanticipated negative event during surgery, which may prejudice separation from CPB.

Conventional postcardiotomy supportive treatment begins with inotropic drugs though prolonged use may augment perioperative ischemic injury. Drugs commonly employed are dopamine, dobutamine, milrinone, and epinephrine. These agents increase stroke work, left ventricular wall tension, and myocardial oxygen consumption, thus depleting energy reserves.[44] High doses may cause endocardial necrosis and impaired diastolic function with an overall negative effect on myocardial recovery. Because of this an IABP or circulatory support system are preferable for patients with moderate to severe hemodynamic compromise.

The principal effects of the IABP are to reduce left ventricular afterload (and MVO_2), improve diastolic coronary blood flow and thereby enhance subendocardial perfusion in patients with elevated LVEDP.[45] The IABP itself does not substantially increase systemic blood flow. Transoesophageal echocardiography indicates that peak diastolic coronary flow velocity increases by a mean of 117% with an increase in mean flow velocity integral of 87%.[46] Blood flow velocities of × 1.5 to × 2.0 baseline have been measured in the stenosed left anterior descending coronary arteries of patients supported by an IABP. Factors that determine the effectiveness of IABP support include balloon volume, location in the aorta, rate of inflation, and deflation and synchrony relative to the events of the cardiac cycle.[47] The optimal inflation timing has been shown to be slightly preceding the diacrotic notch with deflation bordering on isovolumetric systole. Modern IABP controllers are designed to optimize timing during sinus rhythm and in the presence of cardiac arrhythmias. The IABP also has the capacity to improve right heart function through ventricular interdependence mechanisms and augmentation of right coronary blood flow.[48]

In a large series of IABP patients from the Massachusetts General Hospital, multivariate predictors of death in medical and surgical patients included: (a) IABP insertion in the operating room or intensive care unit; (b) transthoracic insertion; (c) advanced age; (d) procedures other than coronary bypass grafting; or (e) percutaneous transluminal coronary angioplasty and insertion for cardiogenic shock.[49] In this series predictors of death were great age, mitral valve replacement, prolonged CPB, urgent or emergency operation, preoperative renal dysfunction, complex ventricular dysrhythmias, right ventricular failure, and emergency resumption of CPB. In the Benchmark Registry and Society of Thoracic Surgeons (USA) National Databases IABP procedures were initiated preoperatively in 52.4% and 63.5%, respectively, of all IABP procedures.[50] Preoperative insertion was associated with a mortality of 18.8–19.6%, intraoperative insertion 27.6–32.3%, and postoperative insertion 39–40.5%. Thus, there is a consensus of opinion that pre-emptive use of the IABP reduces mortality. The absolute risk reduction is around 7%.

Vascular complications are the most frequent cause of morbidity for IABP patients with rates between 9% and 36%.[51] Femoral cannulation may be complicated by leg ischemia caused by mechanical occlusion, thrombosis, or embolism. Factors predisposing to leg ischemia include female gender, diabetes mellitus, and pre-existing peripheral vascular disease. Possible injuries to the aorta include intramural hematoma, dissection, arterial perforation, and arterial thrombus and embolism. The IABP may also cause mesenteric ischemia or acute pancreatitis probably as a result of athero-emboli in the celiac axis. Neurological complications are much less frequent than vascular complications but paraplegia can occur secondary to aortic dissection or adventitial hematoma producing spinal cord infarction. Stroke has occurred after balloon rupture and cerebral helium embolization. Rupture may result in balloon entrapment because blood leaks into the system and forms clots, which block full deflation.

Outcome after circulatory support for postcardiotomy cardiogenic shock

Pae and colleagues from the Pennsylvania State University reviewed combined registry data on the use of first-generation temporary LVADs between 1985 and 1990.[52] Nine hundred and sixty-five patients were treated for postcardiogenic shock, of which 45% were weaned from the system and 25% were discharged from hospital. Notably, 90% of patients who survived to leave hospital were weaned from the pump within one week. Those requiring univentricular support alone fared better irrespective of whether pulsatile pneumatic or non-pulsatile centrifugal pumps were used. The patient age group of over 70 years was the principal determinant of mortality. Irrespective of multiple complications including bleeding, stroke and renal failure, patients who left hospital had 2-year actuarial survival of 82% and 86% were in NYHA Functional Class I or II. In rare incidences of device dependency (4.5%), those patients without contraindications to transplantation were sustained until a donor organ became available. Of the transplanted patients, 62% were discharged from hospital.

Golding and colleagues from the Cleveland Clinic reported a 12-year experience of 91 patients supported with a centrifugal blood pump after failure to wean from CPB.[53] The mean age of postcardiotomy patients was 54.8 years and mean duration of support 3.56 days (range 1 hour to 19 days). Sixty-two percent (62%) of the patients were successfully weaned, but only 25% survived to leave hospital. Patients with biventricular failure and renal failure had worse late outcomes.

DeRose and colleagues from the Columbia Presbyterian Medical Center, New York adopted a policy of early implantation of the ThermoCardioSystems HeartMate XVE LVAD for patients who developed circulatory failure after high-risk cardiac surgery.[54] In a 4-year period, 12 patients received this LVAD for postcardiotomy cardiogenic shock following coronary artery bypass grafting. Of the 12 patients included in the report, one recovered sufficiently for device explantation, while 9 of the remaining 11 patients (82%) survived to undergo transplantation with successful hospital discharge in each case.

From these and other reports, it is clear that less than one third of patients who suffer postcardiotomy heart failure, refractory to the use of the IABP can be salvaged after the onset of cardiogenic shock. Device-related adverse events, particularly bleeding and infection, have so far precluded widespread prophylactic deployment of temporary LVADs for high-risk patients in order to prevent cardiogenic shock.

Elective transfer from cardiopulmonary bypass to centrifugal blood pump support

The decision to pre-emptively deploy an LVAD must balance safety with efficacy. In order to improve outcome in borderline survival situations following high-risk cardiac surgery, the Oxford Group decided to wean directly from CPB to a new temporary centrifugal blood pump designed to reduce bleeding and thromboembolic complications.[55]

The Levitronix Centrimag short-term VAD is an extracorporeal system composed of a single use centrifugal blood pump, a motor, a console, a flow probe, and a tubing circuit. The device is comprised of a bearingless motor, which combines the drive, the magnetic bearing, and the rotor function in a single unit. This device can produce flows up to 10 L/minute under normal physiological conditions with a priming volume of 31 mL. Initial European clinical trials in postcardiotomy cardiogenic shock have been encouraging over mean support periods of 2 weeks, with the longest at 64 days. Overall 30-day mortality was 50%, which compares favorably with that reported for other devices. The system is reliable and versatile so that it can be quickly implemented in situations of rapid deterioration. Device mechanical reliability and relatively low complication rates make the Levitronix pump safe to use for patients who need time for evaluation for cardiac transplantation or a longer-term device.

For elective transfer from CPB to centrifugal blood pump support, the patients at highest risk of postcardiotomy cardiogenic shock are selected before surgery. Candidates may have chronic left ventricular dysfunction with LVEF less than 20%, recent acute myocardial infarction, impaired renal function, or aortoiliac disease precluding IABP use. LVAD implantation is undertaken during a 30-minute reperfusion time before discontinuation of CPB. Conduits for the inflow and outflow cannulas are used to improve the safety of decannulation. A tube of descending aortic homograft (8 cm × 10 mm diameter) is sewn to an incision at the junction of the superior pulmonary vein with the left atrium. Through this conduit is introduced the 32 F right-angled wire reinforced venous cannula into the center of the left atrium. Ligatures are placed around the homograft tube to retain the inflow cannula in position. The distal end of the venous cannula is brought through the skin below the sternotomy wound and then filled by raising left atrial pressure. A Dacron polyester fabric graft (8 mm) is then sewn to the ascending aorta with a side clamp. The straight 22 F arterial inflow cannula is inserted through this graft, secured into place by ligatures and brought out through the skin adjacent to the venous cannula. The system is filled during reperfusion and de-airing of the native heart. The patient is then weaned directly from CPB onto LVAD flow to provide between 3 and 4 liters per minute. Antegrade cardiac ejection continues to provide systemic pulsatility. Combined output from the device and the native left ventricle is around 3.0 L/min/m². Transoesophageal echocardiography is used to confirm the position of the inflow cannula and the efficacy of de-airing.

After protamine administration, the sternotomy wound is closed to allow extubation during support. To minimize bleeding, no anticoagulation is given for 12 hours. Once the chest tube drainage is less than 50 mL/hour heparin infusion is given to provide an activated partial thromboplastin time ratio of 1.5–2.5. For recovery after ischemic arrest the support duration is usually less than 7 days. In this time frame, the Levitronix pump is reliable, safe, and effective. It is readily managed by nursing staff and easily portable. Reoperation for bleeding and decannulation problems are avoided by the use of the conduits.

With a view to explant, myocardial function is assessed daily with the pump flow turned down to 2.0 L/min/m². After sustainable improvement in myocardial function has been achieved, the patient is returned to the operating room, the pump is switched off and the cannulas are withdrawn. The grafts are ligated close to their insertion to prevent thrombus formation. As part of the step-down process, an IABP is used for a further 24–48 hours.

To date the Levitronix Centrimag pump has been used in thousands of patients, of whom around 45% of cases have been salvage postcardiotomy support with a mean of 9 days and 53% survival. It is likely that the 47% mortality could have been reduced substantially by anticipating postoperative deterioration and using the blood pump electively to prevent cardiogenic shock during the duration of reversible post-ischemic stunning.

References

1. **McMurray JJ, Stewart S** (2000). Epidemiology, etiology and prognosis of heart failure. *Heart*, **83**, 596–602.

2. **The CONSENSUS Trial Study Group** (1987). Effects of enalapril on mortality in severe congestive heart failure. Results of the Co-operative Scandanavian Enalapril Survival Study (CONSENSUS). *N Engl J Med*, **316**, 1429–35

3. **Rose EA, Gelijns AL, Moskowitz AJ,** *et al.*; **Randomized Evaluation of Mechanical Assistance for the Treatment of Congestive Heart Failure (REMATCH) Study Group** (2001). Long-term mechanical left ventricular assistance for end-stage heart failure. *N Engl J Med*, **345**, 1435–43.

4. **Adamson PB, Abraham WT, Love C, Reynolds D** (2004). The evolving challenge of chronic heart failure management: a call for a new curriculum for training heart failure specialists. *J Am Coll Cardiol*, **44**, 1354–7.

5. **Dec GW, Fuster V** (1994). Idiopathic dilated cardiomyopathy. *N Engl J Med*, **331**, 1564–75

6. **ACC/AHA** (2001). Guidelines for the evaluation and management of chronic heart failure in adults: executive summary. *J Am Coll Cardiol*, **38**, 2101–13.

7. **Westaby S** (2004). Coronary revascularisation in ischaemic cardiomyopathy. *Surg Clin North Am*, **84**, 179–99.

8. **Yoshida F, Gould KL** (1993). Quantative relation of myocardial infarct size and myocardial viability by positron emission tomography to left ventricular ejection fraction and 3-year mortality with and without revascularisation. *J Am Coll Cardiol*, **22**, 984–97.

9. **Tjan TDT, Kondruweit M, Scheld HH,** *et al.* (2000). The bad ventricle—revascularisation versus transplantation. *J Thorac Cardiovasc Surg*, **48**, 9–14.

10. **Raymond KJ, Edwin W, Allen R** *et al.* (2000). The use of contrast-enhanced magnetic resonance imaging to identify reversible myocardial dysfunction. *New Engl J Med*, **343**, 1445–53.

11. **Hausmann H, Topp H, Siniawski H** *et al.* (1997). Decision making in the end stage coronary artery disease. Revascularisation or heart transplantation. *Ann Thorac Surg*, **64**, 1296–302.

12. **Haas F, Haetinel CJ, Picker W,** *et al.* (1997). Preoperative positron emission tomographic viability assessment and perioperative and postoperative risk in patients with advanced ischemic heart disease. *J Am Coll Cardiol*, **30**, 1693–700.

13. **Luciani GB, Gaggani G, Razzaloni R,** *et al.* (1993). Severe ischemic left ventricular failure: coronary operation or heart transplantation? *Ann Thorac Surg*, **55**, 719–23.

14. **Bax JJ, Visser FC, Poldermans D,** *et al.* (2001). Time course of functional recovery of stunned and hibernating segments after surgical revascularisation. *Circulation*, **104**(Suppl I), 314–18.

15. **Hass F, Jennen L, Heinzmann U,** *et al.* (2001). Ischemically compromised myocardium displays different time course of functional recovery: correlation with morphological alterations. *Eur J Cardiothorac Surg*, **20**, 290–8.

16. **Hickey MS, Smith LR, Muhlbaier LH,** *et al.* (1988). Current prognosis of ischemic mitral regurgitation. Implications for future management. *Circulation*, **78**, 151–9

17. **Dor V, Sabatier M, Di Donato M,** *et al.* (1998). Efficacy of endoventricular patch plasty in large post infarction akinetic scar and severe left ventricular dysfunction: comparison with a series of large dyskinetic scars. *J Thorac Cardiovasc Surg*, **116**, 50–9.

18. **Athanasuleas CL, Stanley AW, Jr, Buckberg GD,** *et al.* (2001). Surgical anterior ventricular endocardial restoration (SAVER) in the dilated remodelled ventricle after anterior myocardial infarction. RESTORE Group. Reconstructive endoventricular surgery, returning torsion original radius elliptical shape to the LV. *J Am Coll Cardiol*, **37**, 1199–209.

19. **Mark DB, Knight JD, Velazquez JG,** *et al.* (2009). Quality of life and economic outcomes with surgical ventricular reconstruction in ischemic heart failure: results from the Surgical Treatment for Ischemic Heart Failure Trial. *Am Heart J*, **157**, 837–44.

20. **Yoon DY, Smedira NG, Nowicki ER,** *et al.* (2010). Decision support in surgical management of ischemic cardiomyopathy. *J Thorac Cardiovasc Surg,* **139,** 283–93.

21. **Deng MC** (2004). Orthotopic heart transplantation: highlights and limitations. *Surg Clin N Am,* **84,** 243–55.

22. **Saito S, Nishinaka T, Westaby S** (2004). Hemodynamics of chronic non-pulsatile blood flow: implications for LVAD development. *Surg Clin North Am,* **84,** 61–74.

23. **Aaronson KD, Patel H, Pagani FD** (2003). Patient selection for ventricular assist device therapy. *Ann Thorac Surg,* **75,** 529–35.

24. **Goldstein DJ, Oz MC** (2000). Mechanical support for post cardiotomy cardiogenic shock. Semin Thorac Cardiovasc Surg, **12,** 220–8.

25. **Samuel LE, Holmes EC, Thomas MP,** *et al.* (2001). Management of acute cardiac failure with mechanical assist: experience with the Abiomed BVS 5000. *Ann Thorac Surg,* **71,** 567–72.

26. **Krishnamani R, DeNofrio D, Korstam MA** (2010). Emerging ventricular assist devices for long term cardiac support. *Nat Rev Cardiol,* **7,** 71–6

27. **Muller J, Wallukat G, Weng Y,** *et al.* (2001). Predictive factors for weaning from a cardiac assist device. An analysis of clinical, gene expression and protein data. *J Heart Lung Transplant,* **20,** 202–7.

28. **Zhang J, Narula J** (2004). Molecular biology of myocardial recovery. *Surg Clin North Am,* **84,** 223–42.

29. **Maybaum S, Kamalakannan G, Murthy S** (2008). Cardiac recovery during mechanical assist device support. *Semin Thorac Cardiovasc Surg,* **20,** 234–46.

30. **Mancini DM, Beniaminovitz A, Levin H,** *et al.* (1988). Low incidence of myocardial recovery after left ventricular assist device implantation in patients with chronic heart failure. *Circulation,* **98,** 2383–9.

31. **Maybaum S, Mancini D, Xydas S,** *et al.* (2007). Cardiac improvement during mechanical circulatory support: a prospective multicentre study of the LVAD working group. *Circulation,* **115,** 2497–505.

32. **Yoon DY, Smedira NG, Nowicki ER,** *et al.* (2010). Decision support in surgical management of ischemic cardiomyopathy. J Thorac Cardiovasc Surg, **139,** 283–93.

33. **Lai VK, Linares-Palomino J, Nadal-Ginard B, Galinanes M** (2009). Bone marrow cell-induced protection of the human myocardium: characterization and mechanism of action. *J Thorac Cardiovasc Surg,* **138,** 1400–8.

34. **Gnechi M, Zhang Z, Ni A, Dzau VJ** (2008). Paracrine mechanisms in adult stem cell signaling and therapy. *Circ Res,* **103,** 1204–9.

35. **Kocher AA, Schuster MD, Szabolcs MJ,** *et al.* (2001). Neovascularisation of ischemic myocardium by human bone-marrow derived angioblasts prevents cardiomyocyte apoptosis, reduces remodeling and improves cardiac function. *Nat Med,* **7,** 430–6.

36. **Amado LC, Saliaris AP, Schuleri KH,** *et al.* (2005). Cardiac repair with intramyocardial injection of allogenic mesenchymal stem cells after myocardial infarction. *Proc Natl Acad Sci USA,* **102,** 11474–9.

37. **Anastasiadis K, Antonitsis P, Argiradou H,** *et al.* (2011). Hybrid approach of ventricular assist device and autologous bone marrow stem cell implantation in end stage ischemic heart failure enhances myocardial perfusion. *J Trans Med,* **9,** 12.

38. **O'Connor GT, Birkmeyer JD, Dacey LJ,** *et al.* (1988). Results of a regional study of modes of death associated with coronary artery bypass grafting. *Ann Thorac Surg,* **66,** 1323–8.

39. **Marso SP, Bhatt DL, Roe MT,** *et al.* (2000). Enhanced efficacy of eptifibatide administration in patients with acute coronary syndrome requiring in-hospital coronary artery bypass grafting. *Circulation,* **102,** 2952–8.

40. **Liu JY, Birkmeyer NJO, Sanders JH** (2000). Risks of morbidity and mortality in dialysis patients undergoing coronary artery bypass surgery. *Circulation,* **102,** 2973.

41. **Goldstein DJ, Oz MC** (2000). Mechanical support for postcardiotomy cardiogenic shock. *Semin Thorac Cardiovasc Surg*, **12**(3), 220–8.

42. **Smedira NG, Blackstone EH** (2001). Postcardiotomy mechanical support: risk factors and outcomes. *Ann Thorac Surg*, **71**(3 Suppl), S60–6.

43. **Westaby S** (2002). League tables, risk assessment and an opportunity to improve standards. Br J Cardiol (Acute Interv Cardiol), **9**, 5–10.

44. **Lazar HL, Buckberg GD, Foglia RP**, *et al.* (1981). Detrimental effects of premature use of inotropic drugs to discontinue cardiopulmonary bypass. *J Thorac Cardiovasc Surg*, **82**, 18–25

45. **Marra C, De Santo LS, Amarelli C**, *et al.* (2002). Coronary artery bypass grafting in patients with severe left ventricular dysfunction: a prospective randomized study on the timing of perioperative intraaortic balloon pump support. *Int J Artif Organs*, **25**, 141–6.

46. **Christenson JT, Simonet F, Badel P**, *et al.* (1999). Optimal timing of properative intra-aortic balloon pump support in high-risk coronary patients. *Ann Thorac Surg*, **68**, 934–9.

47. **Christenson JT, Cohen M, Ferguson III JJ**, *et al.* (2002). Trends in intraaortic balloon counterpulsation complications and outcomes in cardiac surgery. *Ann Thorac Surg*, **74**, 1086–91.

48. **Lim CH, Son HS, Baek KJ**, *et al.* (2006). Comparison of coronary artery blood flow and hemodynamic energy in a pulsatile pump versus a combined nonpulsatile pump and an intra-aortic balloon pump. *ASAIO J*, **52**(5), 595–7.

49. **Torchiana DF, Hirsch G, Buckley MJ**, *et al.* (1997). Intra-aortic balloon pumping for cardiac support: trends in practice and outcome 1968–1995. *J Thorac Cardiovasc Surg*, **113**, 4, 758–69.

50. **Ferguson JJ, Cohen M, Freedman RJ**, *et al.* (2001). The current practice of intra-aortic balloon counterpulsation: results from the Benchmark Registry. *J Am Coll Cardiol*, **38**, 1456–62.

51. **Busch T, Sirbu H, Zenker D** (1999). Vascular complications related to intra-aortic counterpulsation: an analysis of a 10-year experience. *Thorac Cardiovasc Surg*, **45**, 55–9

52. **Pae WE Jr, Miller CA, Matthews Y, Pierce WS** (1992). Ventricular assist devices for postcardiotomy cardiogenic shock. A combined registry experience. *J Thorac Cardiovasc Surg*, **104**(3), 541–52.

53. **Golding LA, Crouch RD, Stewart RW**, *et al.* (1992). Postcardiotomy centrifugal mechanical ventricular support. *Ann Thorac Surg*, **54**(6), 1059–63.

54. **DeRose JJ Jr, Umana JP, Argenziano M**, *et al.* (1997). Improved results for postcardiotomy cardiogenic shock with the use of implantable left ventricular assist devices. *Ann Thorac Surg*, **64**(6), 1757–62.

55. **Westaby S, Balacumaraswami L, Evans BJ**, *et al.* (2007). Elective transfer from cardiopulmonary bypass to centrifugal blood pump support in very high-risk cardiac surgery. *J Thorac Cardiovasc Surg*, **133**(2), 577–8.

Chapter 10

Surgery for atrial fibrillation

Jason O. Robertson, Lindsey L. Saint,
and Ralph J. Damiano, Jr

Introduction

Atrial fibrillation (AF) is the most common of all cardiac arrhythmias and accounts for nearly one-third of all hospital admissions due to heart rhythm irregularities.[1] AF affects nearly 4.5 million people in the European Union and 2.2 million people in the United States. The prevalence of AF increases with age, afflicting 4% of the population over 60 years old and nearly 9% of persons 80 years and older. The most serious complication of AF is thromboembolism and resultant stroke[2]; however, significant morbidity and mortality also result from hemodynamic compromise due to loss of atrial contraction, exacerbations of congestive heart failure from atrioventricular asynchrony, and tachycardia-induced cardiomyopathy. As a result, atrial fibrillation has an enormous socioeconomic impact,[3] and with the aging population in the United States, AF is expected to become an even larger public health burden in the future. A recent study predicted that the number of Americans diagnosed with AF will grow to over 10 million by the year 2050.[4]

The available medical treatments for atrial fibrillation have many shortcomings. Antiarrhythmic drug therapy is complicated by significant side effects and may necessitate warfarin for anticoagulation.[1,5] Moreover, these drugs have limited efficacy. Rate control strategies, conversely, leave the patient in AF and therefore do not address the impaired hemodynamics seen with this arrhythmia.

The Cox-Maze procedure

The first effective surgical procedure for atrial fibrillation was introduced clinically at Washington University in St. Louis in 1987 by Dr. James Cox.[6-8] This operation, now known as the Cox-Maze procedure, was originally developed to interrupt the multiple macro-reentrant circuits that were felt to develop in the atria, thereby precluding the ability of the atrium to flutter or fibrillate. Unlike previous procedures, the Cox-Maze procedure successfully restored both aortic valve (AV) synchrony and sinus rhythm, thereby significantly reducing the risk of thromboembolism, stroke, and hemodynamic compromise.[9] The operation was comprised of a pattern of surgical incisions across both the right and left atria, which were placed so that the sinoatrial node could still direct the propagation of the sinus impulse (Figure 10.1). This allowed for most of the atrial

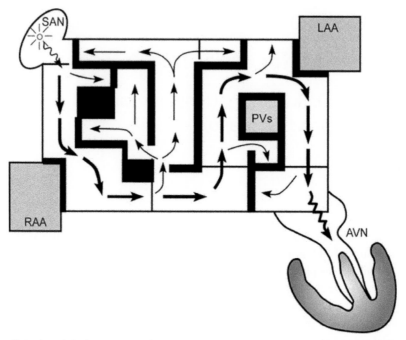

Figure 10.1 The original maze operation was conceptualized as a pattern of surgical incisions that would prevent atrial fibrillation by blocking macro-reentrant circuits while still allowing propagation of a sinus impulse. Both atrial appendages were excised, and the pulmonary veins were isolated.

AVN, atrioventricular node; LAA, left atrial appendage; PVs, pulmonary veins; RAA, right atrial appendage; SAN, sinoatrial node.

myocardium to be activated, resulting in preservation of atrial transport function in most patients.[10]

The first versions of the Cox-Maze procedure were complicated by late chronotropic incompetence resulting in a high incidence of pacemaker implantation, as well as significant surgical complexity. The Cox-Maze III, the third design iteration, became the gold standard for the surgical treatment of AF (Figure 10.2).[7,11] Although the Cox-Maze III procedure was effective in eliminating AF, it did not gain widespread acceptance because it was still technically difficult, and it significantly prolonged time on cardiopulmonary bypass. During the last decade, most groups have replaced the traditional "cut-and-sew" lesions with ablation lines created using various energy sources in an attempt to make the operation simpler and faster to perform.[12] In 2002, our group introduced the Cox-Maze IV operation, which uses a combination of bipolar radiofrequency ablation and cryoablation to effectively replace the majority of lesions that comprise the Cox-Maze III (Figure 10.3).

These ablation-assisted procedures have resulted in widespread adoption of the Cox-Maze and a significant increase in the number of operations that are performed annually for atrial fibrillation.[13] Nationally, as reported in the Society of Thoracic Surgery National Database,

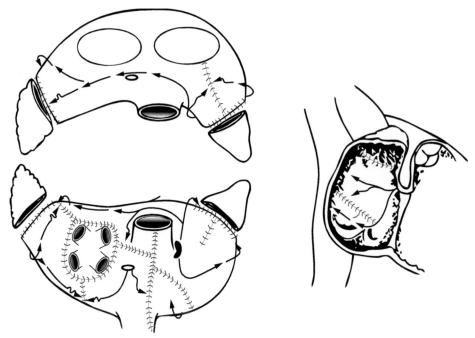

Figure 10.2 The lesion set of the traditional cut-and-sew Cox-Maze III operation.
Reprinted from Cox J.L *et al.* (1995) Modification of the maze procedure for atrial flutter and atrial fibrillation I. Rationale and surgical results, The Journal of Thoracic and Cardiovascular Surgery 110(2):473–84, based on an image first published in Cox J.L (1993) Evolving applications of the maze procedure for atrial fibrillation. The Annals of Thoracic Surgery 55(3):578-580, with permission from Elsevier and the Society of Thoracic Surgeons

representing over 700 institutions, 12,737 patients (5% of cardiac surgery patients) had a surgical procedure performed for AF in 2005, whereas only 3,987 patients had AF surgery in 2004. Prior to 2004, the volume was so low that the operation was not reported.

Surgical ablation technology

The development of surgical ablation technology has transformed a difficult and time-consuming operation into a procedure that is technically easier, shorter, and less invasive. However, incorporation of many new technologies has led to confusion in the literature as to what is the best energy source. It is imperative that the relative advantages and disadvantages of each of the available ablation technologies are understood. Several early energy sources that were clinically available, such as microwave and laser technology, have been removed from the market and will therefore not be discussed further.

The ideal device would meet the following criteria. First, it must reliably produce bidirectional conduction block across the line of ablation. This requires a transmural lesion, as even small gaps in ablation lines can conduct both sinus and fibrillatory wavefronts.[14–16] Second, the ablation device must be safe. This requires a precise definition of dose-response curves to limit excessive or inadequate ablation and potential hazards

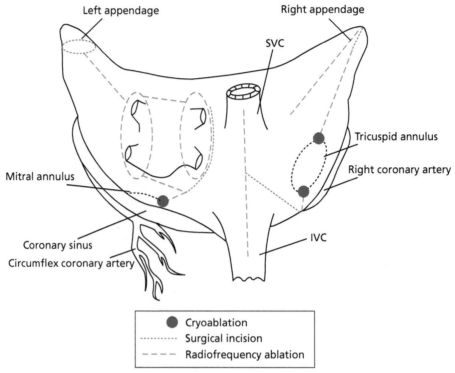

Figure 10.3 Diagram illustrating the Cox-Maze IV procedure.

SVC, superior vena cava; IVC, inferior vena cava.

Reproduced from J Interv Card Electrophysiol., The Cox-maze IV procedure for lone atrial fibrillation: a single center experience in 100 consecutive patients 31(1), 2011, pages 47–54, Weimar T. *et al.* with permission of Springer

to surrounding vital cardiac structures, such as the coronary sinus, coronary arteries, and valvular structures. Third, the ablation device should make AF surgery simpler and require less time to perform. This would require the device to create lesions rapidly, be intuitive to use, and have adequate length and flexibility. Finally, the device should be adaptable to a minimally invasive approach. This would include the ability to insert the device through minimal access incisions or ports. For the treatment of lone AF, there is a further requirement of the device to be able to create a transmural lesion on the beating heart without the need for cardiopulmonary bypass. Failure in this regard has proven to be the biggest shortcoming of unipolar energy sources. As of the present time, no device has met all of these criteria. The following sections will briefly summarize the currently available ablation technologies.

Cryoablation

Cryoablation is unique in that it destroys myocardial tissue by freezing rather than heating. Ice crystals caused by cryoablation cause acute disruption of cell membranes, and microvascular damage leads to chronic local tissue ischemia. This has the benefit of preserving the myocardial fibrous skeleton and collagen structure and is thus safe for use around valvular tissue.[17,18] There is also evidence that the induction of apoptosis plays a role in late lesion expansion.[19] Lesion size and depth depend on the probe temperature, the duration of the ablation, the thermal conductivity and temperature of the tissue, and the choice of cooling agent.[17]

Commercially available sources of cryothermal energy employ nitrous oxide (AtriCure, Cincinnati, OH), or Argon (Medtronic, Minneapolis, MN). At one atmosphere of pressure, nitrous oxide is capable of achieving a temperature of –89.5 °C, whereas argon has a minimum temperature of –185.7 °C. The nitrous oxide technology has a well-defined efficacy and safety profile and is generally safe except around the coronary arteries, where studies have shown late intimal hyperplasia after cryoablation.[18,20] Potential disadvantages of cryoablation are the relatively long time it requires to create lesions (1–3 minutes), and the difficulty encountered in creating transmural lesions on the beating heart. Furthermore, if blood is frozen during epicardial ablation on the beating heart, it may coagulate, creating a potential source for thromboembolism.

Radiofrequency energy

Radiofrequency (RF) energy uses an alternating current at a frequency that is high enough to prevent rapid myocardial depolarization and induction of ventricular fibrillation, yet low enough to prevent tissue vaporization and perforation, ultimately using thermal energy to create a lesion.[21] The lesion size depends on electrode tissue contact area, the interface temperature, the current and voltage (power), and the duration of delivery. Accordingly, the depth of the lesion can be limited by char formation, epicardial fat, myocardial and endocardial blood flow, and tissue thickness. Irrigated devices have been designed to reduce charring.

There have been numerous unipolar RF devices developed for ablation, and some have been modified to use irrigation and suction. Although dry unipolar RF devices have been shown to create transmural lesions on the arrested heart in animals with sufficiently long ablation times, they have not been consistently successful in humans. After 2-minute endocardial ablations during mitral valve surgery, only 20% of the *in vivo* lesions were transmural.[22] Epicardial ablation on the beating heart has been even more problematic. Animal studies have consistently shown that unipolar RF is incapable of creating epicardial transmural lesions on the beating heart,[23] and epicardial RF ablation in humans resulted in only 10% of the lesions being transmural.[24]

To overcome this problem, bipolar RF clamps were developed. With bipolar RF, the electrodes are embedded in the jaws of a clamp to focus the delivery of energy. Shielding the electrodes from the circulating blood pool improves and shortens lesion formation and limits collateral injury. Bipolar ablation has been shown to be capable of creating transmural lesions on the beating heart both in animals and humans with ablation times typically less than 20 seconds.[25–27].

Another advantage of bipolar RF energy over unipolar RF is its safety profile. Several clinical complications of unipolar RF devices have been reported, including coronary artery injuries, cerebrovascular accidents, and esophageal perforation.[28-31] Bipolar RF technology has eliminated this collateral damage by confining the energy within the jaws of the clamp. Moreover, devices by AtriCure and Medtronic employ algorithms capable of predicting lesion transmurality by measuring the tissue conductance between electrodes, whereas the Estech device uses a temperature-controlled algorithm—thus tailoring the energy delivery to the physiological characteristics of tissue. There have been no injuries described with these devices despite extensive clinical use. One drawback of bipolar RF devices is the requirement for the tissue to be clamped. This has limited the potential lesion sets, particularly on the beating heart, and has required the use of adjunctive unipolar technology to create a complete Cox-Maze lesion set.

High-intensity focused ultrasound

High-intensity focused ultrasound, or HIFU, is another modality being applied clinically for surgical ablation (St. Jude Medical, St. Paul, MN). In these devices, ultrasound waves travel through the tissue causing compression, refraction, and particle movement, which are translated into kinetic energy, ultimately creating thermal coagulative tissue necrosis. HIFU is the one unipolar source that produces high-concentration energy in a focused area at a defined distance from the probe, and it is reportedly able to create transmural epicardial lesions through epicardial fat in less than 2 seconds without affecting intervening and surrounding tissue.[32] There is a steep temperature gradient between the focus of energy and collateral tissue with the targeted tissue rapidly raised to 80°C.

An advantage of HIFU technology is its mechanism of thermal ablation. Unlike other energy sources that heat or cool tissue by thermal conduction, which creates a graded response dependent on the distance from the energy source and is susceptible to cooling near blood vessels, HIFU ablates tissue by directly heating it in the acoustic focal volume. It is, therefore, much less vulnerable to this heat sink effect.

A few clinical studies using HIFU have shown good results.[32-35] However, there has been no independent experimental verification of the efficacy of HIFU devices to reliably create transmural lesions, and more recent clinical experience has been much less encouraging.[36] Additionally, the fixed depth of penetration of these devices can be problematic because of the variability of atrial wall thickness in pathological states.

In summary, each ablation technology has its own advantages and disadvantages. It has been the inability of some devices to create reliable linear lesions on the beating heart that has primarily limited their clinical applicability and the development of more minimally invasive procedures for lone AF. Continued research investigating the effects of each surgical ablation technology on atrial hemodynamics, function, and electrophysiology will allow for more appropriate use in the operating room.

Indications for surgical ablation

While there remains controversy over the relative roles of catheter-based ablation and the Cox-Maze procedure in the management of patients with medically refractory, lone AF, there are many patients who are presently undergoing cardiac surgery who have concomitant AF and would benefit from treatment. In a review of our experience at Washington University from 1996 to 2005, the incidence of preoperative AF was 22% in patients referred for valvular surgery and 24% in patients referred for combined valvular/coronary surgery. The role of surgery for AF has been recently clarified and endorsed in a consensus statement.[37] It stated that surgical ablation for atrial fibrillation is indicated for: (1) all symptomatic AF patients undergoing other cardiac surgery; (2) selected asymptomatic AF patients undergoing cardiac surgery in which the ablation can be performed with minimal additional risk; and (3) symptomatic AF patients who prefer a surgical approach, have failed one or more attempts at catheter ablation, or are not candidates for catheter ablation. Thus, surgery is a complimentary, rather than a competitive, approach to catheter ablation.

There are also relative indications for surgery that were not included in the consensus statement. The first is the presence of a contraindication to long-term anticoagulation in patients with persistent AF and a high risk for stroke (CHADS score ≥2). Up to one-third of patients with AF who were screened for participation in clinical trials of warfarin were deemed ineligible for chronic anticoagulation due to a high perceived risk for bleeding complications.[38–40] In one study, the annual rate of intracranial hemorrhage in anticoagulated patients with AF was 0.9% per year, and the overall rate of major bleeding complications was 2.3% per year.[41] In contrast, the stroke rate following the Cox-Maze procedure off anticoagulation has been remarkably low, even in high-risk patients. After a mean follow-up of 6.9 ± 5.1 years, only 5 of 450 patients had a stroke at our institution, and there was no difference in stroke rate between patients with CHADS scores above or below 2.[42] This low risk of stroke after the Cox-Maze procedure has been noted in other series, as well.[9,43] In patients undergoing concomitant valve surgery, studies have shown that adding the Cox-Maze procedure can decrease the late risk of cardiac- and stroke-related deaths.[44,45] However, there have been no prospective, randomized studies demonstrating survival or other benefits in this population.

Finally, surgical treatment for AF with amputation of the left atrial appendage should also be considered in patients with persistent AF who have suffered a cerebrovascular accident despite adequate anticoagulation, as these patients are at high risk for repeat neurologic events. Anticoagulation with warfarin reduces the risk of ischemic and hemorrhagic strokes by more than 60% in patients with AF but does not completely eliminate this serious complication.[2,46] At our institution, 19% of patients who underwent the Cox-Maze III procedure had experienced at least one episode of significant cerebral thromboembolism before undergoing the operation.[47] Less than 1% of patients (2 of 306) had a late stroke after a mean follow-up of 3.8 ± 3.0 years, even with 90% of patients off anticoagulation at last follow-up.[9] Furthermore, a series from Japan has demonstrated a 10% increase in incidence of stroke at 8-year follow-up for patients with chronic AF who underwent mitral valve replacement alone when compared to similar patients who had mitral valve replacement with concomitant Cox-Maze.[48]

Surgical results

The Cox-Maze procedure

The Cox-Maze III procedure has had excellent long-term results. In our series at Washington University, 97% of 198 consecutive patients that underwent the procedure were free from symptomatic AF at a mean follow-up of 5.4 years. There was no difference in the cure rates between patients undergoing a stand-alone Cox-Maze procedure and those undergoing concomitant procedures.[47] Similar results have been obtained from other institutions around the world with the traditional "cut-and-sew" method.[49–51]

Our results using a combination of bipolar RF ablation and cryoablation (the Cox-Maze IV operation) have been encouraging, as well.[12,52] A recent prospective, single-center trial from our institution followed 100 consecutive patients with lone AF between January 2002 and May 2010.[52] The mean follow-up was 17 ± 10 months, and enrolled patients had paroxysmal (31%), persistent (6%) and longstanding persistent (63%) AF. This study demonstrated postoperative freedom from AF of 93%, 90%, and 90% at 6, 12, and 24 months, respectively. Freedom from AF off antiarrhythmic drugs was 82%, 82%, and 84% at the same time points. In a group of 282 patients at our institution, the majority of whom had a Cox-Maze IV procedure with concomitant cardiac surgery, the results were similar with a freedom from AF of 89%, 93%, and 89% at 3, 6, and 12 months, respectively.[53] However, these studies are difficult to compare to the prior Cox-Maze III results due to the more stringent follow-up and endpoints in the present studies. Holter monitor readings were taken at three time points, and AF recurrence was defined as any episode lasting over 30 seconds. A separate propensity analysis performed by our group has shown that there was no significant difference in the freedom from AF at 3, 6, or 12 months between the Cox-Maze III and IV groups.[54]

Interestingly, our group has shown that isolating the entire posterior left atrium by creating a "box" is preferable to isolating the left and right pulmonary veins separately with or without a connecting lesion between the pulmonary veins (Figure 10.4).[52,55] In the Weimer et al. study, 78 patients underwent a "box" lesion, and those patients had higher

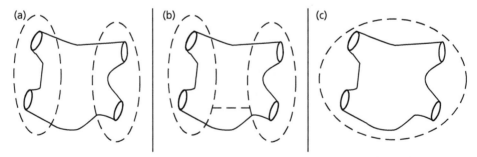

Figure 10.4 Schematic illustration of the methods used to isolate the pulmonary veins, either separately (a), with a connecting lesion (b), or as a "box" isolation of the entire posterior left atrium (c).

freedom from AF (96% *vs.* 86%) and freedom from AF off antiarrhythmic drugs (79% *vs.* 47%) compared to patients that underwent different methods of pulmonary vein isolation. Postoperatively, 7% of patients required a pacemaker for chronotropic incompetence or for slow junction rhythms, and there were zero late strokes. There was only one postoperative death within 30 days (1%).

The Cox-Maze IV procedure has also significantly shortened the mean cross-clamp times for a lone Cox-Maze from 93 ± 34 minutes for the Cox-Maze III to 41 ± 13 minutes for the Cox-Maze IV (*P* <0.001)[52] and from 122 ± 37 minutes for a concomitant Cox-Maze III procedure to 92 ± 37 minutes (*P* <0.005) in those undergoing the Cox-Maze IV procedure concomitantly with another cardiac operation.[25]

Risk factors for late recurrence of AF at 1-year include: enlarged left atrial diameter, failure to isolate the entire posterior left atrium, and early atrial tachyarrhythmias.[53] Increasing left atrial size has been related to operative failure in several studies,[43,56] and our group has clearly demonstrated that the probability of recurrence exceeds 50% once left atrial size is greater than 8 cm.[53] Early atrial tachyarrhythmias were associated with an odds ratio of 3.020 (*P* = 0.01), and it is thought that these might be a marker of more advanced pathology of the atrial substrate in patients with AF of long duration.

Left atrial lesion sets

Several centers have suggested performing lesion sets confined to only the left atrium to cure AF. Deneke and colleagues have provided some evidence in a prospective analysis that suggests a left atrial lesion set is as effective as a biatrial lesion set in patients with chronic AF undergoing concomitant open heart surgical procedures.[57] This concept is supported by the fact that the majority of paroxysmal AF appears to originate around the pulmonary veins and the posterior left atrium. A left atrial lesion set typically involves pulmonary vein isolation with a lesion to the mitral annulus, as well as removal of the left atrial appendage. Many ablation technologies have been used to create these lesion sets with varied degrees of success.[30,58-65]

There have been no randomized trials of biatrial versus left atrial ablation in the surgical population. As a result, the importance of the right atrial lesions of the traditional Cox-Maze procedure has been difficult to define. A meta-analysis of the published literature by Ad and colleagues revealed that a biatrial lesion set resulted in a significantly higher late freedom from AF when compared with a left atrial lesion set alone (87% *vs.* 73%, *P* = 0.05).[66] Moreover, a randomized trial of patients with persistent atrial fibrillation undergoing mitral valve surgery and radiofrequency ablation (RFA) of the left atrium versus mitral valve surgery alone demonstrated that sinus rhythm was only present in 44.4% of RFA patients at one year follow-up (compared to 4.5% in the patients in the valve surgery alone group).[67] However, it is important to note that lesions were created using a monopolar RF device applied from the endocardial surface, which may not have provided transmural ablation. Regardless, it is not surprising that left atrial lesions alone would have lower success rates considering that results of intraoperative mapping of patients with atrial fibrillation from our group, and others have shown that AF originates from the left atrium in approximately 30% of cases.[68–70]

Of the specific left atrial lesions of the Cox-Maze procedure, it is difficult to determine the precise importance of each particular ablation. All surgeons agree on the importance of isolating the pulmonary veins. Work from Gillinov et al. has shown the importance of the left atrial isthmus in a retrospective study.[71] In a rare randomized trial, Gaita and coauthors examined pulmonary vein isolation alone versus two alternate lesion sets that both included ablation of the left atrial isthmus. In this study, normal sinus rhythm at 2-year follow-up was only seen in 20% in the PVI group versus 57% in the other groups (P <0.006).[60] Moreover, as just discussed, we have demonstrated the importance of a "box" lesion around the pulmonary veins. Therefore, most of the left atrial Cox-Maze lesion set is likely needed to ensure a high success rate; however, there has been no randomized trial to conclusively demonstrate the correct left atrial lesion set. It must also be kept in mind that recurrent atrial flutter or tachycardia is a well-known complication of performing only the left atrial lesions, and it has been reported in as many as 13–21% of patients undergoing the procedure.[61,72]

Pulmonary vein isolation

The results of pulmonary vein isolation (PVI) alone have been variable. While most of the triggers for paroxysmal AF originate around the pulmonary veins,[73] over 30% of triggers originate elsewhere.[74] However, PVI is an attractive therapeutic option due to the fact that it can be performed off cardiopulmonary bypass through small or endoscopic incisions. In the first report of surgical PVI, Wolf and colleagues reported that 91% of patients undergoing a video-assisted bilateral PVI and left atrial appendage exclusion were free from AF at three months follow-up.[75] Edgerton et al. reported on 57 patients undergoing PVI with ganglionated plexus (GP) ablation with more thorough follow-up and found 82% of their patients with paroxysmal AF were free from AF at 6 months, with 74% off antiarrhythmic drugs.[76] Subsequent studies have shown encouraging results in patients with paroxysmal AF. McClelland et al. reported 88% freedom from AF at one year without antiarrhythmic drugs in a study involving 21 patients with paroxysmal AF undergoing PVI with GP ablation.[77] A larger, single-center trial recently reported a 65% single procedure success at one year in a series of 45 patients undergoing PVI with GP ablation, including patients with persistent and paroxysmal AF. A multicenter trial reported 87% normal sinus rhythm rate in a more diverse patient population, including some patients with longstanding persistent AF; however, those patients with longstanding persistent AF only had a 71% incidence of normal sinus rhythm.[78]

The success of PVI is highly dependent on patient selection, as results are consistently worse in patients with longstanding persistent AF. In a study from Edgerton and his group, only 56% of patients were free from AF at 6 months (35% off antiarrhythmic drugs).[79] With concomitant procedures, the success rate of PVI is even lower. Of 23 patients undergoing cardiac surgery with concomitant PVI, only 59% of patients were free from AF at their last follow-up (23 ± 15 months).[12] When broken down for patients with paroxysmal versus persistent AF, the percentages were 70% and 43%, respectively. In the setting of mitral valve disease, Tada and colleagues report 61% freedom from AF and only 17% freedom from antiarrhythmic drugs in their series of 66 patients undergoing PVI.[80] These results highlight the need to fully understand the electrophysiological substrate of AF in order to perform an optimal operation for any individual patient.

Ganglionated plexus ablation

Electrophysiologic studies have demonstrated that local autonomic ganglia in ganglionated plexi clustered in the epicardial fat pads play a role in the initiation and maintenance of AF.[81,82] Both pulmonary vein myocardial sleeves and adjacent atrial muscle are innervated by these plexi. As a result, some surgeons have added GP ablation to PVI in hopes of increasing procedural efficacy. Some of the initial surgical results have been encouraging. In 2005, Scherlag and colleagues reported a study of GP ablation combined with catheter PVI in 74 patients with lone AF. After a relatively short median follow-up of 5 months, 91% of patients were free from AF.[82] However, there have not been any direct comparisons as part of randomized clinical trials.

Moreover, the effects of vagal denervation and the long-term efficacy of GP ablation have not been clearly defined. Experimental evidence in our laboratory and others has demonstrated recovery of autonomic function in as few as 4 weeks after GP ablation.[83–85] It is worrisome that the reinnervation may not be homogeneous and could result in a more arrhythmogenic substrate. In a more recent report, Katritsis and colleagues used left atrial GP ablation alone to treat 19 patients with paroxysmal AF. Fourteen of these patients (74%) had recurrent AF during 1-year follow-up.[86] Due to these suboptimal results and the lack of any long-term follow-up of the effects of GP ablation, our practice is not to perform GP ablation to treat AF. GP ablation should be reserved for centers participating in clinical trials.

Surgical techniques

The three categories of surgical procedures currently used in the surgical management of AF are the Cox-Maze procedure, left atrial lesion sets, and pulmonary vein isolation. The important technical details surrounding each of these surgical approaches are discussed in this section.

The Cox-Maze IV procedure

Most centers have replaced the surgical incisions described in the original "cut-and-sew" Cox-Maze III procedure with lines of ablation created by a variety of different energy sources. At our institution, we have successfully used bipolar RF energy to replace most of the surgical incisions of the Cox-Maze III procedure in an operation termed the Cox-Maze IV (Figure 10.3).[87]

The Cox-Maze IV procedure is performed on cardiopulmonary bypass using either a median sternotomy or a less invasive right mini-thoracotomy. Both the right and left pulmonary veins (PVs) are bluntly dissected. If the patient is in AF at the time of surgery, amiodarone is administered and the patient is electrically cardioverted before proceeding with the operation. Pacing thresholds are obtained from each pulmonary vein. The PVs are then isolated using a bipolar RF ablation device, such that a linear line of ablation surrounds a cuff of atrial tissue encompassing the right and left PVs, respectively. The adequacy of electrical isolation is demonstrated by confirming exit and/or entrance block from each PV.

The right atrial lesion set is performed on the beating heart through a small purse-string suture at the base of the right atrial appendage and a single vertical atriotomy (Figure 10.5). A bipolar RF device is used to create most of the lesions. Due to the difficulty in using the bipolar RF clamp in the area of the tricuspid annulus, a unipolar device utilizing either cryoablation or RF energy is used to complete the endocardial ablation lines in this area.

The heart is then arrested by cold cardioplegia. The left atrial appendage is amputated, and bipolar RF ablation is performed through the amputation site into one of the left pulmonary veins. The remaining ablation lines are then created using the bipolar clamp through a standard left atriotomy that extends from the dome of the left atrium to the

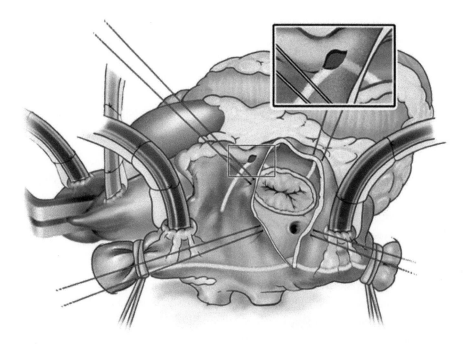

Figure 10.5 Illustration of the right atrial lesion set. Bipolar radiofrequency ablation is indicated by the white lines. Cryoablation is used to complete the ablation lines at the tricuspid valve annulus.

Reproduced from J. Interv. Card. Electrophysiol., The Cox-maze IV procedure for lone atrial fibrillation: a single center experience in 100 consecutive patients 31(1), 2011, pages 47–54, Weimar T. *et al.* with permission of Springer

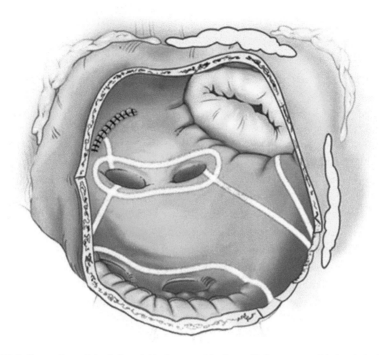

Figure 10.6 Illustration of the left atrial lesion set. Bipolar radiofrequency ablation is indicated by the white lines. Cryoablation is used to complete the ablation line at the mitral valve annulus.
Reproduced from J. Interv. Card. Electrophysiol., The Cox-maze IV procedure for lone atrial fibrillation: a single center experience in 100 consecutive patients 31(1), 2011, pages 47–54, Weimar T. *et al.* with permission of Springer

right inferior PV (Figure 10.6). Connecting lesions into the left superior and inferior pulmonary veins effectively isolate the entire posterior left atrium, and a linear line of ablation is created toward the mitral annulus. Unipolar energy, usually cryoablation, is then used to connect the RF lesion to the mitral annulus and to complete the left atrial isthmus line. An epicardial ablation of the coronary sinus is also performed, typically with a cryoprobe, in line with the endocardial mitral isthmus ablation. In patients undergoing a right mini-thoracotomy, cryoablation is more extensively applied to complete the posterior left atrial isolation.

Left atrial lesion sets

Over the last decade, several left atrial procedures have been introduced in an attempt to find a surgical cure for AF. The individual lesion sets themselves vary widely, and results have been dependent on multiple variables, including the type of ablation device used, the lesion set, and the patient population.[30,63,65,88,89]

From a technical standpoint, all of these procedures have incorporated at least some subset of the left atrial lesion set of the Cox-Maze procedure, and have attempted to electrically isolate the pulmonary veins. A typical left atrial lesion set involves PVI, which can be performed around the right and left PVs individually, with a connecting lesion, or as a "box" isolation of the entire posterior left atrium, along with a lesion to the mitral annulus and removal of the left atrial appendage. Left atrial lesion sets have been performed from both an endocardial and epicardial approach, and have utilized all available ablation technologies.[58–60,62,64,90,91]

Pulmonary vein isolation

Pulmonary vein isolation is an attractive treatment option since the procedure can be added to other open-heart surgeries with minimal impact on operative time, can be performed using minimally invasive techniques, and does not require cardiopulmonary bypass. As previously mentioned, electrical isolation of the pulmonary veins can be performed around the right and left PVs individually, with a connecting lesion, or as a box isolation of the entire posterior left atrium (Figure 10.4). In lone AF, the procedure can be performed via either a mini-thoracotomy or an endoscopic, port-based approach. Although a variety of energy sources have been used successfully in PVI, our institution favors bipolar RF clamps for this procedure.[34,92,93]

Prior to initiating the operation, the patient is intubated using a double-lumen endotracheal tube, and external defibrillator pads are placed. A transesophageal echocardiogram is performed to confirm the absence of thrombus in the left atrial appendage. If thrombus is identified, the procedure is either aborted or converted to an open procedure in order to minimize the risk of systemic thromboembolism. The patient is positioned in a modified left lateral decubitus position, at a 45- to 60-degree angle, with the right arm extended over the head in order to expose the right axilla.

For the more common thoracoscopic approach, a camera port is placed in the sixth intercostal space, and a smaller working port is placed under direct vision in either the third or fourth intercostal space at the mid-axillary line. Upon entering the chest, the right phrenic nerve is identified and a pericardotomy is performed from the superior vena cava to the diaphragm. Care is taken to open the pericardium anterior and parallel to the phrenic nerve in order to protect it from injury. The space above and below the right PVs, including the opening into the oblique sinus and the space between the right superior PV and the right pulmonary artery, is then dissected free. A specialized thoracoscopic dissector and guiding sheath are introduced through a second port, either lateral or medial to the scope port, and the space between the right superior PV and the right pulmonary artery is further dissected. The dissector is removed from the chest, leaving the sheath in place, and the patient is cardioverted into sinus rhythm. Pacing thresholds are obtained for each pulmonary vein in order to ensure appropriate electrical isolation at the end of the procedure. At this point, some surgeons take advantage of the surgical exposure afforded by PVI and also ablate the ganglionated plexi.

A bipolar RF clamp is then introduced into the chest using the previously placed sheath as a guide. The left atrium surrounding the pulmonary veins is clamped and ablated as previously described. Electrical isolation is confirmed with pacing, the instruments are removed, and the right chest is closed.

The patient is repositioned to expose the left chest in the same fashion as the right. A port for the thoracoscopic camera is placed in the sixth intercostal space, slightly posterior to the site on the right chest. The other working ports are introduced into the left chest in the same positions used for the right chest. In a similar fashion, the left phrenic nerve is identified and a pericardotomy is performed, this time parallel and posterior to the structure. The Ligament of Marshall is identified and divided prior to introducing the sheath and dissector. The left PVs are then isolated using a bipolar RF clamp, and exit block is confirmed in identical fashion to the right side. Prior to closing the left chest, the left atrial appendage is typically excluded by either stapling across the base with an endoscopic stapler or using a clip.[94–96] Clip devices are currently favored to address left atrial appendage exclusion since the stapler poses a significant risk of tears and bleeding. While left atrial appendage exclusion is performed to eliminate a potential source of thromboemboli, data is mixed on the effectiveness of the practice.[97]

Future directions in atrial fibrillation surgery

The advent of surgical ablation technology has made the Cox-Maze IV procedure easier and faster to perform while preserving the high success rates of the original lesion set. However, it remains an invasive procedure that requires cardiopulmonary bypass, and there are certain populations, such as patients with enlarged atria, that have high postoperative failure rates.[53] Further modifications based on the most current theoretical mechanisms of AF will be best developed using patient-specific and minimally invasive approaches. Such refinements should preserve normal atrial physiology, incur minimal morbidity, and achieve high success rates in curing AF.

Critical mass hypothesis

In the decades since the introduction of the Cox-Maze procedure, it has been proposed that a "critical mass" of tissue is requisite for fibrillation.[98] The critical mass hypothesis proposes that a certain minimal size of atrial tissue is required for the induction and maintenance of AF, owing to the idea that this area represents the minimum path length necessary for re-entry in sustained AF. The minimum path length, or wavelength, has been quantitatively defined as the product of conduction velocity (CV) and effective refractory period (ERP).[99] *In vitro* studies from our laboratory supporting this model have shown that the probability of sustained AF is dependent on increasing atrial surface area, widths, and weights, as well as the length of the ERP and CV of the tissue.[98] Concordantly, it has been shown that patients with large left atrial surface areas are at disproportionate risk of failing to convert to normal sinus rhythm and of suffering recurrent AF after a Cox-Maze procedure, presumably because the procedure fails to divide the atria into small enough sections to prevent sustained AF.[43,53,56] Based on these data and clinical results, it has been hypothesized that certain patients may benefit from either atrial reduction or additional ablative lines that further subdivide the atria. The initial lesions of a novel AF procedure could be determined by a calculation of the critical area needed to maintain AF in the individual patient.[98]

Electrocardiographic imaging

To calculate the critical mass required to sustain AF in the individual patient, one must be able to derive the minimum wavelength; however, determining CV and ERP, as well as the atrial activation sequence and mechanistic information, has presented a challenge in the past. Because epicardial activation mapping, the traditional gold standard for mapping of AF, is both invasive and time-consuming, a new method of multipoint mapping known as electrocardiographic imaging (ECGI) is currently being evaluated at our institution.[100] When combined with computed tomography (CT) scanning, ECGI uses body surface potential mapping with 250 electrodes representing over 800 epicardial sites to obtain patient-specific heart-torso geometry to create maps of cardiac electrophysiologic activation, which can then be superimposed onto the heart surface.[101–106] This technique has been well-described in patients with AF, and allows activation times to be calculated and displayed as either static or dynamic activation maps on a 3D surface model of an individual patient's atria.[100,107] Previous studies have demonstrated that substrate information can be extracted from this data, allowing ERP to be estimated from the activation intervals calculated at each electrode site, and CV to be calculated from the activation maps.[108,109] Data derived from this technology, which take into account the patient's atrial geometry, electrophysiology, and arrhythmogenic mechanism, may allow a surgeon to design a patient-specific optimal lesion set, thereby leaving the atria unable to sustain AF but able to conduct a normal sinus beat. Additionally, focal trigger mechanisms could be identified using this technique, potentially allowing for targeted ablation strategies in either the electrophysiologic laboratory or operating room.

Minimally invasive techniques

The development of ablation devices not only simplified the formerly complex and technically demanding Cox-Maze procedure, but also introduced the possibility of minimally invasive surgery for AF. Using new ablation technologies, simpler procedures are being developed that can be performed through small incisions without the need for cardiopulmonary bypass.

As discussed previously, there is strong evidence that PVI performed on the beating heart may be effective in the subset of patients with paroxysmal AF.[75] Using minimal access techniques, Edgerton *et al.* have achieved excellent visualization through the transverse sinus in order to develop a new linear lesion set that uses RF ablation to electrophysiologically mimic all of the left atrial lesions of the Cox-Maze procedure on the epicardial surface. This new lesion set, termed the Dallas Lesion Set, uses PVI in combination with connecting lesions created on the dome of the left atrium, and has shown promising results at both 6 and 12 months.[110,111] Two-stage hybrid procedures that combine PVI and resection of the left atrial appendage via a minimally invasive surgery approach with delayed electrophysiology ablation in the area of the biatrial isthmus lines are being performed at some institutions. Similarly, procedures that combine simultaneous epicardial and endocardial ablation have also been performed.[112]

Unfortunately, although new technology has led to advances in the field, the limitations of current ablation devices have impeded the development of a truly minimally invasive procedure. Future advances may be anticipated with new devices and techniques that allow surgeons and electrophysiologists to obtain reproducible complete lines of block.

References

1. **Fuster V, Ryden LE, Cannom DS**, *et al.* (2006). Acc/aha/esc 2006 guidelines for the management of patients with atrial fibrillation. *Europace*, **8**, 651–745.
2. **Hart RG, Halperin JL** (1999). Atrial fibrillation and thromboembolism: a decade of progress in stroke prevention. *Ann Intern Med*, **131**, 688–95.
3. **Valderrama AL, Dunbar SB, Mensah GA** (2005). Atrial fibrillation: public health implications. *Am J Prev Med*, **29**, 75–80.
4. **Miyasaka Y, Barnes ME, Gersh BJ**, *et al.* (2006). Secular trends in incidence of atrial fibrillation in olmsted county, minnesota, 1980 to 2000, and implications on the projections for future prevalence. *Circulation*, **114**, 119–25.
5. **Channer KS** (2001). Current management of symptomatic atrial fibrillation. *Drugs*, **61**, 1425–37.
6. **Cox JL** (1991). The surgical treatment of atrial fibrillation. Iv. Surgical technique. *J Thorac Cardiovasc Surg*, **101**, 584–92.
7. **Cox JL, Boineau JP, Schuessler RB, Jaquiss RD, Lappas DG** (1995). Modification of the maze procedure for atrial flutter and atrial fibrillation. I. Rationale and surgical results. *J Thorac Cardiovasc Surg*, **110**, 473–84.
8. **Cox JL, Schuessler RB, D'Agostino HJ Jr**, *et al.* (1991). The surgical treatment of atrial fibrillation. Iii. Development of a definitive surgical procedure. *J Thorac Cardiovasc Surg*, **101**, 569–83.
9. **Cox JL, Ad N, Palazzo T** (1999). Impact of the maze procedure on the stroke rate in patients with atrial fibrillation. *J Thorac Cardiovasc Surg*, **118**, 833–40.
10. **Feinberg MS, Waggoner AD, Kater KM**, *et al.* (1994). Restoration of atrial function after the maze procedure for patients with atrial fibrillation. Assessment by doppler echocardiography. *Circulation*, **90**, II285–92.
11. **Cox JL** (2000). The minimally invasive maze-iii procedure. *Oper Tech Thorac Cardiovasc Surg*, **5**, 79.
12. **Melby SJ, Zierer A, Bailey MS**, *et al.* (2006). A new era in the surgical treatment of atrial fibrillation: the impact of ablation technology and lesion set on procedural efficacy. *Ann Surg*, **244**, 583–92.
13. **Gammie JS, Haddad M, Milford-Beland S**, *et al.* (2008). Atrial fibrillation correction surgery: lessons from the Society of Thoracic Surgeons National Cardiac Database. *Ann Thorac Surg*, **85**, 909–14.
14. **Inoue H, Zipes DP** (1987). Conduction over an isthmus of atrial myocardium in vivo: a possible model of Wolff-Parkinson-White syndrome. *Circulation*, **76**, 637–47.
15. **Ishii Y, Nitta T, Sakamoto S, Tanaka S, Asano G** (2003). Incisional atrial reentrant tachycardia: experimental study on the conduction property through the isthmus. *J Thorac Cardiovasc Surg*, **126**, 254–62.
16. **Melby SJ, Lee AM, Zierer A**, *et al.* (2008). Atrial fibrillation propagates through gaps in ablation lines: implications for ablative treatment of atrial fibrillation. *Heart Rhythm*, **5**, 1296–301.
17. **Comas GM, Imren Y, Williams MR** (2007). An overview of energy sources in clinical use for the ablation of atrial fibrillation. *Semin Thorac Cardiovasc Surg*, **19**, 16–24.

18. Mikat EM, Hackel DB, Harrison L, Gallagher JJ, Wallace AG (1977). Reaction of the myocardium and coronary arteries to cryosurgery. *Lab Invest*, **37**, 632–41.

19. Baust JG, Gage AA (2005). The molecular basis of cryosurgery. *BJU Int*, **95**, 1187–91.

20. Holman WL, Ikeshita M, Ungerleider RM, *et al.* (1983). Cryosurgery for cardiac arrhythmias: acute and chronic effects on coronary arteries. *Am J Cardiol*, **51**, 149–55.

21. Viola N, Williams MR, Oz MC, Ad N (2002). The technology in use for the surgical ablation of atrial fibrillation. *Semin Thorac Cardiovasc Surg*, **14**, 198–205.

22. Santiago T, Melo JQ, Gouveia RH, Martins AP (2003). Intra-atrial temperatures in radiofrequency endocardial ablation: histologic evaluation of lesions. *Ann Thorac Surg*, **75**, 1495–501.

23. Thomas SP, Guy DJ, Boyd AC, *et al.* (2003). Comparison of epicardial and endocardial linear ablation using handheld probes. *Ann Thorac Surg*, **75**, 543–8.

24. Santiago T, Melo J, Gouveia RH, *et al.* (2003). Epicardial radiofrequency applications: *in vitro* and *in vivo* studies on human atrial myocardium. *Eur J Cardiothorac Surg*, **24**, 481–6; discussion 486.

25. Gaynor SL, Diodato MD, Prasad SM, *et al.* (2004). A prospective, single-center clinical trial of a modified cox maze procedure with bipolar radiofrequency ablation. *J Thorac Cardiovasc Surg*, **128**, 535–42.

26. Prasad SM, Maniar HS, Diodato MD, Schuessler RB, Damiano RJ Jr (2003). Physiological consequences of bipolar radiofrequency energy on the atria and pulmonary veins: a chronic animal study. *Ann Thorac Surg*, **76**, 836–41; discussion 841–32.

27. Prasad SM, Maniar HS, Schuessler RB, Damiano RJ Jr (2002). Chronic transmural atrial ablation by using bipolar radiofrequency energy on the beating heart. *J Thorac Cardiovasc Surg*, **124**, 708–13.

28. Demaria RG, Page P, Leung TK, *et al.* (2003). Surgical radiofrequency ablation induces coronary endothelial dysfunction in porcine coronary arteries. *Eur J Cardiothorac Surg*, **23**, 277–82.

29. Gillinov AM, Pettersson G, Rice TW (2001). Esophageal injury during radiofrequency ablation for atrial fibrillation. *J Thorac Cardiovasc Surg*, **122**, 1239–40.

30. Kottkamp H, Hindricks G, Autschbach R, *et al.* (2002). Specific linear left atrial lesions in atrial fibrillation: intraoperative radiofrequency ablation using minimally invasive surgical techniques. *J Am Coll Cardiol*, **40**, 475–80.

31. Laczkovics A, Khargi K, Deneke T (2003). Esophageal perforation during left atrial radiofrequency ablation. *J Thorac Cardiovasc Surg*, **126**, 2119–20; author reply 2120.

32. Ninet J, Roques X, Seitelberger R, *et al.* (2005). Surgical ablation of atrial fibrillation with off-pump, epicardial, high-intensity focused ultrasound: results of a multicenter trial. *J Thorac Cardiovasc Surg*, **130**, 803–9

33. Groh MA, Binns OA, Burton HG 3rd, *et al.* (2008). Epicardial ultrasonic ablation of atrial fibrillation during concomitant cardiac surgery is a valid option in patients with ischemic heart disease. *Circulation*, **118**, S78–82.

34. Mitnovetski S, Almeida AA, Goldstein J, Pick AW, Smith JA (2009). Epicardial high-intensity focused ultrasound cardiac ablation for surgical treatment of atrial fibrillation. *Heart Lung Circ*, **18**, 28–31.

35. Nakagawa H, Antz M, Wong T, *et al.* (2007). Initial experience using a forward directed, high-intensity focused ultrasound balloon catheter for pulmonary vein antrum isolation in patients with atrial fibrillation. *J Cardiovasc Electrophysiol*, **18**, 136–44.

36. Klinkenberg TJ, Ahmed S, Ten Hagen A, *et al.* (2009). Feasibility and outcome of epicardial pulmonary vein isolation for lone atrial fibrillation using minimal invasive surgery and high intensity focused ultrasound. *Europace*, **11**, 1624–31.

37. Calkins H, Brugada J, Packer DL, *et al.* (2007). Hrs/ehra/ecas expert consensus statement on catheter and surgical ablation of atrial fibrillation: recommendations for personnel, policy,

procedures and follow-up. A report of the heart rhythm society (hrs) task force on catheter and surgical ablation of atrial fibrillation. *Heart Rhythm*, **4**, 816–61.

38. [**No authors listed**] (1991). Stroke prevention in atrial fibrillation study. Final results. *Circulation*, **84**, 527–39.

39. **Rosand J, Eckman MH, Knudsen KA, Singer DE, Greenberg SM** (2004). The effect of warfarin and intensity of anticoagulation on outcome of intracerebral hemorrhage. *Arch Intern Med*, **164**, 880–4.

40. **Schaer GN, Koechli OR, Schuessler B, Haller U** (1996). Usefulness of ultrasound contrast medium in perineal sonography for visualization of bladder neck funneling—first observations. *Urology*, **47**, 452–3.

41. [**No authors listed**] (1996). Bleeding during antithrombotic therapy in patients with atrial fibrillation. The stroke prevention in atrial fibrillation investigators. *Arch Intern Med*, **156**, 409–16.

42. **Pet MA, Damiano RJ, Jr., Bailey MS** (2009). Late stroke following the cox-maze procedure for atrial fibrillation: the impact of chads2 score on long-term outcomes. *Heart Rhythm*, **6**, S14.

43. **Gillinov AM, Sirak J, Blackstone EH**, *et al.* (2005). The cox maze procedure in mitral valve disease: predictors of recurrent atrial fibrillation. *J Thorac Cardiovasc Surg*, **130**, 1653–60.

44. **Bando K, Kasegawa H, Okada Y**, *et al.* (2005). Impact of preoperative and postoperative atrial fibrillation on outcome after mitral valvuloplasty for nonischemic mitral regurgitation. *J Thorac Cardiovasc Surg*, **129**, 1032–40.

45. **Bando K, Kobayashi J, Kosakai Y**, *et al.* (2002). Impact of cox maze procedure on outcome in patients with atrial fibrillation and mitral valve disease. *J Thorac Cardiovasc Surg*, **124**, 575–83.

46. [**No authors listed**] (1994). Risk factors for stroke and efficacy of antithrombotic therapy in atrial fibrillation. Analysis of pooled data from five randomized controlled trials. *Arch Intern Med*, **154**, 1449–57.

47. **Prasad SM, Maniar HS, Camillo CJ**, *et al.* (2003). The cox maze iii procedure for atrial fibrillation: long-term efficacy in patients undergoing lone versus concomitant procedures. *J Thorac Cardiovasc Surg*, **126**, 1822–8.

48. **Bando K, Kobayashi J, Hirata M**, *et al.* (2003). Early and late stroke after mitral valve replacement with a mechanical prosthesis: risk factor analysis of a 24-year experience. *J Thorac Cardiovasc Surg*, **126**, 358–64.

49. **Arcidi JM, Jr., Doty DB, Millar RC** (2000). The maze procedure: the lds hospital experience. *Semin Thorac Cardiovasc Surg*, **12**, 38–43.

50. **McCarthy PM, Gillinov AM, Castle L, Chung M, Cosgrove D 3rd** (2000). The cox-maze procedure: the Cleveland Clinic experience. *Semin Thorac Cardiovasc Surg*, **12**, 25–9.

51. **Schaff HV, Dearani JA, Daly RC, Orszulak TA, Danielson GK** (2000). Cox-maze procedure for atrial fibrillation: Mayo clinic experience. *Semin Thorac Cardiovasc Surg*, **12**, 30–7.

52. **Weimar T, Bailey MS, Watanabe Y**, *et al.* (2011). The cox-maze iv procedure for lone atrial fibrillation: a single center experience in 100 consecutive patients. *J Interv Card Electrophysiol*, **31**, 47–54.

53. **Damiano RJ Jr, Schwartz FH, Bailey MS**, *et al.* (2011). The cox maze iv procedure: predictors of late recurrence. *J Thorac Cardiovasc Surg*, **141**, 113–21.

54. **Lall SC, Melby SJ, Voeller RK**, *et al.* (2007). The effect of ablation technology on surgical outcomes after the cox-maze procedure: a propensity analysis. *J Thorac Cardiovasc Surg*, **133**, 389–96.

55. **Voeller RK, Bailey MS, Zierer A**, *et al.* (2008). Isolating the entire posterior left atrium improves surgical outcomes after the cox maze procedure. *J Thorac Cardiovasc Surg*, **135**, 870–7.

56. **Kosakai Y** (2000). Treatment of atrial fibrillation using the maze procedure: the Japanese experience. *Semin Thorac Cardiovasc Surg*, **12**, 44–52.

57. Deneke T, Khargi K, Grewe PH, *et al.* (2002). Left atrial versus bi-atrial maze operation using intraoperatively cooled-tip radiofrequency ablation in patients undergoing open-heart surgery: safety and efficacy. *J Am Coll Cardiol*, **39**, 1644–50.

58. Benussi S, Nascimbene S, Agricola E, *et al.* (2002). Surgical ablation of atrial fibrillation using the epicardial radiofrequency approach: mid-term results and risk analysis. *Ann Thorac Surg*, **74**, 1050–6; discussion 1057.

59. Fasol R, Meinhart J, Binder T (2005). A modified and simplified radiofrequency ablation in patients with mitral valve disease. *J Thorac Cardiovasc Surg*, **129**, 215–7.

60. Gaita F, Riccardi R, Caponi D, *et al.* (2005). Linear cryoablation of the left atrium versus pulmonary vein cryoisolation in patients with permanent atrial fibrillation and valvular heart disease: correlation of electroanatomic mapping and long-term clinical results. *Circulation*, **111**, 136–42.

61. Imai K, Sueda T, Orihashi K, Watari M, Matsuura Y (2001). Clinical analysis of results of a simple left atrial procedure for chronic atrial fibrillation. *Ann Thorac Surg*, **71**, 577–81.

62. Knaut M, Spitzer SG, Karolyi L, *et al.* (1999). Intraoperative microwave ablation for curative treatment of atrial fibrillation in open heart surgery--the micro-staf and micro-pass pilot trial. Microwave application in surgical treatment of atrial fibrillation. Microwave application for the treatment of atrial fibrillation in bypass-surgery. *Thorac Cardiovasc Surg*, **47**(Suppl 3), 379–84.

63. Kondo N, Takahashi K, Minakawa M, Daitoku K (2003). Left atrial maze procedure: a useful addition to other corrective operations. *Ann Thorac Surg*, **75**, 1490–4.

64. Schuetz A, Schulze CJ, Sarvanakis KK, *et al.* (2003). Surgical treatment of permanent atrial fibrillation using microwave energy ablation: a prospective randomized clinical trial. *Eur J Cardiothorac Surg*, **24**, 475–80; discussion 480.

65. Sie HT, Beukema WP, Misier AR, *et al.* (2001). Radiofrequency modified maze in patients with atrial fibrillation undergoing concomitant cardiac surgery. *J Thorac Cardiovasc Surg*, **122**, 249–56.

66. Barnett SD, Ad N (2006). Surgical ablation as treatment for the elimination of atrial fibrillation: a meta-analysis. *J Thorac Cardiovasc Surg*, **131**, 1029–35.

67. Doukas G, Samani NJ, Alexiou C, *et al.* (2005). Left atrial radiofrequency ablation during mitral valve surgery for continuous atrial fibrillation: a randomized controlled trial. *JAMA*, **294**, 2323–9.

68. Nitta T, Ishii Y, Miyagi Y, *et al.* (2004). Concurrent multiple left atrial focal activations with fibrillatory conduction and right atrial focal or reentrant activation as the mechanism in atrial fibrillation. *J Thorac Cardiovasc Surg*, **127**, 770–8.

69. Sahadevan J, Ryu K, Peltz L, *et al.* (2004). Epicardial mapping of chronic atrial fibrillation in patients: preliminary observations. *Circulation*, **110**, 3293–9.

70. Schuessler RB, Kay MW, Melby SJ, *et al.* (2006). Spatial and temporal stability of the dominant frequency of activation in human atrial fibrillation. *J Electrocardiol*, **39**, S7–12.

71. Gillinov AM, McCarthy PM, Blackstone EH, *et al.* (2005). Surgical ablation of atrial fibrillation with bipolar radiofrequency as the primary modality. *J Thorac Cardiovasc Surg*, **129**, 1322–9.

72. Golovchiner G, Mazur A, Kogan A, *et al.* (2005). Atrial flutter after surgical radiofrequency ablation of the left atrium for atrial fibrillation. *Ann Thorac Surg*, **79**, 108–12.

73. Haissaguerre M, Jais P, Shah DC, *et al.* (1998). Spontaneous initiation of atrial fibrillation by ectopic beats originating in the pulmonary veins. *N Engl J Med*, **339**, 659–66.

74. Lee SH, Tai CT, Hsieh MH, *et al.* (2005). Predictors of non-pulmonary vein ectopic beats initiating paroxysmal atrial fibrillation: implication for catheter ablation. *J Am Coll Cardiol*, **46**, 1054–9.

75. Wolf RK, Schneeberger EW, Osterday R, *et al.* (2005). Video-assisted bilateral pulmonary vein isolation and left atrial appendage exclusion for atrial fibrillation. *J Thorac Cardiovasc Surg*, **130**, 797–802.

76. **Edgerton JR, Jackman WM, Mack MJ** (2007). Minimally invasive pulmonary vein isolation and partial autonomic denervation for surgical treatment of atrial fibrillation. *J Interv Card Electrophysiol*, **20**, 89–93.

77. **McClelland JH, Duke D, Reddy R** (2007). Preliminary results of a limited thoracotomy: new approach to treat atrial fibrillation. *J Cardiovasc Electrophysiol*, **18**, 1289–95.

78. **Beyer E, Lee R, Lam BK** (2009). Point: minimally invasive bipolar radiofrequency ablation of lone atrial fibrillation: early multicenter results. *J Thorac Cardiovasc Surg*, **137**, 521–6.

79. **Edgerton JR, Edgerton ZJ, Weaver T**, *et al.* (2008). Minimally invasive pulmonary vein isolation and partial autonomic denervation for surgical treatment of atrial fibrillation. *Ann Thorac Surg*, **86**, 35–8; discussion 39.

80. **Tada H, Ito S, Naito S**, *et al.* (2005). Long-term results of cryoablation with a new cryoprobe to eliminate chronic atrial fibrillation associated with mitral valve disease. *Pacing Clin Electrophysiol*, **28**(Suppl 1), S73–7.

81. **Po SS, Scherlag BJ, Yamanashi WS**, *et al.* (2006). Experimental model for paroxysmal atrial fibrillation arising at the pulmonary vein-atrial junctions. *Heart Rhythm*, **3**, 201–8.

82. **Scherlag BJ, Nakagawa H, Jackman WM**, *et al.* (2005). Electrical stimulation to identify neural elements on the heart: their role in atrial fibrillation. *J Interv Card Electrophysiol*, **13**(Suppl 1), 37–42.

83. **Mounsey JP** (2006). Recovery from vagal denervation and atrial fibrillation inducibility: effects are complex and not always predictable. *Heart Rhythm*, **3**, 709–10.

84. **Oh S, Zhang Y, Bibevski S**, *et al.* (2006). Vagal denervation and atrial fibrillation inducibility: epicardial fat pad ablation does not have long-term effects. *Heart Rhythm*, **3**, 701–8.

85. **Sakamoto S, Schuessler RB, Lee AM**, *et al.* (2010). Vagal denervation and reinnervation after ablation of ganglionated plexi. *J Thorac Cardiovasc Surg*, **139**, 444–52.

86. **Katritsis D, Giazitzoglou E, Sougiannis D**, *et al.* (2008). Anatomic approach for ganglionic plexi ablation in patients with paroxysmal atrial fibrillation. *Am J Cardiol*, **102**, 330–4.

87. **Damiano RJ Jr, Gaynor SL** (2004). Atrial fibrillation ablation during mitral valve surgery using the atricure device. *Oper Tech Thorac Cardiovasc Surg*, **9**, 24–33.

88. **Onorati F, Mariscalco G, Rubino AS**, *et al.* (2011). Impact of lesion sets on mid-term results of surgical ablation procedure for atrial fibrillation. *J Am Coll Cardiol*, **57**, 931–40.

89. **Sternik L, Schaff HV, Luria D**, *et al.* (2011). Left atrial ablation for atrial fibrillation: creating the "box lesion" with a bipolar radiofrequency device. *Tex Heart Inst J*, **38**, 127–31.

90. **Ad N, Henry L, Hunt S** (2011). The concomitant cryosurgical cox-maze procedure using argon based cryoprobes: 12-month results. *J Cardiovasc Surg (Torino)*, **52**, 593–9.

91. **Albage A, Peterffy M, Kallner G** (2011). Learning what works in surgical cryoablation of atrial fibrillation: results of different application techniques and benefits of prospective follow-up. *Interact Cardiovasc Thorac Surg*, **13**(5), 480–4.

92. **Geuzebroek GS, Ballaux PK, van Hemel NM, Kelder JC, Defauw JJ** (2008). Medium-term outcome of different surgical methods to cure atrial fibrillation: is less worse? *Interact Cardiovasc Thorac Surg*, **7**, 201–6.

93. **Reyes G, Benedicto A, Bustamante J**, *et al.* (2009). Restoration of atrial contractility after surgical cryoablation: clinical, electrical and mechanical results. *Interact Cardiovasc Thorac Surg*, **9**, 609–12.

94. **Healey JS, Crystal E, Lamy A**, *et al.* (2005). Left atrial appendage occlusion study (laaos): results of a randomized controlled pilot study of left atrial appendage occlusion during coronary bypass surgery in patients at risk for stroke. *Am Heart J*, **150**, 288–93.

95. **Salzberg SP, Gillinov AM, Anyanwu A, Castillo J, Filsoufi F, Adams DH** (2008). Surgical left atrial appendage occlusion: evaluation of a novel device with magnetic resonance imaging. *Eur J Cardiothorac Surg*, **34**, 766–70

96. Salzberg SP, Plass A, Emmert MY, *et al.* (2010). Left atrial appendage clip occlusion: early clinical results. *J Thorac Cardiovasc Surg*, **139**, 1269–74.

97. Dawson AG, Asopa S, Dunning J (2010). Should patients undergoing cardiac surgery with atrial fibrillation have left atrial appendage exclusion? *Interact Cardiovasc Thorac Surg*, **10**, 306–11.

98. Byrd GD, Prasad SM, Ripplinger CM, *et al.* (2005). Importance of geometry and refractory period in sustaining atrial fibrillation: testing the critical mass hypothesis. *Circulation*, **112**, I7–13.

99. Wiener N, Rosenblueth A (1946). The mathematical formulation of the problem of conduction of impulses in a network of connected excitable elements, specifically in cardiac muscle. *Arch Inst Cardiol Mex*, **16**, 205–65.

100. Cox JL, Canavan TE, Schuessler RB, *et al.* (1991). The surgical treatment of atrial fibrillation. Ii. Intraoperative electrophysiologic mapping and description of the electrophysiologic basis of atrial flutter and atrial fibrillation. *J Thorac Cardiovasc Surg*, **101**, 406–26.

101. Cuculich PS, Wang Y, Lindsay BD, *et al.* (2010). Noninvasive characterization of epicardial activation in humans with diverse atrial fibrillation patterns. *Circulation*, **122**, 1364–72.

102. Ghanem RN, Jia P, Ramanathan C, Ryu K, Markowitz A, Rudy Y (2005). Noninvasive electrocardiographic imaging (ecgi): comparison to intraoperative mapping in patients. *Heart Rhythm*, **2**, 339–54.

103. Ghosh S, Rudy Y (2005). Accuracy of quadratic versus linear interpolation in noninvasive electrocardiographic imaging (ecgi). *Ann Biomed Eng*, **33**, 1187–201.

104. Intini A, Goldstein RN, Jia P, *et al.* (2005). Electrocardiographic imaging (ecgi), a novel diagnostic modality used for mapping of focal left ventricular tachycardia in a young athlete. *Heart Rhythm*, **2**, 1250–2.

105. Ramanathan C, Ghanem RN, Jia P, Ryu K, Rudy Y (2004). Noninvasive electrocardiographic imaging for cardiac electrophysiology and arrhythmia. *Nat Med*, **10**, 422–8.

106. Wang Y, Rudy Y (2006). Application of the method of fundamental solutions to potential-based inverse electrocardiography. *Ann Biomed Eng*, **34**, 1272–88.

107. Rodefeld MD, Branham BH, Schuessler RB, *et al.* (1997). Global electrophysiological mapping of the atrium: computerized three-dimensional mapping system. *Pacing Clin Electrophysiol*, **20**, 2227–36.

108. Barnette AR, Bayly PV, Zhang S, *et al.* (2000). Estimation of 3-d conduction velocity vector fields from cardiac mapping data. *IEEE Trans Biomed Eng*, **47**, 1027–35.

109. Kim KB, Rodefeld MD, Schuessler RB, Cox JL, Boineau JP (1996). Relationship between local atrial fibrillation interval and refractory period in the isolated canine atrium. *Circulation*, **94**, 2961–7.

110. Edgerton JR, Jackman WM, Mack MJ (2009). A new epicardial lesion set for minimal access left atrial maze: the Dallas lesion set. *Ann Thorac Surg*, **88**, 1655–7.

111. Edgerton JR, McClelland JH, Duke D, *et al.* (2009). Minimally invasive surgical ablation of atrial fibrillation: six-month results. *J Thorac Cardiovasc Surg*, **138**, 109–13; discussion 114.

112. Lee R, Kruse J, McCarthy PM (2009). Surgery for atrial fibrillation. *Nat Rev Cardiol*, **6**, 505–13.

Chapter 11

Mechanical circulatory support

William E. Stansfield, Antigone Koliopoulou,
Stephen H. McKellar, and Craig H. Selzman

Introduction

Over the last half-century, mechanical circulatory support (MCS) for the failing heart has provided a compelling, and often dramatic, story of engineering achievement, pioneering physicians, and brave patients (Table 11.1). The 1950s, 1960s, and 1970s saw the transition of MCS from the necessary extension of cardiopulmonary bypass to the development of durable devices. This era was defined by the occasional case followed by design readjustment. In the late 1980s and moving into the 1990s, the surgical principles as well as improved technology allowed wider adoption by major centers. Within the last 20 years, enhanced pumps as well as surgical and medical experience have allowed MCS to become a routine part of the armamentarium for treating heart failure (HF) patients. Most recently, within the last 10 years, there has been a dramatic shift from the use of large, pulsatile left ventricular assist devices (LVADs) to smaller continuous flow (CF) devices. In fact, the Thoratec XVE, one of the most widely used pulsatile devices, is no longer available or supported. Conversely, several CF LVADs are now available to the heart failure community. In this chapter, we will review the current state of MCS for treating advanced heart failure, as well as detail many of the surgically related issues with LVADs.

General indications

Mechanical circulatory support can be used to salvage the cardiogenic shock patient, bridge a suitable patient for transplant (BTT), or device explantation for myocardial recovery (BTR), and provide lifetime use or destination therapy (DT). In addition, there is a gray zone category of patients that have durable LVADs implanted to determine their eligibility for transplant, also called bridge to eligibility or decision (BTD). Although there is some enthusiasm to investigate the role of durable LVADs in a less sick population,[1] most patients receiving durable LVADs are functional New York Heart Association (NYHA) Class IV or patients in Stage D HF. Classic indications for DT, versus BTT, include—but are not limited to—advanced age and significant comorbidities such as advanced diabetes, pulmonary hypertension, renal dysfunction, and recent malignancy.

The Interagency Registry for Mechanically Assisted Circulatory Support (INTERMACS) follows all FDA-approved pump implants and has created a system to define patient

Table 11.1 Historical milestones in mechanical cardiac support

1813	LeGallois recognizes importance of perfusion for organ survival
1937	Demikov sustains animal on artificial pump
1953	Gibbons introduces heart-lung machine
1958	Atsumi develops hydraulic and roller pump models
1958	Liotta designs first TAH prototype
1963	DeBakey implants first LVAD
1964	President Johnson starts the US Artificial Heart Program
1969	Cooley and Liotta team and perform first human TAH implant
1970	Kolff and Jarvik develop Jarvik-7 prototype
1978	First LVAD as a bridge to transplant
1982	First Jarvik-7 implant
1994	FDA approval of the TCI LVAD for BTT
2001	REMATCH published
2008	FDA approves the continuous axial flow HeartMate II for BTT
2010	FDA approves the continuous axial flow HeartMate II for DT
2012	FDA approves the continuous centrifugal flow HeartWare HVAD for BTT
2017	FDA approves the continuous centrifugal flow HeartWare HVAD for DT
2017	FDA approves the continuous centrifugal flow Heart Mate 3 for short-term support, for BTT (CE Mark in 2015)

Table 11.2 INTERMACS categories. Percentage for each profile in 18,987 primary implants from 2006 to 2016　.

Level 1	Critical cardiogenic shock	15%
Level 2	Progressive decline	37%
Level 3	Stable but inotrope dependent	31%
Level 4	Recurrent advanced HF	13%
Level 5	Exertion intolerant	2%
Level 6	Exertion limited	1%
Level 7	Advanced NYHA III	<1%

Adapted from Kirklin et al. (2010) Second INTERMACS annual report: More than 1,000 primary left ventricular assist device implants. The Journal of Heart and Lung Transplantation 29(1):1–10 with permission from Elsevier.

profiles (Table 11.2). The algorithm for the acute cardiogenic shock patient often involves insertion of non-durable pumps (INTERMACS Profile 1). The majority of LVAD patients are those in progressive decline (INTERMACS Profile 2—inotrope dependent with continuing deterioration) and those stable but inotropic dependent (INTERMACS Profile 3). Recent analysis demonstrates a relative flat rate of implants of Profile 1 patients (~15%), but also a progressive decrease in implants for Profile 2 (41–33%), reflecting the poor outcomes associated with ventricular assist device (VAD) implantation with the most ill patients.[2]

Bridge to recovery

Using mechanical circulatory devices to achieve myocardial recovery is best described by the urgency and length of support needed for a given condition. Most commonly, recovery refers to short-term mechanical support, designed specifically to support patients in postcardiotomy shock, large myocardial infarctions with hemodynamic instability, or cardiogenic shock related to myocarditis. In general, these are INTERMACS Level 1 patients that require urgent/emergent support. Ideally, as the acute insult resolves, the heart recovers, and the pump is removed. This category is markedly different than patients with longstanding HF that have durable pumps implanted, are treated medically, and ultimately are able to have sustained recovery with pump removal.

Short-term recovery—Historically, the first line of defense for most patients requiring mechanical support is the intra-aortic balloon pump (IABP). First described in 1968,[3] the IABP has since undergone numerous improvements that facilitate ease of use, including sensing of the cardiac cycle through both pressure transduction and electrocardiogram (EKG) monitoring. The IABP functions specifically to improve coronary blood flow in diastole and to offload the left ventricle during systole. Several studies have used surrogate measures to evaluate the efficacy of IABP counterpulsation versus pharmacologic therapy alone: for example, in the Kaiser Permanente healthcare system in California, hospitals that were more liberal with IABP therapy had lower mortality for myocardial infarction even when controlling for patient characteristics and other procedures like percutaneous coronary intervention (PCI).[4]

The first randomized trial addressing questions regarding the efficacy and safety of the IABP in addition to early revascularization in patients with cardiogenic shock complicating myocardial infraction, the IABP-SHOCK II trial, was conducted between 2009 and 2012 at 40 centers in Germany.[5,6] Six hundred patients were randomized 1:1 to revascularization by PCI with an IABP and optimal medical therapy (Group 1, 300 patients) and to revascularization by PCI with optimal medical management (Group 2, 300 patients). The primary endpoint was 30-day all-cause mortality. At 30 days, mortality was similar among patients in the IABP group and those in the control group. In addition, there was no significant difference in mortality between the group of patients in whom the balloon pump was inserted before revascularization and the group in whom it was inserted after revascularization. The modest effect on cardiac output and the lack of reducing the infarct size could contribute to those findings. The 6-month and 12 month follow-ups showed that the IABP support did not increase survival compared to the control group, supporting the short-term 30-day follow-up data.[7] Importantly, the functional status and the quality of life for survivors of cardiogenic shock were good at 6 and 12 months. Despite early revascularization and optimal medical therapy in both groups, the mortality of cardiogenic shock complicating myocardial infraction is still higher than 50% at 1-year follow-up.

Patients with chronic systolic heart failure who develop cardiogenic shock are physiologically different than patients who develop cardiogenic shock as a complication of an acute myocardial infraction. In chronic heart failure, the ventricular remodeling has taken place. The IABP increases the coronary blood flow and diastolic blood pressure and reduces isovolumetric contraction and ventricular afterload. As such, any increase in stroke volume is a result of better ventricular performance and not augmentation from the device. In chronic heart failure, IABP reduces arterial impedance and the resultant increase in stroke volume may be enough to rescue patients from severe shock.[8] In this patient population, the IABP inserted through the femoral artery or, in the more recent years, through the axillary artery[9] can provide significant support, hemodynamic improvement, and end-organ recovery in the majority of patients with chronic heart failure who develop heart failure exacerbation or cardiogenic shock. If the patient is unable to be weaned from the device, they can safely be bridged to a durable LVAD or heart transplantation.

Newer percutaneous devices seek to provide support above and beyond balloon counterpulsation. In 2008, the FDA-approved the Impella 2.5 (Abiomed, Danvers, MA). This percutaneously placed, 9 French device spans the aortic valve, drawing blood from the left ventricle and ejecting it into the ascending aorta. The device is capable of providing a theoretical maximum flow of 2.5 lpm. It has been widely used to support high-risk PCI after favorable outcomes in the Protect I and Protect II trials.[10] For the treatment of cardiogenic shock, the Impella 2.5 appears comparable to IABP in efficacy.[11] In 2009 the company gained approval for the Impella 5.0. This device provided reasonable support for postcardiotomy shock patients in the RECOVER I study. [12] The primary limitation is a 21 French deployment system, and therefore it is frequently placed intraoperatively through a graft on the ascending aorta. Most recently, in 2012, Abiomed launched the Impella CP, capable of up to 4 lpm of flow, but able to deployed on the same system as the 2.5.

The Tandem Heart Percutaneous Ventricular Assist Device (pVAD, Cardiac Assist, Inc., Pittsburgh, PA) is another commonly utilized percutaneous device. One cannula is placed through the femoral vein crossing the interatrial septum to drain the left atrium and the return 17 Fr cannula perfuses the aortoiliac system. A centrifugal flow device capable of pumping up to 5 L/min is strapped to the patient's thigh. Early results with this device have been reported by Texas Heart Institute.[13] In their series of 117 patients, all had failed therapy with high-dose inotropes, and 80% had inadequate perfusion with both inotrope and IABP. Nearly half the patients were undergoing cardiopulmonary resuscitation (CPR) at the time the devices were placed. The average duration of therapy was 6 days, and survival was 60% at 30 days, and 55% at 6 months. This led the group to conclude that the pVAD was more effective than the combination of IABP and high-dose inotrope therapy.

Operative placement of a temporary ventricular support device allows for optimal positioning of cannulas, with the opportunity for excellent decompression of the heart and high flow rates that are important in larger patients. Standard approaches for postcardiotomy support include full extracorporeal membrane oxygenation (ECMO) support driven by a centrifugal pump such as the CentriMag (Thoratec, Pleasanton, CA) or the Rotaflow (Maquet, Rastatt, Germany). Either pump can alternately be configured for left, right, or biventricular support. The CentriMag was initially FDA approved as a frictionless pump for cardiopulmonary bypass, but its versatility, compact size, and ease of use paved the way for a transition to temporary extracorporeal support. The CentriMag features a magnetically levitated centrifugal rotor that pumps blood through a device without seals, bearings, vents, or valves. The only connections are the inflow and outflow tubing. The CentriMag is currently FDA 510(k) cleared for use in the US in an investigational capacity for short-term left-sided or biventricular support, and is FDA approved for use as a right ventricular assist device for periods of up to 14 days. Results of an initial safety and efficacy study— the CentriMag ventricular assist system (VAS) Pivotal Trial—revealed a favorable survival profile for cardiogenic shock patients. The three arms of the trial included 12 patients treated with the CentriMag as a temporary right ventricular assist device (RVAD) during permanent LVAD placement, 12 patients with postcardiotomy cardiogenic shock, and 14 patients with postmyocardial infarction cardiogenic shock. In this group of 38, nearly half of the patients were alive 30 days after device explant, with a median duration of support of 15 days.[14] The infection rate was 21%, bleeding 5%, and neurologic dysfunction 11%. Although there was concern for hemolysis given the nature of the pump, the observed rate of significant hemolysis was only 5%. Since this initial trial, the CentriMag has been widely adopted and numerous centers have reported success with this system.[15]

One particular advantage to the CentriMag configuration is the ability to align an oxygenator within the circuit to provide full ECMO support. Indeed, ECMO has long been used to provide cardiopulmonary support for both pediatric and adult patients. Using the femoral vessels, either by cut-down or percutaneously, this approach can be readily accomplished for patients in extremis without having to open the chest. As many of the post-MI patients are on multiple anticoagulants and antiplatelet agents, avoiding bleeding issues with sternotomy can be advantageous. If the patient's end-organ function can be reversed and they demonstrate neurologic recovery, the circulation can either be explanted or transitioned to a more durable device. Alternative access involves cannulating the axillary artery by a graft, and the right atrium through the right internal jugular vein. In this fashion, patients can be on full ECMO support, and have ambulatory potential.[16]

Long-term recovery—Use of durable devices to promote recovery of chronic HF patients is often considered the "holy grail" of the advanced HF field. Although frequently discussed, this is a very rare phenomenon. In the first 1,000 LVADs reported to the INTERMACS database, only 63 (2%) were ultimately explanted. Missing, however, in many of the competing outcomes associated with VAD therapy is the fact that few centers actively look for evidence of myocardial recovery. While one can argue about the pathophysiologic semantics of reverse remodeling, remission of heart failure, and myocardial recovery, the fundamental issue is that the advanced heart failure provider has to look for recovery to see it.[17–19]

The two centers with the largest experience are from Berlin and Harefield. The former group has followed over 100 patients that have had pumps removed. Successful pump removal (freedom from reinsertion and transplant for 5 years) is predicted by off-pump echocardiography demonstrating an ejection fraction more than 45% and an end-diastolic dimension less than 55 mm, as well as patients with shorter duration of HF.[20] The Harefield group has reported a two-phase approach to chronic recovery by first reversing pathologic hypertrophy and remodeling with standard HF meds including high-doses of lisinopril, carvedilol, losartan, spironolactone, and digoxin. When weaning, echocardiography demonstrated an LVIDd less than 60 mm, then the second phase of promoting physiologic hypertrophy was initiated by changing the carvedilol to a beta-1 selective agent and adding clenbuterol, a beta-2 agonist.[21] In their latest report using the CF HeartMate II LVAD, 12 of 20 patients met criteria for explantation with 80% of those free from HF at 3 years.[22] Unfortunately, the promising results from this single center have not been able to be reproduced in a more recent multicenter trial using the Harefield protocol where only 1 out of 17 patients were able to have their LVAD explanted.[23] While the reasons for this disparity in results are unclear, differences related to demographics, chronicity of HF, and medication up-titration point to the difficulty of expanding these demanding studies. That said, when a single institution actively engages in intense medical therapy—with biweekly neurohormonal titration—return of left ventricular (LV) function may be present in a larger proportion of patients.[24,25]

Hence, LVAD-induced cardiac recovery is a real but underrecognized phenomenon. Heart failure teams focusing on this group of patients need to look for it, to adopt a "bridge to recovery strategy," and identify the features of the group of patients amenable to cardiac recovery. The University of Utah recovery program identified six independent predictors of cardiac recovery: age less than 50 years; non-ischemic cardiomyopathy; time from cardiac diagnosis less than 2 years; absence of an implantable cardioverter defibrillators (ICD); serum creatinine level 1.2 mg/dL or less; and left ventricular end diastolic diameter (LVEDD) less than 6.5 cm. On the basis of these results, a prognostic score they labeled the INTERMACS Cardiac Recovery Score (I-CARS) was derived.[26] The score ranged from 0 to 9 and three groups with significantly different prognosis were identified: a low probability group (0 to 3); an intermediate probability group (4 to 6); and a high probability group (7 to 9). The cardiac recovery rates applying I-CARS to a bridge to recovery strategy group and in the non-bridge to recovery group yielded cardiac recovery rates of 0%, 4.9%, and 25.4% for patients in the low, intermediate, and high probability categories, respectively.

The remission from Stage D Heart Failure study (RESTAGE-HF, ClinicalTrials.gov NCT01774656) has since been designed to investigate the influence of aggressive medical intervention, including regular testing of underlying function, on selected patients receiving HeartMate II LVADs. The primary outcome is the proportion of patients in whom their LVADs can be removed and remain free from additional mechanical support or transplant for at least 3 years. Importantly, these patients will be rigorously followed with serial imaging to not only better define predictors of explantation, but to also chart the course of durable recovery after LVAD removal. Forty patients have been enrolled and have finished their initial follow-up. The results of the RESTAGE-HF clinical trial are to be published the spring of 2018, and will offer significant insight on this interesting group of patients.

A discussion of medical therapy would be incomplete without mentioning the vast potential of adjuvant biologic therapy to both enhance reverse remodeling and augment contractile function. Several previous attempts at investigating the role of stem cells in LVAD patients have been abandoned by the National Heart, Lung, and Blood Institute (NHLBI) for administrative reasons. That said, individual centers are injecting both autologous (University of Minnesota, ClinicalTrials.gov NCT00869024) and allogeneic mesenchymal stem cells (MSC) in LVAD patients (AHEPA University Hospital, Greece, ClinicalTrials.gov NCT01759212). The NIH-sponsored Cardiothoracic Surgery Network (CTSN) recently reported a 30-patient pilot trial of intramyocardial MSC injection at the time of LVAD placement. There were no safety issues and potential efficacy signals were observed. A follow-up trial with more centers and a recruitment goal of 169 patients is currently in follow-up (CTSN LVAD MPC-II). Adjuvant therapy studies are not limited to stem cells, but also include growth factor (e.g., SDF) and gene (e.g., SERCA2a) based therapies. Cumulatively, the LVAD patient provides a platform that allows for a multitude of creative, biologic interventions that will provide a robust opportunity for future advances in the field.

Bridge to transplant (BTT)

Although the number of adults with end-stage heart disease continues to increase, the number of heart transplants performed annually remains static. In the United States, there have been roughly 2,400 annual transplants for almost 20 years.[27] To help address deaths on the waiting list, the United Network of Organ Sharing adjusted its allocation strategy in 2006, giving higher priority to patients with a poorer prognosis. This change in the allocation formula, together with improving LVAD therapy for patients in end-stage HF, has helped to significantly reduce wait list deaths in recent years.

LVAD therapy has long offered a way for patients to help survive the wait for a suitable donor heart. Even with the nascent LVAD technology available in the early nineties, Frazier and other investigators demonstrated a doubling in survival to transplant for patients treated with LVADs.[28] The device in the study was the pneumatically driven HeartMate IP (Implantable Pusher Plate). The success of the trial mandated that future BTT LVAD trials could no longer be ethically conducted with a medical treatment arm. This study was followed up in 2001 with the next generation pulsatile device—the HeartMate VE, or vented electric assist device.[29] In this group of 280 patients, 71% survived to either transplant or elective device removal. Although the average creatinine and total bilirubin improved significantly for the population as a whole, hepatic and renal dysfunction were two of the most common complications, with bleeding, infection, neurologic dysfunction, and thrombosis following closely behind. Of these complications, infection and bleeding were the most commonly associated with the device itself. Notably, this was one of the first large-scale papers to report on LVAD patients that were able to live with their LVAD outside of the hospital. Of the 280 patients treated with LVAD, 160 met criteria to participate in a "release program," with 115 achieving full outpatient status. All 160 patients in the release program had improved from an NYHA functional class of III or IV to I or II.[29]

Concurrently, improvements to the HeartMate VE were consolidated and integrated in a newer device, the HeartMate XVE. Mechanistically similar, the XVE incorporated numerous engineering refinements to address issues that had led to mechanical failure. The HeartMate Investigators group published their experience after the XVE became widely available. They observed significantly fewer percutaneous lead fractures, fewer inlet valve failures, and fewer bearing fractures. Trends toward less outflow graft kinking and accidental disconnects were also observed.[30] Overall, freedom from major device malfunction improved from 76% at one year for the VE to 97% for the XVE. This durability and reliability helped establish the HeartMate XVE as the dominant device in the US for much of the early twenty-first century.

Continuous flow devices—At the turn of the century, the next generation of device was just beginning preclinical and clinical trials. These axial flow devices included the Jarvik 2000, HeartMate II, Micromed, and the Berlin devices. The HeartMate II first entered clinical use in 2001,[31] and within a few years, a large scale multicenter trial in BTT patients was initiated. In 2007, the HeartMate II Clinical Investigators published the results of the landmark study investigating this device in status I patients as a BTT.[32] Over 130 patients were enrolled, all of whom were on inotropic therapy and/or IABP. By 180 days, 100 patients had reached the principal outcomes of heart transplantation, cardiac recovery, or survival on device. Twenty-five patients died within the 180-day period, five became ineligible for transplantation, and the last three patients had their device replaced with a different device. Actual survival for patients that continued to receive LVAD therapy was 89% at 1 month, 75% at 6 months, and 68% at 1 year. Although the patients could not be randomized with a medical therapy group for reasons of equipoise, it is likely that this survival pattern was considerably better than that which could have been achieved with medical therapy alone. Additionally, most patients reported an improvement of 2–3 NYHA functional classes at the three-month interval. The six-minute walk, Minnesota Living with Heart Failure score, and the Kansas City Cardiomyopathy score were all significantly better in patients receiving LVAD therapy. Moreover, end-organ perfusion was demonstrably improved on LVAD therapy; the average blood urea nitrogen (BUN) and creatinine decreased from 30 to 18 mg/dL, and 1.4 to 1.1 mcg/dL, respectively. The most common complication was perioperative bleeding, followed by stroke. Eight patients had an ischemic stroke and three had a hemorrhagic stroke. Twenty-eight percent (28%) of patients experienced a localized infection, approximately half of these being driveline infections. Unlike in prior LVAD studies, there were no pump pocket infections. Although not compared directly with the HeartMate XVE, the results of this study were powerful enough to establish axial flow as the new standard in mechanical support.

The HeartMate II Investigator group published again in 2009 with greater patient numbers and extended follow-up.[33] At 18 months, 222 of 281 patients that had been listed status 1A or 1B for heart transplant had either undergone transplantation, LVAD removal for cardiac recovery, or had ongoing VAD support. Survival was 72% at 18 months, and 83% of patients had recovered from NYHA Stage IV to Stage I or II. Complication profiles were consistent with those previously reported, including death from sepsis in 4% of patients, stroke in 6% of patients, and right heart failure in 3% of patients. Deaths directly attributable to the LVAD totaled 3%, including pump thrombosis, kinking of the inflow graft in implantation, disconnect of the outflow graft, and driveline fracture with power loss. This study helped further cement axial or CF as the new standard in left ventricular assist technology.

One of the criticisms of the axial flow devices is that they contain bearings, and this is a potential source of thrombosis, device wear, and shearing of blood components like the von Willebrand factor (vWF) multimer. To address these design issues, the newest generation of devices are centrifugal flow, using a magnetically levitated impeller—conceptually identical to the CentriMag. This allows for a bearingless device with zero wear and possibly less thrombosis risk. The two most commonly implanted centrifugal pumps to date include the DuraHeart (Terumo Heart, Inc, Ann Arbor, MI), and the HeartWare HVAD (HeartWare Intl, Framingham, MA). European centers have achieved greater experience with the DuraHeart, and have published their trial experience and early postmarket surveillance data.[34] The study population included 68 patients with heart failure that had been listed for heart transplant; the first 33 patients were part of the European multicenter clinical trial and the next 35 were from the postmarket launch surveillance. Adverse event rates were comparable to those of axial flow devices. Bleeding requiring surgery was less than expected in axial flow support, while driveline and pocket infection were comparable. Overall neurological events were higher than expected for axial flow devices at 0.56 per patient year of support, with a high rate of fatal hemorrhagic stroke. This was recognized early in the trial and the anticoagulation regimen was reduced.[34]

The HeartWare HVAD gained rapid popularity in part because of its small size. Although it uses the same blood acceleration principle as the DuraHeart, its overall displacement is small enough to allow the body of the pump to be placed intrapericardially, thus avoiding the need for a preperitoneal pocket.[35] The ADVANCE BTT trial, published in 2012, enrolled 140 patients in 30 centers. ADVANCE demonstrated that 92% of the patients successfully made it to transplant or survived to 6 months. The adverse event profile was favorable compared to an INTERMACS propensity matched cohort. Patients had a marked improvement in functional capacity and quality of life that matched those obtained with heart transplant.[36] Initial concerns with stroke incidence were addressed halfway through recruitment in the trial with an improved ventricular coring device and a sintered inflow cannula. This decreased ischemic strokes with permanent deficits by nearly half.[37] FDA approval of the HVAD for BTT in 2012 allowed widespread use of both the HVAD and the HeartMate II in North American BTT patients.

The adverse clinical events related to mechanical circulatory support, infection, neurologic complications, and pump thrombosis are pushing the field toward innovation and engineering improvements. The HeartMate 3 is a new centrifugal flow pump engineered to optimize fluid dynamics. It involves a magnetically levitated rotor and wide blood-flow passages the are designed with the intent to reduce blood shear stress exposure. In addition, the wide blood-flow passages facilitate rapid rotor speed changes, allowing for the introduction of an artificial pulse with intend to disrupt regions of stasis within the pump and provide a degree of native pulsatility. Initial studies in Europe allowed for CE Mark approval.[38] In the United States, The Multicenter Study of MagLev Technology in patients undergoing mechanical circulatory support therapy with Heart Mate3 (MOMENTUM 3) trial began in September 2014. It has as primary objective to evaluate the safety and effectiveness of the HM3 Left Ventricular Assist System by demonstrating non-inferiority to the HeartMate II. Secondary objective includes the assessment of adverse events, quality of life, functional status, device malfunction rates. The study population includes a short-term cohort (6-month follow-up) and a long-term cohort of a total of 1,028 patients for evaluation of the secondary end-points of pump replacement at 2 years.[39]

The 6-month report demonstrated that the HeartMate 3 was associated with a higher rate of survival free of disabling stroke or survival free of reoperation to replace or remove the device.[40] The hemocompatibility profile of the HeartMate 3 was superior and was associated with the absence of medically or surgically managed pump thrombosis and marked reduction in non-disabling strokes. In 289 patients, survival free of any hemocompatibility related clinical adverse events was achieved in 69% of the HM3 group and in 55% of the HMII group ($P = 0.012$). There was no difference between the two left ventricular assist system (LVAS) in disabling strokes, which typically represent a devastating non-surgical bleeding complication.[41] The results of two-year follow-up will be published in 2018.

Biventricular support—Patients requiring biventricular support can be categorized in two classes: those requiring temporary support during the placement of a durable LVAD and those requiring long-term biventricular support. The former group often utilizes an extracorporal pump (i.e., CentriMag or Thoratec percutaneous ventricular assist device (PVAD)) in the hope that LVAD support will satisfactorily unload the pulmonary circulation and thus allow the RVAD to be removed within a relatively short-period of time (days–weeks). In an INTERMACS report of 10,542 patients, 579 patients required biventricular support.[42] Although it is difficult to discern if some of these patients only required short-term RVADs, it is thought that 5–10% of HF patients will require this level of support. The Thoratec paracorporeal or intracorporeal VADs are the most commonly used devices for this situation. More recently, use of tandem CF devices—one for the RV, the other for the LV—has been successfully reported with both the HeartWare and Jarvik devices.[43,44]

In the latest INTERMACS report, 396 total artificial hearts (TAH) were reportedly implanted with a 12-month survival less than 60%.[2] Although used somewhat rarely, the TAH—its development and use—has played a vital role in the history of mechanical support (Table 11.1).[45] The most complete set of data on the Cardiowest comes from Copeland and his colleagues from University of Arizona.[46] Five centers enrolled 130 patients in a prospective, non-randomized study from 1993 to 2002. Nearly 80% of patients receiving the Cardiowest survived to transplant compared with only 46% in the control group. The overall one-year survival rate of patients receiving TAH was 70% compared to 31% of controls. In comparing the 1- and 5-year survival rates in patients who received an organic transplant, those bridged to transplant with the TAH group had 86% and 64% survival rates, respectively, while the controls were 69% and 34%, respectively. As would be expected, infection and bleeding were the most common adverse early events. However, only two patients died secondary to these complications. Ultimately, this study provides reassuring evidence for the potential use and standardization of the TAH as a successful means to bridge patients to transplantation with improved survival rates and improved outcomes in quality of life. This latter point has become even less of an issue, as a portable driver is now available.

Destination therapy (DT)

Fundamentally, destination therapy is an evolution of bridge to transplant. BTT was designed to provide life-sustaining support for patients awaiting transplantation. To even consider a device as a permanent therapy for a patient, a device must enable a patient to be discharged from the hospital. At minimum, it must be implantable, it must grant the patient mobility, and must be reasonably straightforward to care for and manage. Device requirements are further complicated by the nature of the DT patient population. Because they are not transplant candidates, they are either older than, or have more comorbidities than, the BTT population. In the mid to late 1990s, device technology matured to the point where clinical trials of devices for DT could begin. With the publication of the Randomized Evaluation of Mechanical Assistance for the Treatment of Congestive Heart Failure (REMATCH) in 2001, DT therapy began in earnest.

From 1998 to 2001, 129 patients with NYHA Stage IV heart disease that were not eligible for transplantation were randomized to either optimal medical management or LVAD therapy with the HeartMate VE vented electrical device. The survival benefit of LVAD therapy was both statistically significant and clinically relevant: LVAD patients had a 48% reduction in the risk of death from any cause compared to optimal medical therapy. Quality of life was also assessed with numerous measures, with most demonstrating a significant improvement over medical therapy. Perhaps most importantly, those patients treated with LVAD achieved on average a NYHA level II, while those treated medically remained level IV. Despite this incredible survival advantage, LVAD therapy was associated with several major limitations including an infection rate of 28% by 3 months and a bleeding rate of 42% at 6 months. Device failure among patients that lived 24 months was 35%. The neurologic dysfunction rate, including stroke, TIA, and encephalopathy, was 0.39 events per patient year, approximately 4.35 times that of the medical group.[47] Summarily, REMATCH was the first major study to demonstrate the viability of LVADs as a meaningful therapeutic option for severe heart failure patients, and in doing so, set the minimum criteria for DT VAD therapy (Figure 11.1).

In 2005, the four largest centers from the Thoratec DT registry pooled their results from 2003 and 2004 and reported significantly improved results relative to REMATCH, using the HeartMate XVE device. They demonstrated less neurologic dysfunction, fewer infections, less bleeding, and overall improved survival, reporting a 40% reduction in mortality relative to the REMATCH LVAD therapy group.[48] These improvements were likely related to the institutional experience at these high-volume centers, as well as some technical modifications to the HeartMate device.

By establishing a clear superiority of LVAD over optimal medical management for end-stage heart failure patients, REMATCH has redefined the way in which new devices are trialed for DT. Most recently, the CF HeartMate II was compared to its predecessor in a 2:1 head-to-head trial for DT.[49] Similar 1- and 2-year survival with the XVE during REMATCH was observed (55% and 24%, respectively). Comparatively, HM II survival at 1 and 2 years was markedly improved (68% and 58%, respectively). Of the patients surviving 2 years in the pulsatile flow group, 18 had had their device changed to a HeartMate II during the trial for reasons of mechanical failure or infection. Quality of life was also better in the HMII arm of the trial, with 40 (of 50 surviving) patients achieving a NYHA functional class of I or II at 24 months. By comparison, only one of the 55 patients implanted with the HM XVE was both still alive and still had his device at 2 years. All of the

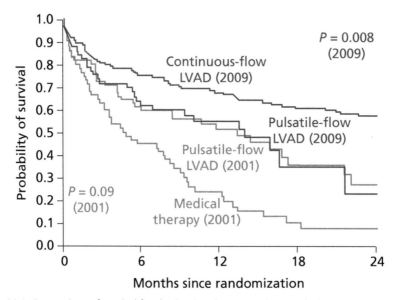

Figure 11.1 Comparison of survival for destination therapy patients with the HeartMate I (pulsatile) and HeartMate II (continuous flow) pumps.

Reproduced from Fang JC. Rise of the machines--left ventricular assist devices as permanent therapy for advanced heart failure. *N Engl J Med* 2009;361:2282–5 © 2009 Massachusetts Medical Society. Reprinted with permission from the Massachusetts Medical Society.

complications reviewed favored patients with the HM II CF device, with significant benefits in pump replacement, infection including sepsis, right heart failure requiring extended inotropic support, arrhythmia, respiratory failure, and renal failure. Thrombosis was the only major comorbidity in which the CF LVAD was worse, with 4% of patients having a thrombosis event, whereas none of the pulsatile flow patients experienced thrombosis. Overall, the HeartMate II has demonstrated a clear benefit over the HeartMate XVE, and has evolved to become the new standard to beat.

The ENDURANCE trial randomized 297 patients ineligible for transplant from 48 US sties to either a centrifugal flow LVAD (HeartWare, study device) or an axial flow LVAD (Heart Mate II, control device).[50] The 2-year follow-up analysis of the primary end point showed that the study device was non-inferior to the control device with respect to survival free from disabling stroke or need for device replacement. There was also a sustained improvement in functional and quality-of-life measures. Importantly, the HVAD had more strokes, predominately hemorrhagic, occurring within the first 6 months, after which the rate of stroke decreased (29.7% *vs.* 12.1%, *P* <0.001). Changes in the protocol to mandate strict blood pressure control with a mean arterial pressure of 90 mmHg or lower was accompanied with a subsequent 34% decrease of risk of stroke among those patients. Finally, no significant difference between the two devices in the rate of pump exchange because of device thrombosis was identified. Based on results from the ENDURANCE and ENDURANCE Supplement trials (which enrolled 465 patients to be followed up for a total of 5 years) the FDA approved the HeartWare HVAD system for destination therapy in patients for whom subsequent transplantation is not planned, in September 2017.

Extended survival with the current and newer generation of cardiac assist devices, HeartWare, and HM3, has helped providers to the following terms: bridge to decision (BTD) or bridge to candidacy (BTC). This is a subset of destination therapy patients that are not too old to receive a transplant, but instead are prohibited by comorbidities that are consequences of their heart failure. With the rehabilitation facilitated by their device, and the improved end-organ perfusion they achieve, they are able to reach a state where they may actually be considered for transplant. Most commonly, this has been observed in patients with pulmonary hypertension refractory to inotropic challenge. Several papers have documented regression of pulmonary hypertension with chronic unloading of the left atrium by assist device, to the point where transplant becomes feasible.[51,52]

Surgical implantation

Despite the variety of pumps available, issues related to surgical implantation remain the same. That is, most devices use the apex of the left ventricle as the inflow site to the pump that subsequently gives off an outflow graft to the aorta, thus bypassing the ailing left ventricle. Herein, we will describe some of the issues related to implantation of LVADs. Although there are many types of devices currently available, the general approaches are similar.

Patient selection—Although most patients listed for transplant are at some level candidates for mechanical circulatory support, there are several compelling issues that might lead a group to go straight to transplant. These include multiple reoperations, congenital heart anomalies, restrictive heart disease with small ventricles, and other surgical issues (i.e., previous pericardectomy). These are all relative contraindications. The most important contraindication to LVAD therapy is the ability of the right ventricle to support LVAD flows. Although it is not unusual (<10% of implants) to require temporary RVAD support at the time of LVAD, if one has a high suspicion of RV failure (severe dysfunction, low right ventricular stroke work index, high right atrial pressures, low pulmonary artery pulsatility index)[53,54] then the best options are either biventricular assist devices, total artificial heart, or transplant. The emergence of destination therapy has a created a different set of issues as many of these patients are older with end-organ dysfunction and seen as last-option or even heroic implants. Rigorous assessment of their ability to survive and thrive after LVAD needs to be seriously evaluated by a multidisciplinary team.

Perioperative considerations—Standard cardiac surgery anesthesia is utilized with LVAD procedures. Although most procedures are done with the use of cardiopulmonary bypass, many centers will maintain low tidal volume ventilation during bypass to theoretically decrease post-pump pulmonary vascular resistance. Antifibrinolytic therapy is usually used and blood products are used as indicated. Some centers rely heavily on thromboelastography and more recently rotational thromboelastometry (ROTEM) for guiding replacement therapy.

Most LVAD procedures can be performed without systemic cooling and routine measures for cardiopulmonary bypass are used. As most of the HF patients are fluid overloaded, perfusionists should utilize ultrafiltration, if possible, and avoid excessive hemodilution. Cell saver should be replaced with concomitant, liberal use of fresh frozen plasma (2–3:1). In patients with heparin-induced thrombocytopenia, successful LVAD implants have been performed, albeit with additional risk, using alternative anticoagulants such as bivalrudin or argatroban.[55] Additional strategies to minimize perioperative bleeding complications include the use of desmopressin acetate (DDAVP), discontinuation of aspirin for elective LVAD placement, a strong focus on a short pump run, synthetic factor replacement, and delayed primary closure, although none of these strategies have been studied explicitly.

Postinsertion attention is focused on decreasing pulmonary vascular resistance and protecting right ventricular function. Some centers will routinely use nitric oxide or inhaled epoprostenol on each case. All efforts are aimed at reducing transfusion requirements as well as avoidance of hypoxia, hypercarbia, and acidosis. Several preoperative risk factors are associated with right ventricular (RV) failure including female sex, non-ischemic cardiomyopathies, elevated central venous pressure, right ventricular stroke work index, and previous cardiac surgery.[56,57] More sophisticated echocardiographic measurements, including an increased RV-to-LV end-diastolic ratio (>0.72) can also predict postoperative RV failure.[58] Intravenous pulmonary vasodilators are used routinely, including nitrates and phosphodiesterase inhibitors (milrinone). Inotropic support for the right ventricle is also routinely used (milrinone, epinephrine, dobutamine). There is recent enthusiasm to use sildenafil both pre- and perioperatively in these patients. For very sick right ventricles, it might be necessary to support the RV mechanically for several days (e.g., RVAD with CentriMag device).

Surgical implantation—Although individual surgeons and centers have different methods of inserting the device, the fundamental concepts outlined remain true for all. The sequence of implantation can vary also from patient to patient depending on their particular situation.

The majority of LVADs are placed in the supine position standard to any cardiac surgery operation. This standard position can be used for several non-sternotomy approaches as well. For example, some pumps (notably the Jarvik 2000) have been placed through a left subcostal incision with the outflow to the supracoeliac aorta.[59] Others have used a left subcostal incision and tunneled the outflow graft to the ascending aorta through a counterincision in the right third interspace or mini upper sternotomy. A left thorocotomy approach can alternatively have the outflow graft anastomosis to the descending thoracic aorta. This latter technique has been most often used with the off-cardiopulmonary by-pass approach using the Jarvik 2000 LVAD, but has been successfully used for several other small pumps as well.[60] In these cases, the patient should be positioned in the left lateral position with the hips turned back to give access to the left femoral vessels if needed.

After anesthesia, monitoring lines, and positioning, median sternotomy is performed. In many cases, this will be a redo-sternotomy. If the patient has a hostile mediastinum (multiple surgeries, recent surgery, congenital heart disease, right ventricular enlargement, or substernal grafts), alternative forms of cannulation for cardiopulmonary bypass should be considered. Arterial inflow can be accessed through the subclavian or femoral arteries (we usually sew a side-armed graft on the vessel) and venous return is through a long femoral venous cannula placed under transesophageal echocardiography (TEE) guidance with the tip in the superior vena cava (SVC).

Before full heparinization and sternal re-entry, many will try to develop the LVAD pocket. For the HeartMate 2 device, full creation of the pocket is made easier when the sternum is open. Two schools of thought regarding the pocket creation exist: within the preperitoneal space or between the posterior rectus sheath and the rectus abdominis muscle. The latter was routinely performed with the larger pumps to avoid peritoneal erosion. That said, with the smaller pumps, requiring smaller pockets, many have gone back to the preperitoneal approach just under the diaphragm. Most will take down the anterior slip of diaphragm laterally to allow the inflow cannula to orient correctly. Either electrocautery or a vascular endoscopic stapler can be used to divide this muscle. Be sure to check this transection line prior to closure as it often will have points of bleeding. With the emergence of the HeartWare, Jarvik, HeartMate 3, and other small size pumps, each of which can be placed inside the pericardium, many of the pocket problems will become obsolete.

The pericardium is opened, and the LV apex is identified. One of the nice features of the HeartMate II device is its inflow elbow. Theoretically this allows good placement without having to go as lateral on the pocket. The prospective sight for driveline exit is then identified. This is usually in the typical right upper quadrant position but can vary according to the patient's need. A tunneling device is then brought through the rectus sheath. Enough subfascial dissection should be performed on the right side to allow for tension-free closure as well as space for driveline exit.

On the backtable, the pump is prepared according to the device manufacturer. Some outflow grafts need to be prepared. Some devices require some reinforcement as well. Others are taken out of the package and are ready to go. It is beyond the scope of this review to discuss individual pump preparation especially with the excellent training provided by all the respective VAD companies with regards to their specific pump.

Depending on the pump, the outflow anastomosis can either be done before or after the inflow. The outflow graft is stretched and cut to size with a slight bevel. A side-biting aortic cross-clamp is placed and an aortotomy is created. Many will round the two ends of the aortotomy with a 4.5 mm proximal coronary punch. The distal anastomosis is sewn with any number of techniques. Some will place individual pledgeted mattresses or running sutures over felt or pericardium. After removal of the cross clamp, hemostasis is checked, and repair sutures are placed as necessary.

Aortic and right atrial cannulas are placed and, often, an aortic vent needle as well. The patient is placed on cardiopulmonary bypass and maintained at normothermia. As mentioned before, it is possible, even from a sternotomy approach, to perform this without the use of cardiopulmonary bypass.[61] That said, most centers perform the remainder of the operation on bypass. The heart is elevated with the assistance of laparotomy packs in the posterior mediastinum. The left anterior descending artery is identified, thus marking the intraventricular grove. With larger ventricles, identification of the apex is fairly straightforward. On smaller ventricles, some will core a little more anterior to provide a reasonable angle. Conversely, with the newer intrapericardial devices, some will take a more inferior and posterior approach. The core is excised, the LV cavity is inspected, and further debridement of trabeculae or thrombus is performed as necessary. The alignment along the interventricular septum is examined. Large plegeted sutures are then passed full thickness. Sutures are then mattressed to get the edge of the epicardium. Usually 12–14 sutures are required, although some use less. These are attached to the sewing ring and tied. Many surgeons will put a very thin layer of BioGlue over the insertion site and pledgets.

The prospective driveline site is cored and the tunneling device is passed subcutaneously and then through the rectus at the inferior margin of the incision. The controller and pump are brought to the table. The driveline is passed and connected to the controller. During this time, we insufflate CO_2 into the LV cavity to evacuate air. The inflow stabilizing ring is removed. The LV cavity is inspected to make sure the inflow is clear. The inflow cannula is inserted and secured with the sewing rings suture. Tie-Bands can also be placed to further secure the cannula. Others will place several large suture ties.

At this point, the anesthesiologist and perfusionist have had ample timing for weaning. Inotropic support is going, full ventilation ensues, calcium is repleted, and the acid-base status is corrected. Some will routinely use nitric oxide or inhaled epoprostenol to assist with reduction of pulmonary vascular resistance. The aortic graft is backbled. Volume is left in the heart and the outflow cap is loosened to help de-air the ventricle. The unkinked outflow graft is then connected. The patient is weaned off cardiopulmonary bypass or to 1–2 liters/minute of flow. The LVAD is started at its lowest RPM with the aortic clamp on to continue de-airing. With the aortic vent on, the outflow graft clamp is removed. Often there is a small rush of air bubbles visible on the long axis view of the TEE that is air around the clamp. Usually this last for less than 5 seconds and is removed with the aortic vent.

LVAD flows are slowly increased while monitoring right-sided function, pressures, and septal motion. Often no flow will be recorded on the monitor, but the patient will be doing just fine. Avoid the temptation to quickly increase RPMs to get high flows. Most centers will leave the operating room without full decompression as long the hemodynamics are suitable. Often the "final" settings on the pump are often not made for days after the implant. Protamine is administered, and all of the cannulas are removed. Chest and mediastinal tubes are placed.

Final position of the LVAD within the chest, especially without the retractor, should be viewed under TEE. In particular, the inflow cannula should be directed slightly posterior toward the mitral valve. TEE is crucial for this procedure. In addition to evaluating cannula location, TEE can identify valvular problems (see next). Importantly, a bubble study needs to be performed with the LVAD on in order to identify a patent foramen ovale (PFO). With heart failure patients with high left-sided pressures, these defects can be difficult to detect until the left side is decompressed. If identified, the PFO needs to be repaired.

Some centers have advocated an aggressive policy of leaving the chest open for 1 day to allow for stability prior to chest closure. Our approach is to leave the chest open if there are ongoing bleeding concerns or if we are worried about RV functional decline associated with sternal compression. Leaving the sternum open can be an excellent strategy for the marginal patients.

At the beginning of 2011, an increase on the incidence of pump thrombosis with the Heart Mate 2[62] led to the PREVENtion of Heart Mate II Pump Thrombosis Through Clinical Management (PREVENT) prospective, multicenter, non-randomized study. Strict adherence to surgical recommendations, anticoagulation, and antiplatelet management, pump speed management, and blood pressure control with the Heart Mate II implantation demonstrated lower rate of confirmed pump thrombosis at 3 months post implant (2.9%), lower than what was hypothesized (4%).[63]

For BTT, it is helpful to prepare for the re-entry that will occur with transplant. For starters, attention to spacing of the aortic cannulation site and outflow graft can help leave space for recannulation, aortic cross clamp, and a cuff of sewable aorta. Some will place vessel loops around the SVC and inferior vena cava (IVC) to allow for the identification. We have done this with some reoperative LVAD patients, yet, if possible, we try not to create dissection planes if not necessary. We take a piece of spare graft to cover the outflow graft from the edge of the bend relief to the aorta. We then place a piece of 1 mm GoreTex to the base of the pericardium on the left side where it joins the diaphragm and use interrupted sutures to reconstruct the pericardium and isolate the LVAD. In particular, we try to separate the left lung from the device as this can be quite traumatic at the time of explant. Other barrier products (CorMatrix) can also be used to help with transplant reentry.

Increasingly, VAD surgeons are tunneling further through the abdomen in order to bury more of the driveline. One approach is to bring the driveline out first through a counterincision in the right upper quadrant and then retunnel to exit in the patient's left upper quadrant. Alternately, the counterincision can be made in the right lower quadrant, and the driveline then brought back up and out in the right upper quadrant. Thoratec recently presented registry results for patients in which the entire velour component of the driveline is buried, showing an 85% freedom from driveline infection at two years compared to 65% in the HeartMate II DT Trial. [64] At operation, we use two #1 Prolene sutures to provide traction relief around the exit site that are removed 4–6 weeks after surgery.

Other considerations

Several issues require additional commentary that can complicate what often can be a very straightforward operation.

- *Coronary artery disease and prior grafts*: Coronary artery disease for LVAD patients is mostly related to the right ventricle. In a right dominant system with significant right coronary artery (RCA) disease, a bypass graft to that coronary would be advisable. If possible, protect all patent grafts at the time of reentry.

- *Valvular disease*: Many patients have either had prior valve operations or have concomitant and significant valvular disease. The risks and benefits of additional valve procedures remain controversial.[65] Some general, but valve-specific guidelines include:

  - *Aortic stenosis*: Generally, not a problem and can be left alone.
  - *Aortic insufficiency*: Needs to be fixed if anything more than mild. Options include bioprosthetic aortic valve replacement (AVR), oversewing the valve with a Hemashield patch, and approximation of the Nodes of Arantius.[66] The particular option is debatable between multiple centers. Although there is much enthusiasm for the relatively ease of oversewing the valve, this makes the patient completely LVAD dependent for LV ejection.

  - *Prosthetic AVR*: No problem if bioprosthetic; currently no data on what to do with mechanical AVR. Some think it would be best to oversew or replace with a bioprosthetic (especially if DT or BTR). The sandwich plug technique is also a simple, safe, and effective way to close the valve.[67] Others might consider leaving it in place.

  - *Mitral stenosis*: This needs to be repaired to allow for LV inflow. Options include tissue valve replacement or, if amenable, valvuloplasty.

  - *Mitral regurgitation*: Mitral valve repair can be done at the time of implantation either transatrially with placement of a mitral annuloplasty ring, or an Alfieri stitch can be placed through the ventriculotomy. Valve repair has been shown to assist with decreasing pulmonary vascular resistance,[68] but to date there is no conclusive evidence that overall outcomes are improved with repair. This may be most beneficial in bridge to transplant (or BTC) patients with high pulmonary vascular resistance.

- *Prior mitral valve replacement (MVR)*: Can be left in place.
- *Tricuspid regurgitation*: Some centers have demonstrated improved outcomes with tricuspid valve annuloplasty or replacement in the setting of moderate to severe regurgitation[69] and/or annular dilatation (>4.2 cm) at time of LVAD implantation.[70] Other centers have been unable to demonstrate similarly conclusive findings,[71] so the standard of care is yet to be defined.

- *Anticoagulation*: Most centers will administer warfarin when the patient is extubated and taking oral medications with an ultimate goal of 2.0–3.0. If a delay in anticoagulation is anticipated, heparin is administered. Some patients with the HeartMate II LVAD have been successfully managed either off coumadin or with lower target INRs.[72] All patients receive aspirin, either low- or high-dose. Many will add other antiplatelet agents such as dipyridamole or clopidogrel. Some centers will also use outpatient thromboelastography to help drive their therapy. The intensity of anticoagulation has recently come under increased scrutiny in the VAD community. Recently, three major implant centers published findings of dramatically increased pump thrombosis in the HeartMate II device. At 18 months, thrombosis rates increased from 5% in 2011 to 15% in 2013.[62] Until the reasons for this finding are further clarified, clinicians may return to erring on the side of more anticoagulation. More concerning, these findings have led some centers to slow recruitment into trials of early LVAD therapy for Stage IIIB heart failure patients.

- Other circumstances can alter surgical strategies and need to be planned for including previous heart operations, congenital heart disease, and prior ventricular reconstruction.

Importantly, the success of the LVAD implantation is more than the technical performance of the operative procedure. Judicious preoperative evaluation and preparation must be combined with vigilant postoperative management, both for the usual issues in the intensive care unit, as well as those as an outpatient. We cannot overstate the importance of an active and engaged multidisciplinary team.

Complications

Advances in patient management, as well as technical advances in miniaturization, pump, efficiency, and battery power have made LVAD therapy safer and more applicable to a wider range of patients than ever before. Still, LVAD therapy continues to be associated with significant morbidity and mortality. Table 11.3 lists some of the major adverse events and their general incidence based on the recent HeartMate II and HeartWare CF device data.[32,35,49] The operative mortality for these patients ranges between 2% and 30%, mostly dependent on the INTERMACS level of the patient as well as if the device is placed for

Table 11.3 Common adverse events associated with LVAD therapy

Infection	
LVAD related	18–35%
Non-LVAD related	14–46%
Neurologic dysfunction	
Stroke (ischemic or hemorrhagic)	8–18%
Other (TIA)	5–17%
Bleeding requiring reoperation	15%
Right heart failure	
Prolonged inotropes	20–30%
RVAD	3–5%
Pump replacement	7–10%
Hepatic dysfunction	3%
Renal dysfunction	8–15%

BTT or DT. Well-known complications include bleeding requiring reoperation or transfusion, neurologic events including stroke (both ischemic and hemorrhagic), infections (LVAD related, and remote), arrhythmia, respiratory failure, renal failure, hepatic dysfunction, hemolysis, pump thrombosis, and rehospitalization. In addition, many of these patients will be readmitted for heart failure as diuretic and right ventricular dysfunction is managed.

Several particular intraoperative complications should be noted. Foremost is right ventricular failure. There is a trend by many centers to take an aggressive approach for temporary RVAD support. Rather than leave the operative suite on high-doses of multiple inotropes and vasoconstrictors, many would rather place a temporary RVAD to allow for hemodynamics and coagulopathic stabilization. This pump can usually be removed within 5 days. Another potentially catastrophic intraoperative complication is related to air embolism. Although some air is to be expected, especially as pumping is initiated, persistent air entrainment should lead to suspicion for apical disruption of the inflow cannula.

Three particular long-term complications are becoming more problematic as more patients are being supported and for longer periods of time:

1. *Aortic insufficiency*: The native aortic valve is under a different pattern of shear stress with CF valves and is prone to develop leaflet fusion and hemodynamically significant aortic insufficiency.[73] As just discussed, an aggressive approach to aortic valve pathology is important, especially with long-term use patients. Postoperatively, there is evidence to suggest that aggressive blood pressure control and intermittent aortic

valve opening may decrease the progression of aortic insufficiency (in addition to decreasing the frequency of neurologic events).[74] For symptomatic severe aortic insufficiency, reoperation for valve closure, valve replacement, and the use of transcatheter valve replacement have been shown to be reasonable and effective.[75]

2. *Acquired von Willebrand syndrome*: As mentioned previously, axial flow is associated with the development of acquired von Willebrand syndrome.[76] The breakdown of the vWF multimers appears to be one of many different factors associated with major bleeding issues including subarachnoid hemorrhages, epistaxsis, and importantly, gastrointestinal bleeding.[77,78] HeartMate 2 and HeartWare have shown the same degree of vWF factor brake down and large multimers loss. However, the HeartMate 3 centrifugal pumps demonstrated a significantly lower level of high-molecular-weight multimers degradation compared with the Heart Mate II. This finding did not translate to functional difference in von Willebrand factor (VWF) activity between these devices.[79] How bleeding and thrombotic complications will be affected by the engineering changes of the HeartMate3 will require further study.

3. *Driveline infections*: As the durability of the actual pump has increased, more attention has focused on issues related to the power source. Driveline infections as well as cable damage are important causes for pump exchange, are associated with worse transplant outcomes, and cause significant psychologic stress on the patients. Transcutaneous energy transfer technology is still actively being investigated. The skull pedestal implant of the Jarvik 2000 LVAD is one novel approach to dealing with driveline issues that has been particularly successful in over 110 European patients.

The future

The evolution of technology, along with the development of dedicated care teams, has allowed LVAD therapy to become an integral and highly effective component of any advanced HF center. Perioperative and long-term medical strategies will continue to be refined. Peripheral components are becoming lighter, and more user-friendly. Removing the driveline component of VADs, as demonstrated by the actively used skull pedestal implant with the Jarvik 2000, or the ongoing development of transcutaneous energy technology will provide even more freedom for patients that require these pumps for lifetime use. The next generation of pumps from multiple different vendors will be smaller and more efficient (i.e., CircuLite, HeartMate 3, HeartWare's MVAD).[80] This detail will be important as the field moves to implant mechanical devices in patients that are less ill and perhaps do not require full replacement of their cardiac output. Broadening indications to class III patients will necessitate pumps that can be placed, and potentially removed, less invasively. This latter point is further highlighted in the enthusiasm to promote myocardial recovery. Device technology has progressed so much that providers and patients feel comfortable with its routine use (not to say improvements to the morbidity profile are not needed). As such, less attention will be focused on the study of the pumps, but rather on the study of the heart. Indeed, mechanical circulatory device companies have traditionally focused on whether or not their pump will work or not; how they handle blood, or how long the pump will last. With newer, smaller devices, physicians will again be able to focus on the biology of the heart and use these pumps to provide pressure/volume relief while simultaneously delivering adjuvant biologic therapies. This latter direction within the field remains in its infancy.

References

1. **Meyns BP, Simon A, Klotz S,** *et al.* (2011). Clinical benefits of partial circulatory support in New York Heart Association Class IIIB and Early Class IV patients. *Eur J Cardiothorac Surg*, **39**, 693–8.

2. **Kirklin JK, Pagani FD, Kormos RL,** *et al.* (2017). Eighth annual INTERMACS report: special focus on framing the impact of adverse events. *J Heart Lung Transplant*, **36**, 1080–6.

3. **Laird JD, Madras PN, Jones RT,** *et al.* (1968). Theoretical and experimental analysis of the intra-aortic balloon pump. *Trans Am Soc Artif Intern Organs*, **14**, 338–43.

4. **Chen EW** (2003). Relation between hospital intra-aortic balloon counterpulsation volume and mortality in acute myocardial infarction complicated by cardiogenic shock. *Circulation*, **108**, 951–7.

5. **Thiele H, Schuler G, Neumann FJ,** *et al.* (2012). Intraaortic balloon counterpulsation in acute myocardial infarction complicated by cardiogenic shock: design and rationale of the Intraaortic Balloon Pump in Cardiogenic Shock II (IABP-SHOCK II) trial. *Am Heart J*, **163**, 938–45.

6. **Thiele H, Zeymer U, Neumann FJ,** *et al.* (2012). Intraaortic balloon support for myocardial infarction with cardiogenic shock. *N Engl J Med*, **367**, 1287–96.

7. **Thiele H, Zeymer U, Neumann FJ,** *et al.* (2013). Intra-aortic balloon counterpulsation in acute myocardial infarction complicated by cardiogenic shock (IABP-SHOCK II): final 12 month results of a randomised, open-label trial. *Lancet*, **382**, 1638–45.

8. **Sintek MA, Gdowski M, Lindman BR,** *et al.* (2015). Intra-aortic balloon counterpulsation in patients with chronic heart failure and cardiogenic shock: clinical response and predictors of stabilization. *J Card Fail*, **21**, 868–76.

9. **Nwaejike N, Son AY, Milano CA, Daneshmand MA** (2017). Is there a role for upper-extremity intra-aortic balloon counterpulsation as a bridge-to-recovery or a bridge-to-transplant in the treatment of end-stage heart failure? *Interact Cardiovasc Thorac Surg*, **25**, 654–8.

10. **O'Neill WW, Kleiman NS, Moses J,** *et al.* (2012). A prospective, randomized clinical trial of hemodynamic support with Impella 2.5 versus intra-aortic balloon pump in patients undergoing high-risk percutaneous coronary intervention: the PROTECT II study. *Circulation*, **126**, 1717–27.

11. **Seyfarth M, Sibbing D, Bauer I,** *et al.* (2008). A randomized clinical trial to evaluate the safety and efficacy of a percutaneous left ventricular assist device versus intra-aortic balloon pumping for treatment of cardiogenic shock caused by myocardial infarction. *J Am Coll Cardiol*, **52**, 1584–8.

12. **Griffith BP, Anderson MB, Samuels LE,** *et al.* (2013). The RECOVER I: a multicenter prospective study of Impella 5.0/LD for postcardiotomy circulatory support. *J Thorac Cardiovasc Surg*, **145**, 548–54.

13. **Kar B, Gregoric ID, Basra SS, Idelchik GM, Loyalka P** (2011). The percutaneous ventricular assist device in severe refractory cardiogenic shock. *J Am Coll Cardiol*, **57**(6), 688–96.

14. **John R, Long JW, Massey HT,** *et al.* (2011). Outcomes of a multicenter trial of the Levitronix CentriMag ventricular assist system for short-term circulatory support. *J Thorac Cardiovasc Surg*, **141**, 932–9.

15. **Loforte A, Montalto A, Ranocchi F,** *et al.* (2011). Levitronix CentriMag third-generation magnetically levitated continuous flow pump as bridge to solution. *ASAIO J*, **57**, 247–53.

16. **Abrams DC, Brodie D, Rosenzweig EB**, *et al*. (2013). Upper-body extracorporeal membrane oxygenation as a strategy in decompensated pulmonary arterial hypertension. *Pulm Circ*, **3**, 432–5.

17. **Drakos SG, Kfoury AG, Stehlik J**, *et al*. (2012). Bridge to recovery: understanding the disconnect between clinical and biological outcomes. *Circulation*, **126**, 230–41.

18. **Selzman CH, Madden JL, Healy AH**, *et al*. (2015). Bridge to removal: a paradigm shift for left ventricular assist device therapy. *Ann Thorac Surg*, **99**, 360–7.

19. **Drakos SG, Mehra MR** (2016). Clinical myocardial recovery during long-term mechanical support in advanced heart failure: insights into moving the field forward. *J Heart Lung Transplant*, **35**, 413–20.

20. **Dandel M, Weng Y, Siniawski H**, *et al*. (2011). Heart failure reversal by ventricular unloading in patients with chronic cardiomyopathy: criteria for weaning from ventricular assist devices. *Eur Heart J*, **32**, 1148–60.

21. **Birks EJ, Tansley PD, Hardy J**, *et al*. (2006). Left ventricular assist device and drug therapy for the reversal of heart failure. *N Engl J Med*, **355**, 1873–84.

22. **Birks EJ, George RS, Hedger M**, *et al*. (2011). Reversal of severe heart failure with a continuous-flow left ventricular assist device and pharmacological therapy: a prospective study. *Circulation*, **123**, 381–90.

23. **Aaronson KD, Pagani FD, Maybaum SW**, *et al*. (2011). Combination therapy with pulsatile left ventricular assst device, heart failure medication and clenbuterol in chronic heart failure: results from HARPS. *J Heart Lung Transplant*, **30**, S8–S9.

24. **Drakos SG, Wever-Pinzon O, Selzman CH**, *et al*. (2013). Magnitude and time course of changes induced by continuous-flow left ventricular assist device unloading in chronic heart failure: insights into cardiac recovery. *J Am Coll Cardiol*, **61**, 1985–94.

25. **Patel SR, Saeed O, Murthy S**, *et al*. (2013). Combining neurohormonal blockade with continuous-flow left ventricular assist device support for myocardial recovery: a single-arm prospective study. *J Heart Lung Transplant*, **32**, 305–12.

26. **Wever-Pinzon O, Drakos SG, McKellar SH**, *et al*. (2016). Cardiac recovery during long-term left ventricular assist device support. *J Am Coll Cardiol*, **68**, 1540–53.

27. **Lund LH, Khush KK, Cherikh WS**, *et al*. (2017). The registry of the international society for heart and lung transplantation: thirty-fourth adult heart transplantation report 2017; focus theme: allograft ischemic time. *J Heart Lung Transplant*, **36**, 1037–46.

28. **Frazier OH, Rose EA, McCarthy P**, *et al*. (1995). Improved mortality and rehabilitation of transplant candidates treated with a long-term implantable left ventricular assist system. *Ann Surg*, **222**, 327–36; discussion 36–8.

29. **Frazier OH, Rose EA, Oz MC**, *et al*. (2001). Multicenter clinical evaluation of the HeartMate vented electric left ventricular assist system in patients awaiting heart transplantation. *J Thorac Cardiovasc Surg*, **122**, 1186–95.

30. **Pagani FD, Long JW, Dembitsky WP, Joyce LD, Miller LW** (2006). Improved mechanical reliability of the HeartMate XVE left ventricular assist system. *Ann Thorac Surg*, **82**, 1413–8.

31. **Griffith BP, Kormos RL, Borovetz HS**, *et al*. (2001). HeartMate II left ventricular assist system: from concept to first clinical use. *Ann Thorac Surg*, **71**, S116–20; discussion S4–6.

32. **Miller LW, Pagani FD, Russell SD**, *et al*. (2007). Use of a continuous-flow device in patients awaiting heart transplantation. *N Engl J Med*, **357**, 885–96.

33. **Pagani FD, Miller LW, Russell SD**, *et al*. (2009). Extended mechanical circulatory support with a continuous-flow rotary left ventricular assist device. *J Am Coll Cardiol*, **54**, 312–21.

34. **Morshuis M, El-Banayosy A, Arusoglu L**, *et al*. (2009). European experience of DuraHeart magnetically levitated centrifugal left ventricular assist system. *Eur J Cardiothorac Surg*, **35**, 1020–7; discussion 7–8.

35. **Strueber M, O'Driscoll G, Jansz P,** *et al.* (2011). Multicenter evaluation of an intrapericardial left ventricular assist system. *J Am Coll Cardiol,* **57,** 1375–82.

36. **Aaronson KD, Slaughter MS, Miller LW,** *et al.* (2012). Use of an intrapericardial, continuous-flow, centrifugal pump in patients awaiting heart transplantation. *Circulation,* **125,** 3191–200.

37. **Slaughter MS, Pagani FD, McGee EC,** *et al.* (2013). HeartWare ventricular assist system for bridge to transplant: combined results of the bridge to transplant and continued access protocol trial. *J Heart Lung Transplant,* **32,** 675–83.

38. **Netuka I, Sood P, Pya Y,** *et al.* (2015). Fully magnetically levitated left ventricular assist system for treating advanced HF: a multicenter study. *J Am Coll Cardiol,* **66,** 2579–89.

39. **Heatley G, Sood P, Goldstein D,** *et al.* (2016). Clinical trial design and rationale of the Multicenter Study of MagLev Technology in Patients Undergoing Mechanical Circulatory Support Therapy with HeartMate 3 (MOMENTUM 3) investigational device exemption clinical study protocol. *J Heart Lung Transplant,* **35,** 528–36.

40. **Mehra MR, Naka Y, Uriel N,** *et al.* (2017). A fully magnetically levitated circulatory pump for advanced heart failure. *N Engl J Med,* **376,** 440–50.

41. **Uriel N, Colombo PC, Cleveland JC,** *et al.* (2017). Hemocompatibility-related outcomes in the MOMENTUM 3 Trial at 6 months: a randomized controlled study of a fully magnetically levitated pump in advanced heart failure. *Circulation,* **135,** 2003–12.

42. **Kirklin JK, Naftel DC, Pagani FD,** *et al.* (2014). Sixth INTERMACS annual report: a 10,000-patient database. *J Heart Lung Transplant,* **33,** 555–64.

43. **Saito S, Sakaguchi T, Sawa Y** (2011). Clinical report of long-term support with dual Jarvik 2000 biventricular assist device. *J Heart Lung Transplant,* **30,** 845–7.

44. **Strueber M, Meyer AL, Malehsa D, Haverich A** (2010). Successful use of the HeartWare HVAD rotary blood pump for biventricular support. *J Thorac Cardiovasc Surg,* **140,** 936–7.

45. **Gray NA Jr, Selzman CH** (2006). Current status of the total artificial heart. *Am Heart J,* **152,** 4–10.

46. **Copeland JG, Smith RG, Arabia FA,** *et al.* (2004). Cardiac replacement with a total artificial heart as a bridge to transplantation. *N Engl J Med,* **351,** 859–67.

47. **Rose EA, Gelijns AC, Moskowitz AJ,** *et al.* (2001). Long-term use of a left ventricular assist device for end-stage heart failure. *N Engl J Med,* **345,** 1435–43.

48. **Long JW, Kfoury AG, Slaughter MS,** *et al.* (2005). Long-term destination therapy with the HeartMate XVE left ventricular assist device: improved outcomes since the REMATCH study. *Congest Heart Fail,* **11,** 133–8.

49. **Slaughter MS, Rogers JG, Milano CA,** *et al.* (2009). Advanced heart failure treated with continuous-flow left ventricular assist device. *N Engl J Med,* **361,** 2241–51.

50. **Rogers JG, Pagani FD, Tatooles AJ,** *et al.* (2017). Intrapericardial left ventricular assist device for advanced heart failure. *N Engl J Med,* **376,** 451–60.

51. **Alba AC, Rao V, Ross HJ,** *et al.* (2010). Impact of fixed pulmonary hypertension on post-heart transplant outcomes in bridge-to-transplant patients. *J Heart Lung Transplant,* **29**(11), 1253–8.

52. **Mikus E, Stepanenko A, Krabatsch T,** *et al.* (2011). Reversibility of fixed pulmonary hypertension in left ventricular assist device support recipients. *Eur J Cardiothorac Surg,* **40,** 971–7.

53. **Drakos SG, Janicki L, Horne BD,** *et al.* (2010). Risk factors predictive of right ventricular failure after left ventricular assist device implantation. *Am J Cardiol,* **105,** 1030–5.

54. **Kang G, Ha R, Banerjee D** (2016). Pulmonary artery pulsatility index predicts right ventricular failure after left ventricular assist device implantation. *J Heart Lung Transplant,* **35,** 67–73.

55. **Christiansen S, Jahn UR, Meyer J,** *et al.* (2000). Anticoagulative management of patients requiring left ventricular assist device implantation and suffering from heparin-induced thrombocytopenia type II. *Ann Thorac Surg,* **69,** 774–7.

56. **Dang NC, Topkara VK, Mercando M**, *et al.* (2006). Right heart failure after left ventricular assist device implantation in patients with chronic congestive heart failure. *J Heart Lung Transplant*, **25**, 1–6.

57. **Fitzpatrick JR, 3rd, Frederick JR, Hsu VM**, *et al.* (2008). Risk score derived from pre-operative data analysis predicts the need for biventricular mechanical circulatory support. *J Heart Lung Transplant*, **27**, 1286–92.

58. **Kukucka M, Stepanenko A, Potapov E**, *et al.* (2011). Right-to-left ventricular end-diastolic diameter ratio and prediction of right ventricular failure with continuous-flow left ventricular assist devices. *J Heart Lung Transplant*, **30**, 64–9.

59. **Gregoric ID, La Francesca S, Myers T**, *et al.* (2008). A less invasive approach to axial flow pump insertion. *J Heart Lung Transplant*, **27**, 423–6.

60. **Selzman CH, Sheridan BC** (2007). Off-pump insertion of continuous flow left ventricular assist devices. *J Card Surg*, **22**, 320–2.

61. **Sun BC, Firstenberg MS, Louis LB**, *et al.* (2008). Placement of long-term implantable ventricular assist devices without the use of cardiopulmonary bypass. *J Heart Lung Transplant*, **27**, 718–21.

62. **Starling RC, Moazami N, Silvestry SC**, *et al.* (2014). Unexpected abrupt increase in left ventricular assist device thrombosis. *N Engl J Med*, **370**, 33–40.

63. **Maltais S, Kilic A, Nathan S**, *et al.* (2017). PREVENtion of HeartMate II Pump Thrombosis Through Clinical Management: the PREVENT multi-center study. *J Heart Lung Transplant*, **36**, 1–12.

64. **Dean D, Ewald GA, Tatooles A**, *et al.* (2014). Reduction in driveline infection rates: results from the HeartMate II Multicenter Silicone-Skin-Interface (SSI) Registry. *J Heart Lung Transplant*, **33**, S11–S2.

65. **John R, Naka Y, Park SJ**, *et al.* (2014). Impact of concurrent surgical valve procedures in patients receiving continuous-flow devices. *J Thorac Cardiovasc Surg*, **147**, 581–9; discussion 9.

66. **McKellar SH, Deo S, Daly RC**, *et al.* (2014). Durability of central aortic valve closure in patients with continuous flow left ventricular assist devices. *J Thorac Cardiovasc Surg*, **147**, 344–8.

67. **Cohn WE, Demirozu ZT, Frazier OH** (2011). Surgical closure of left ventricular outflow tract after left ventricular assist device implantation in patients with aortic valve pathology. *J Heart Lung Transplant*, **30**, 59–63.

68. **Taghavi S, Hamad E, Wilson L**, *et al.* (2013). Mitral valve repair at the time of continuous-flow left ventricular assist device implantation confers meaningful decrement in pulmonary vascular resistance. *ASAIO J*, **59**, 469–73.

69. **Piacentino V 3rd, Troupes CD, Ganapathi AM**, *et al.* (2011). Clinical impact of concomitant tricuspid valve procedures during left ventricular assist device implantation. *Ann Thorac Surg*, **92**, 1414–8; discussion 8–9.

70. **Goldraich L, Kawajiri H, Foroutan F**, *et al.* (2016). Tricuspid valve annular dilation as a predictor of right ventricular failure after implantation of a left ventricular assist device. *J Card Surg*, **31**, 110–6.

71. **Song HK, Gelow JM, Mudd J**, *et al.* (2016). Limited utility of tricuspid valve repair at the time of left ventricular assist device implantation. *Ann Thorac Surg*, **101**, 2168–74.

72. **Boyle AJ, Russell SD, Teuteberg JJ**, *et al.* (2009). Low thromboembolism and pump thrombosis with the HeartMate II left ventricular assist device: analysis of outpatient anti-coagulation. *J Heart Lung Transplant*, **28**, 881–7.

73. **Cowger J, Pagani FD, Haft JW**, *et al.* (2010). The development of aortic insufficiency in left ventricular assist device-supported patients. *Circ Heart Fail*, **3**, 668–74.

74. **Lampert BC, Eckert C, Weaver S**, *et al.* (2014). Blood pressure control in continuous flow left ventricular assist devices: efficacy and impact on adverse events. *Ann Thorac Surg*, **97**, 139–46.

75. **Atkins BZ, Hashmi ZA, Ganapathi AM**, *et al.* (2013). Surgical correction of aortic valve insufficiency after left ventricular assist device implantation. *J Thorac Cardiovasc Surg*, **146**, 1247–52.

76. **Meyer AL, Malehsa D, Budde U**, *et al.* (2014). Acquired von Willebrand syndrome in patients with a centrifugal or axial continuous flow left ventricular assist device. *JACC Heart Fail*, **2**, 141–5.

77. **Geisen U, Heilmann C, Beyersdorf F**, *et al.* (2008). Non-surgical bleeding in patients with ventricular assist devices could be explained by acquired von Willebrand disease. *Eur J Cardiothorac Surg*, **33**, 679–84.

78. **Uriel N, Pak SW, Jorde UP**, *et al.* (2010). Acquired von Willebrand syndrome after continuous-flow mechanical device support contributes to a high prevalence of bleeding during long-term support and at the time of transplantation. *J Am Coll Cardiol*, **56**, 1207–13.

79. **Netuka I, Kvasnicka T, Kvasnicka J**, *et al.* (2016). Evaluation of von Willebrand factor with a fully magnetically levitated centrifugal continuous-flow left ventricular assist device in advanced heart failure. *J Heart Lung Transplant*, **35**, 860–7.

80. **Fang JC** (2009). Rise of the machines--left ventricular assist devices as permanent therapy for advanced heart failure. *N Engl J Med*, **361**, 2282–5.

Chapter 12

Current status of heart transplantation

Ayyaz Ali and Robert L. Kormos

Introduction

Cardiac transplantation represents one of the major medical advances of the twentieth century. Since its introduction it has extended and improved the lives of patients suffering from severe heart failure. Despite advances in medical therapy, cardiac transplantation remains the definitive treatment for end-stage heart disease. The success of heart transplantation was made possible by prior landmark achievements in the transplantation of other solid organs, primarily renal transplantation. Extensive laboratory research provided the foundation for the development of this procedure. Surgical techniques for organ procurement and implantation, development of appropriate methods for preserving the heart, and understanding the immunological challenges associated with transplantation were among the many areas which required focused investigation. In the current era, heart transplantation is associated with a low operative mortality and excellent long-term survival.[1,2] Furthermore, alleviation of symptoms of heart failure following transplantation has transformed the lives of patients with severely impaired cardiac function.[3,4] A major obstacle to the more widespread application of heart transplantation is a shortage of suitable donor organs.[5] Consequently, strategies aimed at expanding the donor pool have been actively implemented. The use of marginal donor organs describes a policy where criteria used to describe adequate function of the organ are made less stringent. Consequently, organs which may previously have been discarded on the basis of borderline performance or adverse characteristics, such as left ventricular hypertrophy or depressed left ventricular ejection fraction, have been utilized for transplantation.[6-8]

History of cardiac transplantation

Alexis Carrel and Charles Claude Guthrie were responsible for pioneering early techniques for transplantation of the heart, lungs, and other organs. In 1905 Carrel reported the first successful heterotopic heart transplant in a canine model.[9,10] In 1933, Frank C. Mann and James T. Priestley described survival of up to 8 days in a canine model of heterotopic heart transplantation.[11] They observed that explanted hearts were infiltrated with lymphocytes, mononuclear cells, and neutrophils. They correctly suggested that the success of transplantation was limited not by technical factors but by unidentified biological factors, later identified as allograft rejection. The next advance in cardiac transplantation was made by Vladimir Demikhov who performed the first intrathoracic heterotopic cardiac transplant, once again using a canine model.[12] He reported survival of up to 32 days. In the 1960s Norman Shumway and Richard Lower established a dedicated research program at Stanford University which they aimed to translate into a clinical program of human cardiac transplantation. They reported that the major obstacle to long-term survival of cardiac allografts was rejection and that without immunosuppression, extended graft survival would be impossible.[13] Adrian Kantrowitz and Yoshio Kondo, working at Downstate Medical Center in Brooklyn, New York, demonstrated prolonged survival of up to 112 days after heart transplantation in puppies without any immunosuppressive therapy.[14] The suggestion that newborn animals may possess an immunological advantage encouraged Kantrowitz to later attempt cardiac transplantation in infants.

The first heart transplant operation in a human was performed in 1964 by James Hardy on the background of several years of laboratory research.[15-17] The donor heart was obtained from a chimpanzee. Their intention had been to use a human heart, but the condition of their recipient did not permit them to wait for a human organ to become available. The decision to use a chimpanzee heart was based on an experience of transplantation of kidneys from chimpanzees into humans.[18] Although the xenograft demonstrated good function within the recipient, it was unable to support the circulation after separation of the recipient from cardiopulmonary bypass.

On December 3, 1967, the first human-to-human heart transplant was performed by Christiaan Barnard in Cape Town, South Africa.[19] The recipient was a 53-year-old male with ischemic cardiomyopathy named Louis Washkansky, suffering from severe biventricular failure. The donor was a 25-year-old female who had suffered severe head injuries after being hit by a speeding car. At that time in South Africa there was no legislation for the designation of brain death as being synonymous with circulatory death. Therefore, cardiac arrest was awaited after withdrawal of life support and was deemed necessary for declaration of death. Immediately after the heart had stopped the donor was placed on cardiopulmonary bypass (CPB) and the coronary circulation was reperfused with oxygenated blood to resuscitate the heart. Hypothermia was established to facilitate preservation and protection of the heart prior to transplantation. The patient survived the operation but died of pneumonia on the eighteenth postoperative day. The transplant attracted the attention of the entire world and was one of the most publicized medical events in history. Three days after the transplant in South Africa, Adrian Kantrowitz performed the second human heart transplant in Brooklyn.[20] This was undertaken in an 18-day-old infant with severe cardiac failure due to congenital heart disease. The donor heart was obtained from an anencephalic infant. The recipient died 5 hours after implantation of the heart due to poor graft function. Toward the end of 1968, 102 heart transplant operations had been performed in 17 different countries around the world. The results of the procedure were disappointing with a 60% early mortality rate and a mean survival of 29 days.[21] By 1970 this had led to a wide-scale abandonment of the procedure with only a few institutions continuing with clinical cardiac transplantation. Dr. Shumway persisted with the procedure with intensive efforts directed toward improving outcomes, principally through continued research efforts. His dedication was rewarded by an improvement in the 1-year survival of heart transplant patients at Stanford from 22% to 65%.[22]

Recipient selection

Patients with end-stage cardiac disease need careful evaluation to determine their suitability for transplantation. Most patients considered for transplantation suffer from ischemic or dilated cardiomyopathy. Causes of dilated cardiomyopathy include viral infection, inflammatory, toxic, metabolic, and genetic etiologies. Valvular and congenital heart disease are less common indications for transplantation.

Patient evaluation begins with history and physical examination. Investigations include a chest X-ray and routine blood tests. Exercise tolerance is determined by exercise testing and quantified by measurements of maximal oxygen consumption (VO_2). The patient is screened for viral disease and the presence of reactive antibodies to human leukocyte antigen (HLA). Right heart catheterization and coronary angiography are performed before the patient is placed on the waiting list. This allows determination of pulmonary artery pressure and the presence of coronary artery disease. Further tests include thyroid function, blood glucose, creatinine clearance, electrocardiography, echocardiography, and pulmonary function testing. Final selection of patients is based on subjective and objective criteria. If the patient's one-year survival without transplantation is judged to be less than 50%, transplantation is deemed to be an effective treatment option.

Contraindications to heart transplantation include advanced age. Comorbidity increases with age and is associated with reduced post-transplant survival. Elevated pulmonary vascular resistance (PVR) is an absolute contraindication to orthotopic heart transplantation. If the PVR is fixed above six wood units and the pressure drop across the pulmonary circulation (transpulmonary gradient) is greater than 15 mmHg without evidence of reversibility with vasodilators, the patient is not suitable for transplantation. Elevated PVR predicts post-transplant right heart failure which can be fatal. These patients may be candidates for heart-lung transplantation. Diabetes is a contraindication if there is end-organ damage such as retinopathy, neuropathy, or nephropathy. Active infection, hepatic dysfunction, malignancy, advanced lung disease, and peripheral vascular disease are largely considered to be contraindications to transplantation. The patient's psychosocial condition is also important as they are required to adhere to a strict regimen of medical therapy and regular medical follow-up.

Recipient management

Patients awaiting a cardiac transplant should receive optimal medical therapy for heart failure. Angiotensin-converting-enzyme (ACE) inhibitors, beta blockers, and diuretics are used in varying combinations. Patients in severe heart failure can be stabilized hemodynamically with inotrope therapy. The use of an intra-aortic balloon pump can further augment hemodynamics in critically ill patients with heart failure. A selected group of patients with severe refractory heart failure may be candidates for mechanical circulatory support with a ventricular assist device (VAD). Such devices are indicated if patients remain unstable despite a period of conventional support. VAD's are used to stabilize or "bridge" a patient until a suitable donor heart becomes available. In patients with a history of inducible ventricular tachycardia or fibrillation, the placement of an automatic implantable cardioverter-defibrillator may reduce the likelihood of sudden cardiac death. Sudden cardiac death is the commonest cause of death in patients awaiting heart transplantation and is most common in the first 3 months after listing.

Organ procurement and preservation

Routine evaluation of the cardiac donor includes a review of biographical data such as height, weight, gender, and blood type. Laboratory tests are taken for serology, hematological, and biochemical analysis. Hemodynamic status of the donor is scrutinized, and specific investigations include an electrocardiogram (EKG), chest X-ray, and echocardiography. Swan-Ganz catheterization can be undertaken for more detailed assessment of hemodynamic function. Coronary angiography is recommended in male donors aged greater than 45 and females older than 50. In donors with risk factors for coronary artery disease or history of cocaine abuse angiography is obtained regardless of age.

Brainstem death results in physiological derangements which culminate in hemodynamic instability. The culprit is an increase in serum catecholamines in response to brainstem ischemia. An initial hyperdynamic phase with hypertension, tachycardia, and subendocardial ischemia is followed by vasodilatation, autonomic dysfunction, and dysrhythmia. The severity of this response is proportional to the extent of brain injury. Aims in management of the donor are to restore stable hemodynamics with a mean arterial pressure greater than 60 mmHg and a central venous pressure in the range of 6–10 mmHg. Swan-Ganz catheterization allows for more accurate assessment, evaluation, and control of hemodynamics. Exogenous catecholamine administration is minimized as it can deplete ATP stores in the donor heart which may impair post-transplant function. Vasopressin is used for maintenance of blood pressure and to treat coexisting diabetes insipidus. Hormonal replacement, with insulin, triiodothyronine, and steroid therapy, is also commonly administered. Volume replacement and maintenance of fluid, electrolyte, and acid-base balance are important in maintaining cardiovascular stability within the organ donor.

Final assessment of the donor heart is undertaken in the operating room. A median sternotomy is performed and visual assessment of cardiac function is undertaken. The superior vena cava (SVC) is dissected and encircled with a tie. The azygos vein is identified and ligated. The inferior vena cava (IVC) can be encircled between finger and thumb which facilitates its separation from the right inferior pulmonary vein. Heparin is administered intravenously (300 units/kg). Prior to the application of a cross-clamp across the ascending aorta, the SVC is ligated close to its junction with the innominate vein. The donor heart is vented to prevent distension by incising the IVC and left superior pulmonary vein. Alternatively, the left atrial appendage is transected if the lungs are being procured. The aorta is clamped and cardioplegia is infused into the aortic root. Cold saline solution or slushed ice is copiously applied around the donor heart to augment preservation. The donor left atrium is incised; if the lungs are being procured, care is taken to preserve a cuff of left atrial tissue incorporating the pulmonary veins, otherwise the left atrium can be incised at the pulmonary veins. The ascending aorta, pulmonary artery, SVC, and IVC are transected and the donor heart removed and placed into a container with cold preservation solution. Further packaging is undertaken using sterile bags and the organ is surrounded by ice and transported.

Preservation of the donor heart relies on methods of myocardial protection to minimize injury during procurement, storage, transportation, and implantation of the organ. Hypothermia remains the cornerstone of most preservation strategies. Crystalloid cardioplegic solutions (4–10°C) are most commonly utilized for perfusion of the aortic root and their composition can vary widely. These solutions are categorized based on their constituents as either intracellular or extracellular solutions. Intracellular solutions have higher concentrations of potassium and lower sodium content; their purported benefits relate to avoidance of cellular edema. Bretschneider (HTK), University of Wisconsin, and Euro-Collins solutions are commonly used intracellular solutions. Extracellular solutions have higher concentrations of sodium with lower potassium levels due to concerns over cell damage secondary to hyperkalemia. This category includes St. Thomas's hospital solution, Celsior, and Krebs solutions. Cardiac distension is avoided during administration of the preservative by insuring that the both the right and left heart are vented as described just now. The maximal tolerable cold ischemic period is between 4 and 6 hours. Increasing cold ischemic times are associated with a higher incidence of donor organ dysfunction and primary graft failure. After removal from cold storage, the organ is subjected to warm ischemia as it is exposed to room temperature. Cardioplegic solutions are often administered into the aortic root immediately following removal of the organ from its storage container. Further doses can be administered intermittently during the course of implantation.

Machine perfusion and continuous delivery of preservative solutions have been advocated as a means of improving myocardial preservation. Such methods may allow an extension of the maximum period of cold ischemia to which the donor organ can be exposed. Concerns remain over the development of myocardial edema due to the large volumes of perfusate that may be infused. More recently, the development of devices that allow for continuous warm perfusion of the donor heart with oxygenated blood has been suggested as a means to improve organ preservation. These devices may also offer the potential for resuscitation and biochemical and functional assessment prior to implantation. The use of machine perfusion remains largely experimental and substantial clinical experience is lacking. However, it is feasible that this technology may play an important role in the future of organ preservation.

Surgical procedure

Recipient operation

Standard antiseptic preparation and draping is undertaken and the thoracic cavity is accessed via a median sternotomy. A proportion of patients will have had a prior sternotomy for previous cardiac surgical procedures such as coronary artery bypass grafting. Increasingly, patients with left ventricular assist devices are being bridged to heart transplantation. In both of these patient groups and particularly in the latter, dissection of the heart and institution of cardiopulmonary bypass can be difficult (CPB). Peripheral CPB can be used as an alternative if there are concerns about being able to safely institute extracorporeal circulation. Bicaval cannulation is necessary with separate drainage of the SVC and IVC. Ascending aortic cannulation is most commonly used for CPB inflow. Following the initiation of bypass, core temperature is often reduced to achieve moderate hypothermia (28°C). Both vena cavae are snared and a cross-clamp is applied across the ascending aorta. The recipient cardiectomy is then performed. An incision is made into the right atrium (RA) close to the aortic valve (AV) groove and continued along the AV groove toward the coronary sinus. The classical biatrial technique described by Lower and Shumway is less commonly performed and has been replaced by the bicaval technique, where the recipient RA is incised circumferentially to create a cuff for the IVC anastomosis. The SVC is also dissected and mobilized and divided from the recipient RA to allow for a separate SVC anastomosis. An incision is made across the atrial septum and the left atrium (LA) is incised along the AV groove leaving a cuff for anastomosis to the donor LA. Both the pulmonary artery and ascending aorta are divided above the commissures of their respective semi-lunar valves. Both vessels are separated from one another proximally to facilitate anastomosis to the donor great vessels. It is important to ensure that the recipient and donor cardiotomies are coordinated in a manner to minimize allograft ischemic time. The donor heart is removed from cold storage and prepared for implantation. Prior to this, cardioplegia can be administered to the donor heart via the aortic root. If the pulmonary vein orifices are intact, incisions are made to connect them to open the LA. Excess atrial tissue is trimmed to create a cuff for anastomosis to the recipient LA. If an RA anastomosis is undertaken as opposed to separate caval anastomoses an incision is made from the IVC toward the RA appendage. If a patent foramen ovale is identified it should be oversewn.

Implantation

The LA anastomosis is constructed with a 3-0 Prolene suture and is commenced near the left superior pulmonary vein of the recipient. The suture is passed through the corresponding area of the donor LA and the donor heart is parachuted into the pericardial cavity. Both left atria are aligned via retraction of the donor heart to facilitate the anastomosis. The suture line is continued inferiorly toward the left inferior pulmonary vein, then medially toward the septum. The second arm of the suture is used to complete the superior aspect of the anastomosis. A vent can be inserted at this time into the left ventricular (LV) via the right superior pulmonary vein to drain collateral blood entering the

LV via the pulmonary veins. The pulmonary artery anastomosis is constructed next in an end-to-end fashion using a continuous 4-0 Prolene suture. The donor pulmonary artery can be trimmed to a point about 1 cm above the pulmonary valve. If the pulmonary artery is left too long it can predispose to kinking in the region of the anastomosis. The donor and recipient aorta are anastomosed to one another using 3-0 or 4-0 Prolene, prior to tying this suture the heart is initially deaired through this anastomosis. Prior to releasing the cross-clamp warm blood "hot shot" cardioplegia may be administered to promote re-covery of anerobic myocardial metabolism. An aortic root vent can be inserted to further facilitate the de-airing process after the cross-clamp is released. After the aortic cross-clamp is removed the allograft is reperfused. Using the biatrial technique, a continuous 3-0 Prolene suture is used to anastomose the donor and recipient right atria. Currently the bicaval technique is preferred as it is associated with a lower incidence of arrythmias, atrioventricular valve insufficiency, and conduction disturbances. Also, it has been asso-ciated with less right ventricular (RV) failure, shorter hospital stay, and improved 1-year survival.[23–26] The IVC and SVC are anastomosed separately to the recipient cavae in an end-to-end fashion. The implantation procedure can vary significantly depending upon surgeon preference. Some prefer to complete the RA or IVC anastomosis prior to anas-tomosing the great vessels. Releasing the cross-clamp prior to the caval/RA connections minimizes warm ischemic time and allows time for reperfusion of the donor heart while implantation is completed. Ischemic time can further be minimized by undertaking the pulmonary artery anastomosis and even the LA anastomosis after the aortic anastomosis, although these maneuvers are technically more challenging.

Heterotopic heart transplantation

This technique of implantation is less commonly used in the current era. Recipient cardiectomy is not performed and the donor heart is anastomosed to the recipient heart with the two organs working in tandem. The principal indications for this procedure are when the donor heart is judged to be too small to support the circulation in isolation or in patients with fixed pulmonary hypertension. A left atriotomy is made in the Sondergaards groove in the recipient. A corresponding incision is made in the donor LA to connect the left inferior and superior pulmonary veins. The donor and recipient atriotomies are anastomosed such that the allograft lies to the right of the native heart. Both the donor aorta and pulmonary artery are anastomosed to the recipient great vessels in an end-to-side fashion. An interposition graft may be required to connect the donor and recipient pulmonary arteries. The donor SVC is then connected to the RA. Despite its infrequent application, heterotopic transplantation is associated with satisfactory outcomes which are comparable to those of orthotopic transplantation.[27,28]

Postoperative management

Inotropic support is usually required in the postoperative period due to impaired myocar-dial contractility. Myocardial dysfunction in this setting is often transient and secondary to injury sustained prior to procurement, during cold storage, and in association with warm ischemia during implantation. The RV is particularly susceptible to injury and this can result in RV failure, especially in the presence of elevated PVR. Inotropic support with beta-agonists and phosphodiesterase inhibitors is often utilized and is gradually discontinued after hemodynamic stability and satisfactory cardiac function are confirmed. Nitric oxide can be introduced to ameliorate RV dysfunction by reducing the PVR. As the donor heart is denervated due to transection of its autonomic nerve fibers, it has an intrinsic resting heart rate of between 90 and 110 beats per minute. The absence of reflex control of heart rate can interfere with normal cardiovascular physiology and can result in adverse effects such as orthostatic hypotension and an increased sensitivity to inotropic and chronotopic agents.[29]

Primary allograft dysfunction is one of the commonest causes of perioperative mortality. The underlying cause for severe donor organ dysfunction is not always easily identified and is often multifactorial. Common causes include ischemic myocardial injury due to inadequate preservation, acute rejection, or pulmonary hypertension with severe RV failure. After maximal inotropic support has been instituted, ongoing donor organ dysfunction requires mechanical support. An intra-aortic balloon pump can be used to support cardiac function. More aggressive forms of mechanical circulatory support include extracorporeal membrane oxygenation (ECMO) and the use of VAD to support the failing heart. Retransplantation can be considered in rare circumstances but is often not feasible due to limited availability of donor organs. Irrespective of the different treatment options, the mortality associated with early allograft failure is high and accounts for one-fifth of perioperative deaths following heart transplantation.[30] As mentioned earlier, RV failure is an important cause of mortality early after cardiac transplantation and is due to inability of the RV to function in the presence of an elevated PVR. The RV can be supported by administering agents that reduce the PVR such as prostaglandin E1, prostacyclin, inhaled nitric oxide, and nitroglycerin.[31,32] If pharmacological therapy is insufficient, mechanical support of the RV can be instituted using a right ventricular assist device.[33]

Antiarrythmic therapy should be initiated if clinically indicated to reduce rhythm-related complications. Hypertension should be controlled with medical therapy to reduce afterload. Patients should be followed up in the outpatient clinic and echocardiography can be used to evaluate cardiac structure and function. Endomyocardial biopsies are performed for the detection of acute rejection.

Immunosuppression

Induction therapy

Immunization of animals with human lymphocytes leads to the production of polyclonal antibodies that can destroy immune cells. They are potent agents which can markedly reduce the number of circulating T cells. Thymoglobulin is comprised of purified IgG immunoglobulins derived from rabbits after exposure to human thymocytes. Polyclonal antibodies have been utilized for induction of immunosuppression in the perioperative period as prophylaxis against rejection and evidence indicates that they reduce early acute rejection.[34,35] They are also used for the treatment of acute rejection which is unresponsive to steroid therapy. Monoclonal antibodies have also been developed and are also used for induction therapy and treatment of refractory rejection.[36] OKT3 is a murine monoclonal antibody, which was the first to be used in clinical practice. By interacting with the T-cell recognition complex it inhibits the function of naïve as well as cytotoxic T cells. Its use for induction therapy has decreased significantly due to an increased incidence of infection and post-transplant lymphoproliferative disorders.[37,38] Administration can also lead to the development of human antimouse antibodies which reduce its efficacy. IL-2 receptor blockers such as basiliximab and daclizumab confer more selective immune suppression as they target only activated T cells which express CD25 antigen. These chimeric antibodies have a greater human component reducing the production of antimouse antibodies after exposure. Doses given at induction produce a protracted effect which markedly reduces the rates of acute rejection early after heart transplantation. This has been confirmed in randomized studies,[39] although concerns have been raised over a possible increased risk of infection and graft dysfunction. Alemtuzumab is a rat-derived chimeric monoclonal antibody directed against CD52 on mature lymphocytes. We currently use this agent for induction therapy in cardiac transplantation at our center and its potent activity against T cells has allowed us to withdraw corticosteroids from our immunosuppression regimen.[40]

Perioperative and maintenance therapy

Cyclosporine inhibits the calcium-calcineurin pathway which is involved in the activation of transcription factors that lead to the expression of important molecules involved in the immune response, such as IL-2, CD154, and CD25. Inhibition of this signal transduction pathway impairs proliferation of cytotoxic T-lymphocytes. Other components of the immune response are less affected conferring a degree of selectivity. Its introduction is responsible for the improvement in long-term survival following heart transplantation observed over the last three decades, attributed largely to an associated reduction in infective complications. Renal insufficiency is the major adverse effect associated with its use. Its evolution into a microemulsion formulation has improved its pharmacokinetics and therapeutic index. Tacrolimus (FK506) is a macrolide antibiotic that binds to FK506-binding protein. This complex is a more potent inhibitor of the calcineurin pathway than cyclosporine. Tacrolimus has been demonstrated to produce less hyperlipidemia and hypertension compared to cyclosporine, although the incidence of rejection and death after heart transplantation has been similar.[41,42] Recent reports indicate that tacrolimus is now the most commonly used calcineurin inhibitor in the current era. Antiproliferative agents interfere with cell replication and lymphocyte proliferation in response to antigen. Mycophenolate mofetil (MMF) is an ester prodrug of mycophenolic acid which interferes with purine synthesis. Azathioprine impairs DNA synthesis. Randomized trials of the two agents have demonstrated that the former reduces mortality and rejection and is therefore more commonly administered.[43] Serolimus and everolimus prevent T-cell proliferation by interfering with signal transduction following IL-2 receptor activation. Similar to tacrolimus, these agents bind to FK-506-binding protein but in contrast do not inhibit calcineurin; alternatively, they inhibit cytoplasmic proteins necessary for normal progression of the cell cycle. Both agents may also attenuate the development and progression of coronary allograft vasculopathy. Corticosteroids have been used since the early era of transplantation and are powerful inhibitors of the immune response. They are used for induction and maintenance therapy as well as being the most common first-line agents for treatment of acute rejection. Side effects associated with steroid use have been the impetus for using reduced doses or even withdrawing these agents from current regimens. However, most centers continue to use steroids for long-term maintenance therapy.

Acute rejection

Rejection of the allograft remains a significant cause of morbidity and mortality after heart transplantation.[44] Cell-mediated immune responses are primarily responsible for this process but antibody mediated rejection can also occur. In the modern era, acute rejection can be reliably diagnosed and adequately treated in most patients.

Constitutional symptoms include lethargy, malaise, and low-grade pyrexia. Cardiac dysfunction can result in low cardiac output and congestive heart failure. Arrythmias are also a manifestation of acute rejection. However, patients may remain asymptomatic despite advanced rejection, particularly with current immunosuppressive regimens. Endomyocardial biopsies from the RV are routinely obtained to identify rejection.[45] Right heart catheterization also allows assessment of hemodynamic function. In patients with hemodynamic compromise inotropic agents may be necessary and occasionally mechanical circulatory support is required for extreme situations. Biopsies are performed frequently in the initial few weeks after transplantation and then less often after the first postoperative year. Grading of rejection from biopsy specimens is undertaken by examining the extent of lymphocyte infiltration and the presence of myocyte necrosis. Gene expression profiling from peripheral blood samples may allow for non-invasive identification of acute rejection in the future. Rejection episodes within the first 3 months are treated with 1 gram of intravenous methylprednisolone administered daily for 3 days. Later episodes are treated with high doses of oral prednisone. Response to therapy is assessed by biopsy approximately a week after completion of treatment. Refractory rejection can be treated with a second steroid pulse. Polyclonal or monoclonal antibody therapy is reserved for severe steroid-resistant rejection associated with hemodynamic instability. If rejection is mild in severity it can be monitored with repeat biopsies as in most instances it does not progress. Myocyte necrosis is an indicator of severe rejection and requires aggressive treatment.

Humoral immune responses are associated with vascular rejection and often result in severe cardiac dysfunction.[46] The diagnosis can be made by light microscopy and immunoflourescence of biopsy specimens. Treatment involves the use of plasmapheresis, high dose corticosteroid therapy, heparin, immunoglobulins, and cyclophosphamide. The mortality is high despite aggressive treatment. Repeated and recurrent episodes predispose to the development of coronary allograft vasculopathy.

Allograft vasculopathy

The coronary arteries of the transplanted heart develop cardiac allograft vasculopathy (CAV). This process is characterized by intimal proliferation with stenosis of the epicardial coronary arteries and occlusion of smaller vessels leading to myocardial ischemia.[47] The onset of CAV is variable and it can develop early after heart transplantation. CAV reduces long-term survival and is the primary cause of death after the first post-transplant year.[48] Approximately 50% of patients have evidence of CAV on angiography within 5 years.[49] In contrast to conventional atherosclerosis, luminal narrowing is concentric and diffuse as opposed to eccentric and proximal. Both immunologic and non-immunologic factors contribute to its development.[50] The presence of circulating anti-HLA antibodies and episodes of acute rejection are associated with CAV. Additional risk factors include advanced donor age and recipient hypertension, hyperlipidemia, and diabetes.[51] Inflammation of the endothelium following injury may be an early trigger for CAV.[52] Myocardial ischemia associated with CAV is silent due to cardiac denervation and consequently the disease often manifests as congestive cardiac failure, arrythmias, or sudden cardiac death. Surveillance and screening can be achieved with either coronary angiography or intravascular ultrasound (IVUS).[53] Percutaneous or surgical interventions are difficult due to the diffuse pattern of disease.[54] Minimizing cold ischemia, optimizing cardiac preservation, and modifying risk factors for atherosclerosis can attenuate its development and progression. Calcium channel blockers, ACE inhibitors, and statin therapy have been demonstrated to decrease the incidence of CAV.[55,56] The only definitive treatment for established CAV is retransplantation.

Infection

Infection is a major cause of morbidity and mortality following heart transplantation. Prophylactic treatment with antimicrobial agents is instituted to minimize infectious complications. Although a variety of pathogens can produce infection, cytomegalovirus (CMV) is the predominant cause of infection related mortality and morbidity in cardiac transplant recipients.[57] In addition CMV has been implicated in allograft vasculoathy and post-transplant lymphoproliferative disease (PTLD).[57] Infection can result from reactivation of latent infection in the recipient or due to transmission from the donor. Patients who are seropositive for CMV may also become re-infected by a different viral strain. Ganciclovir is used for prophylaxis, as well as for treatment of symptomatic CMV infections.[58] Valganciclovir has greater bioavailability than ganciclovir and has also been demonstrated to be effective for both prophylaxis and treatment of active infection. Fungal infections can result from species such as candida and aspergillus, the latter being associated with a high mortality. Aspergillus pneumonia develops in up to 10% of patients early after heart transplantation.[59] Pneumonia can also be caused by protozoal organisms such as Pneumocystis carinii.[60] Toxoplasmosis can result from reactivation of latent disease, with toxoplasma gondii often implicated.[61]

Late complications

Renal insufficiency is common among late survivors of heart transplantation.[62] Nephrotoxicity associated with the use of calcineurin inhibitors such as cyclosporine is the most important predisposing factor.[63] Modification of immunosuppressive regimens aimed at minimizing or avoiding calcineurin inhibitors may reduce renal dysfunction.[64] Hypertension is also extremely common among cardiac transplant recipients. Altered activity of the sympathetic nervous system and cyclosporine nephrotoxicity are implicated in its progression.[65] Pharmacological therapy includes the use of calcium channel blockers, diuretics, and beta blockers. Hyperlipidemia is also prevalent and is controlled through dietary modification and lipid-lowering therapy. The incidence of malignancy among heart transplant patients is 100-fold greater than that of the general population.[66] Its incidence is rising, and it represents an increasingly important obstacle to long-term survival. Lymphoproliferative disorders and skin cancers are the most common malignant processes.[67] Treatment can be undertaken with chemotherapy, radiotherapy, and surgery, however mortality remains high despite intervention.

Clinical outcome following cardiac transplantation

Since its inception 40 years ago heart transplantation has become an established treatment for severe heart failure. The evolution and success of this procedure over this time period can be appreciated in a recent report of the 1,446 heart transplant operations performed at Stanford University between 1968 and 2007.[1] Over this time the 1-year survival of patients undergoing heart transplantation has increased from 43.1% to 90.2%. Very long-term survival (20 years) was achieved in 12.5% of patients transplanted before 1988. The commonest causes of death in heart transplant patients were identified as allograft vasculopathy (56.3%) and malignancy (25.0%). Since 1983 approximately 85,000 heart transplants performed worldwide have been reported to the registry of the International Society for Heart and Lung Transplantation (ISHLT).[2] There has been a steady decline in the number of procedures performed over the last 15 years. The number of procedures performed worldwide peaked in 1994 at 4,460, following which there has been a steady decline toward just over 3,000 heart transplants per year over the last 3 years. This decline is largely due to a decrease in the number of brainstem-dead organ donors.

The primary indication for adult heart transplantation over the past decade has been divided equally between ischemic and non-ischemic cardiomyopathy. Recently patients with non-ischemic cardiomyopathy have become the predominant group presenting for transplantation.[2] The mean age of adults currently undergoing heart transplantation is 51.1 years. The average recipient age continues to increase, with patients over the age of 60 representing 25% of all patients receiving heart transplants over the last 5 years. There has also been a 10-fold increase in the number of patients aged 70 and older undergoing heart transplantation.[2] Consequently, with continued refinement of the procedure of heart transplantation and its associated pre- and postoperative management, the number of individuals to whom this treatment can be offered is expanding. This further magnifies the relative shortage of donor organs in the face of increasing demand. Accordingly, criteria used for selection of organ donors have been made less stringent in order to accommodate for the reduction in organ supply. The mean age of donors for heart transplantation has increased from 23 years in 1983 to 33.6 years in 2009. Donors aged 50 or greater were exceedingly rare prior to 1986. Currently this age group accounts for 12% of donors, with donors over the age of 60 representing 1.4% of all donors.[2]

The transplant half-time is the time at which 50% of transplanted patients remain alive (median survival). For patients transplanted between 1982 and 2007, the transplant half-time for all patients having undergone adult and pediatric heart transplantation is currently 10 years. For patients who survived the first postoperative year the transplant half-life is 13 years. Survival for adult recipients has improved successively for each 5–10-year era. This increase in survival during each progressive era has been observed during the first postoperative year. The attrition of transplant recipients over the longer term has remained relatively unchanged over the entire history of heart transplantation. The transplant half-life for recipients transplanted between the year 2000 and 2007 is approximately 11 years. This increase in long-term survival has occurred despite more frequent utilization of marginal organs from "higher risk" organ donors and despite performing transplantation in recipients with a higher preoperative risk. In a risk-adjusted analysis undertaken by the ISHLT registry there was a 5% increase in 1-year predicted survival between patients transplanted in 1998 and in 2002 and a 9% increase observed in the 5-year survival.

A range of risk factors are associated with increased 1-year mortality following heart transplantation. These include the need for temporary circulatory support prior to transplantation, congenital heart disease as the indication, preoperative mechanical ventilation, or hemodialysis, female sex, recent treatment for infection with intravenous antibiotics, and ischemic cardiomyopathy. Increasing recipient age, body mass index (BMI), serum creatinine, and PVR are associated with reduced 1-year survival.[2] With regards to donor characteristics, increasing age and organ ischemic time along with decreasing BMI were predictive of an increase in 1-year mortality.[2] The mortality during the first year following heart transplantation is greater than the next 4 years combined. Accordingly, risk factors for 1-year mortality are also important predictors of longer-term outcome. In those patients surviving the first postoperative year, risk factors for subsequent 5-year mortality include the development of CAV within the first postoperative year, the need for retransplantation, mechanical ventilation prior to transplantation and treatment for rejection during the first postoperative year. Recipients with diabetes, increasing age, and a diagnosis of ischemic cardiomyopathy had reduced conditional 5-year survival. An increase in age of the donor also imparted a higher 5-year mortality risk in those patients who had survived for 1 year following transplantation.[2]

The leading cause of death within the first 30 days after heart transplantation is primary graft failure, accounting for 41% of deaths followed by multiorgan failure (13%) and infection (13%). After the first month infection is the predominant risk factor for death during the first year following transplantation, accounting for 30% of deaths during this period with graft failure being responsible for 18% and acute rejection for 12%. Over the longer-term allograft coronary artery disease was responsible for 32% of deaths 5 years after transplantation, followed by malignancy (23%) and infection (10%).[2] During the most recent era of transplantation, there has been a modest yet significant reduction in the incidence of CAV.

The future

Cardiac transplantation remains an established and effective treatment for patients with advanced heart failure. Clinical outcomes after transplantation continue to improve despite an increase in the risk profiles of both recipients and donors. Furthermore, the incidence of CAV, renal dysfunction, malignancy, and other barriers to prolonged survival have been decreasing.[2] Advances in immunosuppression, diagnostic testing, medical management, and mechanical support are likely to have a favorable impact on outcomes after heart transplantation. As mentioned earlier, the major limitation toward increasing the availability of this procedure for patients with heart disease has been the limited numbers of organs available. Donor organ shortage is the most prominent obstacle preventing heart transplantation from being offered to a substantial population of patients who may benefit from this procedure. The number of patients listed for heart transplantation is approximately two times greater than the number of suitable donor hearts. Consequently, approximately 8% of patients die while awaiting a heart transplant.[2]

Despite a more aggressive approach toward the utilization of "borderline" donor organs, a considerable number of organs continue to be declined on the basis of suboptimal function or other unfavorable characteristics related to the organ or donor. The development of more rigorous methods for organ assessment, resuscitation, recuperation, and preservation may allow for such organs to be utilized. New sources of organ donation may also allow for expansion of the donor pool. Donation of organs after circulatory arrest within the organ donor has led to significant increases in the number of organs available for renal, liver, and lung transplantation.[68-70] Although there are concerns over injury incurred to the donor heart during warm ischemia, historical experience and scientific investigation supports the possibility that cardiac donation from DCD (donation after circulatory death) donors may be possible.[19,71] Machine perfusion and *ex-vivo* evaluation of donor hearts may represent a means to objectively evaluate the function of such extended criteria donor hearts. The potential for recovering organs initially identified as having inadequate function for transplantation will require robust methods of measurement of cardiac function, and machine perfusion devices may provide the ideal platform to allow repeated assessment and evaluation of donor organ function. Furthermore, there may be scope for the application of therapeutic measures to improve donor heart function in this setting. The potential for eliminating cold ischemia by maintaining perfusion of organs during transportation promises to enhance donor heart viability and favorably influence logistical considerations associated with cardiac transplantation.

The worldwide decline in heart transplant activity since the mid-1990s is a concerning trend. Despite an overall decrease in heart transplant volumes the short and long-term results of heart transplantation continue to be satisfactory, improving the lives of thousands of patients with severe heart failure. The early era of heart transplantation was plagued with poor clinical outcomes, but through persistence and dedication the therapy became an outstanding success. Similar efforts may be necessary in the current era to revitalize heart transplantation, primarily through high-caliber scientific investigation and through the optimal utilization of the existing donor pool and the identification of new donor sources.

References

1. **Deuse T, Haddad F, Pham M**, *et al.* (2008). Twenty-year survivors of heart transplantation at Stanford University. *Am J Transplant*, **8**(9), 309–17.
2. **Taylor DO, Stehlik J, Edwards LB**, *et al.* (2009). Registry of the international society for heart and lung transplantation: twelfth official adult heart transplant report-2009. *J Heart Lung Transplant*, **28**(10), 1007–22.
3. **Petroski RA, Grady KL, Rodgers S**, *et al.* (2009). Quality of life in adult survivors greater than 10 years after pediatric heart transplantation. *J Heart Lung Transplant*, **28**(7), 661–6.
4. **Politi P, Piccinelli M, Poli PF**, *et al.* (2004). Ten years of "extended" life: quality of life among heart transplantation survivors. *Transplantation*, **78**(2), 257–63.
5. **Large SR** (2002). Is there a crisis in cardiac transplantation? *Lancet*, **359**(9308), 803–4.
6. **Wheeldon DR, Potter CD, Oduro A, Wallwork J, Large SR** (1995). Transforming the "unacceptable" donor: outcomes from the adoption of a standardized donor management technique. *J Heart Lung Transplant*, **14**(4), 734–42.
7. **Wittwer T, Wahlers T** (2008). Marginal donor grafts in heart transplantation: lessons learned from 25 years of experience. *Transpl Int*, **21**(2), 113–25.
8. **Menkis AH, Novick RJ, Kostuk WJ**, *et al.* (1991). Successful use of the "unacceptable" heart donor. *J Heart Lung Transplant*, **10**, 28–32.
9. **Carrel A, Guthrie CC** (1905). The transplantation of veins and organs. *Am Med*, **10**, 1101–2.
10. **Carrel A** (1907). The surgery of blood vessels. *Johns Hopkins Hosp Bull*, **18**, 18–28.
11. **Mann FC, Priestly JT, Markowitz J, Yater WM** (1953). Transplantation of the intact mammalian heart. *Arch Surg*, **66**, 179–91.
12. **Demikhov VP** (1962). *Experimental Transplantation of Vital Organs*. New York, NY, Consultants Bureau.
13. **Shumway NE, Lower RR** (1964). Special problems in transplantation of the heart. *Ann NY Acad Sci*, **120**, 773–7.
14. **Kondo Y, Gridel F, Kantrowitz A** (1965). Heart transplantation in puppies: long-term survival without immunosuppressive therapy. *Circulation*, **32**(Suppl 1), 181.
15. **Hardy JD, Chavez CM** (1968). The first heart transplant in man. *Am J Cardiol*, **22**, 772–81.
16. **Hardy JD, Chavez CM, Eraslan S, Adkins JR, Williams RD** (1966). Heart transplantation in dogs. Procedures, physiologic problems and results in 142 experiments. *Surgery*, **60**, 361.
17. **Hardy JD, Kurrus FD, Chavez CM, Webb WR** (1964). Heart transplantation in infant calves; evaluation of coronary perfusion to preserve organs during transfer. *Ann NY Acad Sci*, **120**, 766.
18. **Reemtsma K, McCracken BH, Schlegel JU, Pearl M** (1964). Heterotransplantation of the kidney: two clinical experiences. *Science*, **143**, 700–2.

19. **Barnard CN** (1967). The operation. A human cardiac transplant: an interim report of a successful operation performed at Groote Schuur Hospital, Cape Town. *S Afr Med J*, **31**(48), 1271–4.

20. **Kantrowitz A, Huller JD, Joos H, Cerutti MM, Carstensen HE** (1968). Transplantation of the heart in an infant and an adult. *Am J Cardiol*, **22**, 782–90.

21. **Cooley DA, Bloodwell RD, Hallman GI**, *et al.* (1969). Organ transplantation for advanced cardiopulmonary disease. *Ann Thorac Surg*, **8**, 30–46.

22. **Griepp RB** (1979). A decade of human heart transplantation. *Transplant Proc*, **1191**, 285–92.

23. **Milano CA, Shah AS, Van Trigt P**, *et al.* (2000). Evaluation of early postoperative results after bicaval versus standard cardiac transplantation and review of the literature. *Am Heart J*, **140**(5), 717–21.

24. **Park KY, Park CH, Chun YB, Shin MS, Lee KC** (2005). Bicaval anastomosis reduces tricuspid regurgitation after heart transplantation. *Asian Cardiovasc Thorac Ann*, **13**, 251.

25. **Meyer SR, Modry DL, Bainey K**, *et al.* (2005). Declining need for permanent pacemaker insertion with the bicaval technique of orthotopic heart transplantation. *Can J Cardiol*, **21**(2), 159–63.

26. **Aziz T, Burgess M, Khafagy R**, *et al.* (1999). Bicaval and standard techniques in orthotopic heart transplantation: medium-term experience in cardiac performance and survival. *J Thorac Cardiovasc Surg*, **118**, 115–22.

27. **Newcomb AE, Esmore DS, Rosenfeldt FL, Richardson M, Marasco S** (2004). Heterotopic heart transplantation: an expanding role in the twenty-first century? *Ann Thorac Surg*, **78**, 1345–50.

28. **Ridley PD, Khagani A, Musumeci F**, *et al.* (1992). Heterotopic heart transplantation and recipient heart operation in ischemic heart disease. *Ann Thorac Surg*, **54**, 333–7.

29. **Gerber BL, Bernard X, Melin KA**, *et al.* (2001). Exaggerated chronotropic and energetic response to dobutamine after orthotopic cardiac transplantation. *J Heart Lung Transplant*, **20**(8), 824–32.

30. **Kirklin JK, Naftel DC, Bourge RC**, *et al.* (2003). Evolving trends in risk profiles and causes of death after heart transplantation: a ten-year multi-institutional study. *J Thorac Cardiovasc Surg*, **125**, 881–90.

31. **Kieler-Jensen N, Lundin S, Ricksten E** (1995). Vasodilator therapy after heart transplantation: effects of inhaled nitric oxide and intravenous prostacyclin, prostaglandin E1, and sodium nitroprusside. *J Heart Lung Transplant*, **14**(3), 436–43.

32. **Ardehali A, Hughes K, Sadeghi A**, *et al.* (2001). *Transplantation*, **72**(4), 638–41.

33. **Arafa OE, Geiran OR, Andersen K**, *et al.* (2000). Intraaortic balloon pumping for predominantly right ventricular failure after heart transplantation. *Ann Thorac Surg*, **70**, 1587–93.

34. **Carrier M, White M, Perrault LP**, *et al.* (1999). A 10-year experience with intravenous thymoglobulin immunosuppression following heart transplantation. *J Heart Lung Transplant*, **18**(12), 1218–23.

35. **Chien NC, Lin FL, Chou NK**, *et al.* (2000). Rabbit antithymocyte globulin induction immunosuppression in heart transplantation. *Transplant Proc*, **32**(7), 2380–2.

36. **Frist WH, Gerhardt EB, Merrill WH**, *et al.* (1990). Therapy of refractory, recurrent heart rejection with multiple courses of OKT3. *J Heart Transplant*, **9**(6), 724–6.

37. **Swinnen LJ, Costanzo-Nordin MR, Fisher SG**, *et al.* (1994). Increased incidence of lymphoproliferative disorders and immunsuppression with the monoclonal antibody OKT3 in cardiac transplant recipients. *Am J Cardiol*, **74**(3), 261–6.

38. **Johnson MR, Mullen GM, O'Sullivan EJ**, *et al.* (1994). Risk/benefit ratio of perioperative OKT3 in cardiac transplantation. *Am J Cardiol*, **74**(3), 261–6.

39. **Mehra MR, Zucker MJ, Wagoner L**, *et al.* (2005). A multicenter, prospective, randomized, double-blind trial of basiliximab in heart transplantation. *J Heart Lung Transplant*, **24**(9), 1297–304.

40. **Teuteberg JJ, Shullo MA, Zomak R**, *et al.* (2010). Alemtuzumab induction prior to cardiac transplantation with lower intensity maintenance immunosuppression: one-year outcomes. *Am J Transplant*, **10**(2), 382–8.

41. **Reichart B, Meiser B, Viganò M**, *et al.* (2001). European multicenter tacrolimus heart pilot study: three-year follow-up. *J Heart Lung Transplant*, **20**(2), 249–50.

42. **Taylor DO, Barr ML, Radovancevic B**, *et al.* (1999). A randomized, multicenter comparison of tacrolimus and cyclosporine immunosuppressive regimens in cardiac transplantation: decreased hyperlipidemia and hypertension with tacrolimus. *J Heart Lung Transplant*, **18**(4), 336–45.

43. **Eisen HJ, Kobashigawa J, Keogh A**, *et al.*; **Mycophenolate Mofetil Study Investigators** (2005). Three-year results of a randomized, double-blind, controlled trial of mycophenolate mofetil versus azathioprine in cardiac transplant recipients. *J Heart Lung Transplant*, **24**(5), 517–25.

44. **Sharples LD, Caine N, Mullins P**, *et al.* (1991). Risk factor analysis for the major hazards following heart transplantation—rejection, infection, and coronary occlusive disease. *Transplantation*, **52**(2), 244–52.

45. **Caves PK, Coltart J, Billingham ME**, *et al.* (1975). Transvenous endomyocardial biopsy. Application of a method for diagnosing heart disease. *Postgrad Med J*, **51**, 286.

46. **Miller LW, Wesp A, Jennison SH**, *et al.* (1993). Vascular rejection in heart transplant recipients. *J Heart Lung Transplant*, **12**(2), S147–52.

47. **Billingham ME** (1992). Histopathology of graft coronary disease. *J Heart Lung Transplant*, **11**, S38.

48. **Taylor DO, Edwards LB, Boucek MM**, *et al.* (2005). Registry of the International Society for Heart and Lung Transplantation: twenty-second official adult heart transplant report—2005. *J Heart Lung Transplant*, **24**, 945–55.

49. **Costanzo MR, Naftel DC, Pritzker MR**, *et al.* (1998). Heart transplant coronary artery disease detected by coronary angiography: a multi-institutional study of preoperative donor and recipient risk factors. Cardiac Transplant Research Database. *J Heart Lung Transplant*, **17**, 744–53.

50. **Caforio AL, Tona F, Fortina AB**, *et al.* (2004). Immune and nonimmune predictors of cardiac allograft vasculopathy onset and severity: multivariate risk factor analysis and role of immunosuppression. *Am J Transplant*, **4**, 962–70.

51. **Valantine H** (2004). Cardiac allograft vasculopathy after heart transplantation: risk factors and management. *J Heart Lung Transplant*, **23**, S187–93.

52. **Day JD, Rayburn BK, Gaudin PB**, *et al.* (1995). Cardiac allograft vasculopathy: the central pathogenic role of ischemia-induced endothelial cell injury. *J Heart Lung Transplant*, **14**, S142–9.

53. **Bocksch W, Wellnhofer E, Schartl M**, *et al.* (2000). Reproducibility of serial intravascular ultrasound measurements in patients with angiographically silent coronary artery disease after heart transplantation. *Coronary Artery Dis*, **11**, 555–62.

54. **Redonnet M, Tron C, Koning R**, *et al.* (2000). Coronary angioplasty and stenting in cardiac allograft vasculopathy following heart transplantation. *Transplant Proc*, **32**, 463–5.

55. **Mehra MR, Ventura HO, Smart FW**, *et al.* (1995). Impact of converting enzyme inhibitors and calcium entry blockers on cardiac allograft vasculopathy: from bench to bedside. *J Heart Lung Transplant*, **14**, S246–9.

56. **Kobashigawa JA, Katznelson S, Laks H**, *et al.* (1995). Effect of pravastatin on outcomes after cardiac transplantation. *New Engl J Med*, **333**, 621–7.

57. **Rubin RH** (2000). Prevention and treatment of cytomegalovirus disease in heart transplant patients. *J Heart Lung Transplant*, **19**, 731–5.

58. **Wiltshire H, Hirankarn S, Farrell C**, *et al.* (2005). Pharmacokinetic profile of ganciclovir after its oral administration and from its prodrug, valganciclovir, in solid organ transplant recipients. *Clin Pharmacokinet*, **44**, 495–507.

59. **Montoya JG, Chaparro SV, Celis D**, *et al.* (2003). Invasive aspergillosis in the setting of cardiac transplantation. *Clin Infect Dis*, **37**, S281–92.

60. **Cardenal R, Medrano FJ, Varela JM**, *et al.* (2001). *Pneumocystis carinii* pneumonia in heart transplant recipients. *Eur J Cardiothorac Surg*, **20**, 799–802.

61. **Speirs GE, Hakim M, Wreghitt TG** (1988). Relative risk of donor transmitted *Toxoplasma gondii* infection in heart, liver and kidney transplant recipients. *Clin Transplant*, **2**, 257–60.

62. **Senechal M, Dorent R, du Montcel ST** (2004). End-stage renal failure and cardiac mortality after heart transplantation. *Clin Transplant*, **18**, 1–6.

63. **Sivathasan C** (2004). Experience with cyclosporine in heart transplantation. *Transplant Proc*, **36**, 346S–8S.

64. **Angermann CE, Stork S, Costard-Jackle A** (2004). Reduction of cyclosporine after introduction of mycophenolate mofetil improves chronic renal dysfunction in heart transplant recipients: the IMPROVED multicentre study. *Eur Heart J*, **25**, 1626–34.

65. **Starling RC, Cody RJ** (1990). Cardiac transplant hypertension. *Am J Cardiol*, **65**, 106–11.

66. **Ippoliti G, Rinaldi M, Pellegrini C,** *et al.* (2005). Incidence of cancer after immunosuppressive treatment for heart transplantation. *Crit Rev Oncol Hematol*, **56**, 101–13.

67. **Opelz G, Dohler B** (2004). Lymphomas after solid organ transplantation: a collaborative transplant study report. *Am J Transplant*, **4**, 222–30.

68. **Alonso A, Fernandez-Rivera C, Villaverde P,** *et al.* (2005). Renal transplantation from non-heart beating donors: a single-center 10-year experience. *Transplant Proc*, **37**(9), 3658–60.

69. **Abt PL, Desai NM, Crawford MD, Forman LM, Markmann JF** (2004). Survival following liver transplantation from non-heart beating donors. *Am Surg*, **239**(1), 87–92.

70. **De Vleeschauwer S, Van Raemdonck D, Vanaudenaerde B,** *et al.* (2009). Early outcome after lung transplantation from non-heart beating donors is comparable to heart-beating donors. *J Heart Lung Transplant*, **28**(4), 380–7.

71. **Ali AA, White P, Xiang B,** *et al.* (2011). Hearts from DCD donors display acceptable biventricular function after heart transplantation in pigs. *Am J Transplant*, **11**(8), 1621–32.

Chapter 13

Current status of lung transplantation

Varun Puri and G. Alexander Patterson

Introduction

Since the first successful human lung transplant by the Toronto Lung Transplant Group in 1983[1] over 16,000 lung transplants have been performed. Donor shortage and chronic allograft rejection continue to be the biggest hurdles preventing lung transplantation from reaching its full potential.

Recipient selection

General selection criteria are listed in Box 13.1.[2] Patients over age 65 or with failure of another organ system are generally not eligible for transplantation due to an elevated risk of mortality.[3] A history of malignancy within the prior 5 years generally precludes pulmonary transplantation. A potential exception is a patient with bilateral bronchoalveolar carcinoma or a recent extrathoracic malignancy judged to be cured.[4,5] Serious psychological dysfunction, active smoking, and high-dose corticosteroid therapy (≥20 mg prednisone) are other contraindications. Ventilator dependency is also not a contraindication but has been identified as a risk factor for increased mortality.[3]

Patients considered for transplantation participate in a monitored exercise rehabilitation program while awaiting transplantation. Patients experience an improvement in strength and exercise tolerance without any measurable change in pulmonary function thus better enabling patients to withstand the rigors of a transplant procedure and subsequent convalescence.

Prior to 2005, lung allocation in the US was based on time spent on the waiting list, regardless of medical urgency or deterioration in medical condition. This system favored recipients well enough to survive on the transplant list while sicker patients, who may benefit most from the operation, risked death while waiting. An ideal system balances organ allocation based on clinical necessity while selecting recipients able to recover from a transplant operation. The United Network for Organ Sharing (UNOS) Thoracic Organ Committee revised the listing algorithm by assigning each patient a lung allocation score (LAS), based on the need for transplant and the probability of post-transplant survival. Details of the new allocation system are found on the Organ Procurement and Transplantation Network website, https://optn.transplant.hrsa.gov/learn/about-transplantation/how-organ-allocation-works/.[6] The highest scores are listed first for

---

Box 13.1 Recipient selection criteria

Clinically and physiologically severe disease

Medical therapy ineffective or unavailable

Substantial limitations in activities of daily living

Limited life expectancy

Adequate cardiac function without significant coronary disease

Ambulatory with rehabilitation potential

Acceptable nutritional status

Satisfactory psychosocial profile and emotional support system

Data sourced from Maurer JR, Frost AE, Estenne M, *et al*: International guidelines for selection of lung transplant candidates. J Heart Lung Transplant 1998; 17: 703–9.

---

transplantation. Several recent studies have analyzed data obtained a short-to-moderate length of time after the LAS implementation. In general, the results have been promising and have achieved the goals of the change in the allocation system (i.e., a decrease in waiting list times, decreased waiting list mortality, and an increased number of lung transplants performed),[7-11] with an increase in the urgency of those transplanted, which is particularly reflected in the group of idiopathic pulmonary fibrosis (IPF) patients. Longer follow-up will be needed to confirm these findings and determine the non-inferiority of long-term survival of patients.

Single- versus double-lung transplantation

Double-lung transplantation is the norm for septic lung disease. A significant number of patients worldwide receive single-lung transplants for COPD (Chronic Obstructive Pulmonary Disease) and IPF but registry data indicate that double-lung transplantation is rising in popularity for these indications.[12] The advantages of a single-lung transplant include a technically easier operation, shorter ischemic time, and a societal benefit with two recipients benefiting from each donor. On the other hand, double-lung transplant recipients have better lung function and better quality of life than single-lung recipients.[13,14] The long-term survival of double-lung transplant recipients is also better with median survival improving from 4.5 to 6.0 years.[15] Our preference is to perform a bilateral sequential lung transplant for all patients if possible.

Specific indications

COPD has previously been the most common indication for lung transplantation, accounting for 46% of the adult lung transplantations reported in the 2007 Registry of the UNOS/ISHLT.[3] When evaluating patients with emphysema for surgical therapy, consideration should be given to lung volume reduction surgery (LVRS) in ideal patients: hyperinflation, heterogeneous distribution of disease, forced expiratory volume in 1 s (FEV1) of more than

20%, and normal pco2.[16] Preliminary LVRS does not jeopardize subsequent successful lung transplantation.[17] Patients with rapid decline of FEV1 to less than 25% predicted, progressive hypercarbia (Paco2 ≥55 mmHg), increasing oxygen requirement, secondary pulmonary hypertension, or frequent life-threatening infections are better suited for transplantation.[2]

Cystic fibrosis is now the most common indication for bilateral lung transplantation.[3] An FEV_1 of less than 30% predicted, elevated $PaCO_2$, requirement for supplemental oxygen, frequent admissions to the hospital for control of acute pulmonary infection, and failure to maintain weight are reliable predictors of early mortality in these patients.[18] Patients with multidrug-resistant organisms, especially Burkholderia cepacia, are considered high risk, and many centers consider this a contraindication to transplantation.[19,20] If preoperative testing reveals no effective antibiotic regimen on synergy testing, we do not proceed with transplantation.

With the LAS system, UNOS data from 2008 show that more lung transplants were performed for pulmonary fibrosis than for obstructive lung disease.[21] Moderate pulmonary hypertension is common in these patients.

With the use of prostacyclins, endothelin receptor antagonists and phosphodiesterase inhibitors, an improvement in pulmonary artery pressures and relief of symptoms are seen in most patients with primary pulmonary hypertension.[22,23] Transplantation may be delayed as long as patients remain clinically stable on vasodilatory therapy.

Donor selection

Since many conditions resulting in brain death (trauma, spontaneous intracerebral hemorrhage) also lead to significant pulmonary parenchymal pathologic change because of lung contusion, infection, aspiration, or neurogenic pulmonary edema, only 20% of otherwise multiorgan donors have lungs satisfactory for transplantation by standard criteria (Box 13.2).

Although a significant smoking history (≥30 pack years) in the donor is a concern, it is not an absolute contraindication. Histocompatibility antigen (HLA) matching currently

---

Box 13.2 Ideal lung donor selection criteria

Age <55 years

No history of pulmonary disease

Normal serial chest radiograph

Adequate gas exchange—PaO_2 >300 mmHg; F_{IO2} 1.0; positive end-expiratory pressure 5 cm H_2O

Normal bronchoscopic examination

Negative serologic screening for hepatitis B and human immunodeficiency virus (HIV)

Recipient matching for ABO blood group

Size matching

is not performed between donor and recipient unless the patient has an elevated panel reactive antibody or known HLA antibodies from prior sensitization.

Size matching between donor and recipient is a significant consideration. The most reliable method of size matching predicts donor and recipient lung volumes using standard nomograms based on age, sex, and height. Implantation of a large allograft is easily achieved in a patient with obstructive lung disease because of the enormous size of the recipient pleural space. Conversely, in patients with pulmonary fibrosis or pulmonary vascular disease, the pleural spaces are reduced or normal in size, respectively. It is therefore inadvisable to oversize these patients. Donor lungs that are larger than the recipient's chest cavity but are otherwise usable should be accepted. A minor degree of pulmonary infiltrate may be accepted in donor lungs being used for a bilateral transplantation.[24]

Novel techniques to optimize donor usage have been introduced. The first is a split-lung technique that bipartitions the left lung of a large cadaveric donor and uses the two lobes to perform a bilateral lobar transplant in the smaller recipient. It requires significant expertise but has been performed successfully with good outcomes.[25,26]

Another technique is the use of non-heart-beating donors.[27–30] Results from this group of DCD donors (donation after cardiac death), where withdrawal of support is under controlled circumstances, have been published in some series over the last 3–4 years. Some series show excellent early results.[29,30] DCD lung transplantation should continue to be used cautiously at experienced centers.[28]

Steen and colleagues from Sweden have advocated extracorporeal perfusion and *ex-vivo* assessment of donor lung function in non-heart beating donors by reconditioning initially unacceptable lungs.[31] The lungs are perfused *ex vivo* with Steen solution, mixed with red blood cells to a hematocrit of 15%. An oxygenator maintains a normal mixed venous blood gas level in the perfusate. The lungs are ventilated and evaluated through analyses of pulmonary vascular resistance, oxygenation capacity, and arterial carbon dioxide pressure minus end-tidal carbon dioxide difference. The technique has also been outlined by the Toronto Lung Transplant Group.[32] Since then, a growing body of literature is looking at clinical results from such approaches.[29,33]

In the living lobar donation strategy, two healthy donors donate one lobe each. Donor right lower lobe and left lower lobe are implanted in the recipient on the respective side. In a large series, the operation provided recipient results comparable to conventional transplantation with no donor mortality but a morbidity rate of 20%.[34] With the new LAS the need for this approach has dropped off dramatically as patients who would benefit most from it, namely decompensated sicker patients, now have much reduced waiting periods for cadaveric organs.

Donor procurement

Brain-dead donor

Once a donor is determined to be suitable, the procuring team is activated. The procuring surgeon has the ultimate responsibility in making the final assessment of suitability of lungs and in ensuring the safe and expeditious conduct of the operation. The procuring team ensures appropriate ABO compatibility (including two separate blood group analyses on the donor), cross-checks the declaration of brain death and confirms appropriate permission for lung procurement. A flexible bronchoscopy is performed to assess anatomy and evaluate secretions. Clear communication between the heart and lung procurement teams is important. The sites of left and right heart venting, division of the left atrial cuff and the site of cannulation and division of the main pulmonary artery (PA) should be discussed and agreed upon.

Via a standard median sternotomy, the pericardium and both pleural spaces are widely opened. The lungs are palpated and a compliance check is performed. The pericardium is retracted with heavy sutures. At this point the quality of lungs and any concerns are communicated with the implantation team.

The superior vena cava (SVC) is encircled caudal to the azygous vein with heavy silk suture. The plane between the anterior surface of the right PA and the back of the SVC and the ascending aorta is developed. The aortopulmonary window is dissected and the aorta encircled with an umbilical tape that is useful in placement of the cross-clamp. The SVC and the aorta are gently retracted, posterior pericardium is incised above the right PA, and the plane around the trachea is developed bluntly. After all the procurement teams are ready, the donor is heparinized (250–300 units/kg iv). An aortic cardioplegia cannula is placed if the heart is being procured. A U-stitch is placed just proximal to the bifurcation of the main PA and a Sarns (Sarns, Ann Arbor, MI) 6.5-mm curved metal cannula is placed into the main PA (Figure 13.1)

A 500-microgram bolus of prostaglandin-E1 (PGE1) is injected directly into the PA. Hypotension ensues. Next the SVC is ligated, and the left atrial appendage is incised venting the left side of the heart. The inferior vena cava (IVC) is divided, thus venting the right heart. The aorta is cross-clamped and cardioplegia initiated. The pulmonary preservation solution consisting of several liters (50–75 cc/kg) of cold (4°C) Perfadex (Vitrolife, Goteborg, Sweden) is initiated via the PA cannula. Ice slush is generously used to topically cool the heart and both pleural spaces. We continue gentle ventilation to prevent atelectasis and homogenously distribute the perfusate. Clear perfusate exiting the left atriotomy confirms adequate lung flushing. After completion of the antegrade flush, the cannulae are removed. The IVC is now freed posteriorly and dissected up to the level of the right atrium avoiding injury to the right inferior pulmonary vein. Division of the left atrium ensues with the cooperation of the heart and lung teams. The heart is retracted toward the right and an incision is made in the left atrium midway between the coronary sinus and the left inferior pulmonary vein. The opening is extended superiorly and inferiorly while visualizing the orifices of the left sided pulmonary veins from inside the atrium. The remaining cuff of left atrium is transected while visualizing the orifice of right pulmonary veins from within the atrium. An appropriate residual atrial cuff should have a rim of atrial muscle around each of the pulmonary vein orifices (Figure 13.2).

The SVC is transected between ties. This is followed by division of the aorta proximal to the cross-clamp and the PA at the site of cannulation. The heart is then passed off the

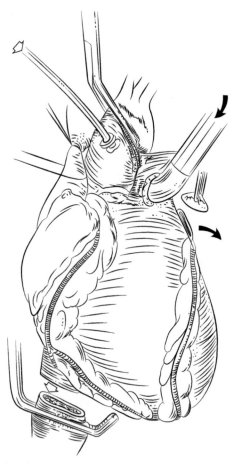

Figure 13.1 Cross clamping during procurement. Cardioplegia cannula in place in the ascending aorta and a cannula in the main pulmonary artery (PA). Venting of blood is via the inferior vena cava and the left atrial appendage.

Reproduced from Sundaersan S, Trachiotis GD, Aoe M, *et al*: Donor lung procurement: Assessment and operative technique. Ann Thorac Surg 56:1409–1413, © 1993 WB Saunders with permission from Elsevier.

field. Next, we use a Foley catheter to deliver about 250 cc of retrograde pulmonary flush via each of the pulmonary vein orifices.

The mediastinal contents are now removed en bloc. This avoids injury to the hilar structures and preserves maximal soft tissue for collateral flow to the airway. The superior mediastinal tissues are divided and the trachea encircled several cm above the carina. The endotracheal tube is backed into the proximal trachea. The trachea is divided between staple lines. The esophagus is also divided using a stapler (Figure 13.3).

The lungs are retracted inferiorly and superior mediastinal tissue divided down to the spine. Staying directly on the spine the posterior mediastinal tissue is divided to the level of the mid-thoracic spine. Now the dissection shifts inferiorly. The pericardium

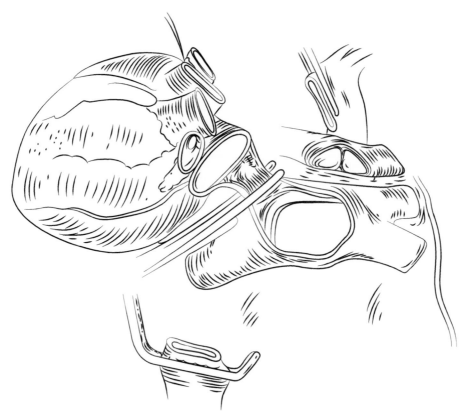

Figure 13.2 The heart is being explanted leaving a rim of atrium around each pulmonary vein orifice.

Reproduced from Sundaersan S, Trachiotis GD, Aoe M, et al: Donor lung procurement: Assessment and operative technique. Ann Thorac Surg 56:1409–1413, © 1993 WB Saunders with permission from Elsevier.

just superior to the diaphragm and the inferior pulmonary ligaments are divided. The supradiaphragmatic esophagus is divided with the linear stapler followed by division of the posterior mediastinal tissue including the aorta. Now the dissection is connected with the superior dissection and the lungs are removed en bloc.

If the lungs are to be used at separate institutions, they are separated on the back table. The donor esophagus and aorta are removed and the pericardium is excised. The lungs are separated by division of the posterior pericardium, left atrium between the pulmonary veins, division of the main PA at the bifurcation, and division of the left bronchus close to the carina. The lungs are placed in three layers of plastic bags, with cold preservation solution and transported on ice. The hila are prepared by dissecting the pulmonary arteries back to their first branches. The donor bronchus is divided one ring proximal to the upper lobe orifice while minimizing proximal peribronchial dissection to preserve collateral flow.

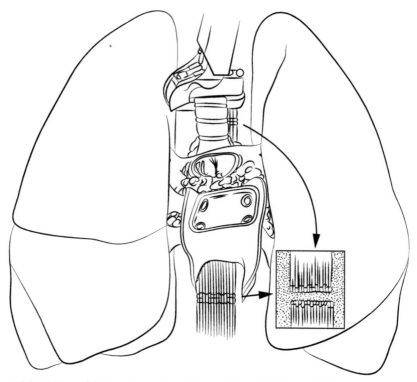

Figure 13.3 Division of the trachea and esophagus prior to double-lung bloc extraction after cardiectomy.

From Sundaersan S, Trachiotis GD, Aoe M, et al: Donor lung procurement: Assessment and operative technique. Ann Thorac Surg 56:1409–1413, © 1993 WB Saunders with permission from Elsevier

Non-heart beating donor

DeAntonio *et al.* have published their procurement technique with uncontrolled non-heart beating donors.[35] After systemic heparinization, the donor is placed on arterio-venous extracorporeal membrane oxygenation via a femoral approach. A fogarty catheter is placed in the supradiaphragmatic aorta for better abdominal organ perfusion and bi-lateral chest tubes are placed for topical lung cooling with cold Perfadex. Bronchoscopy is performed and the chest is opened. Ventilation is now resumed with 100% FiO_2 and 5 cm of positive end-expiratory pressure (PEEP). The pleural spaces are drained and pericar-dium opened. The aorta is clamped and both venae cavae ligated. Antegrade lung perfu-sion is performed with 5–6 L of Perfadex followed by infusion of 300 cc of donor blood through the PA. A blood gas analysis is performed on the left atrial effluent. Retrograde perfusion and the lung procurement are now performed in routine fashion.

For the controlled non-heart beating donor, support is withdrawn by extubation in the intensive care unit (ICU) or the OR. Once cardiac activity ceases, the donor is de-clared dead, endotracheal intubation done, and a bronchoscopy performed. A median sternotomy is performed and the lungs expeditiously evaluated. If the lungs are deemed suitable, the remaining operation proceeds as for a brain-dead donor. If the donor does not expire within 60 min of withdrawal of support, the procurement is abandoned. A thorough evaluation of institutional guidelines is mandatory prior to initiating a DCD lung transplantation program.

Procurement problems

Injuries often involve the right inferior pulmonary vein, occurring during the division of the left atrial cuff or division of the IVC, due to excessive dissection of the inferior pulmonary ligament or unnecessary dissection of the atrial cuff within the pericardium.

Several novel techniques have been described for salvage in this situation.[36]

A bronchus suis (i.e., a tracheal upper lobe bronchus) is a common anomaly and may represent a segmental or a lobar bronchus. If the bronchus is determined to be a segmental bronchus, it may be simply overseen. If the entire upper lobe bronchus arises as an abnormal tracheal bronchus, the options are donor right upper lobectomy, left single-lung transplantation, or incorporating the bronchus intermedius and the aberrant upper lobe bronchus into a modified anastomosis with the recipient bronchus.

Recipient implantation

Recipient anesthesia and intraoperative conduct

An experienced anesthesia team well-versed with double lumen tube management, bronchoscopy, and transesophageal echocardiography (TEE) is invaluable to the conduct of the operation. An epidural catheter is placed unless systemic heparinization for cardiopulmonary bypass is anticipated. Patients with cystic fibrosis undergo therapeutic bronchoscopy and suctioning via a large single lumen endotracheal tube. Radial and femoral arterial lines, a PA catheter, TEE probe, and an infraumbilical heating blanket are routine. The patient is placed supine with arms tucked. We employ vasopressors as indicated and avoid excessive volume resuscitation.[37]

We use epoprostenol and/or nitric oxide for acute refractory pulmonary hypertension in the perioperative period with inhaled nitric oxide also being used for poor oxygenation.

Operative approach

Bilateral anterolateral thoracotomy without sternal division is our preferred incision for bilateral lung transplant.[38] The chest cavity is entered in the fourth interspace (Figure 13.4).

A transverse sternothoracotomy (clamshell incision) additionally involves division of the sternum (Figure 13.5). This incision provides excellent exposure and requires the division of both mammary arteries. A clamshell incision is used for providing added exposure when a concomitant cardiac procedure is performed or when cardiomegaly, or a relatively small chest cavity, make hilar exposure difficult. The sternum is reapproximated using two figure-of-eight #5 sternal wires.

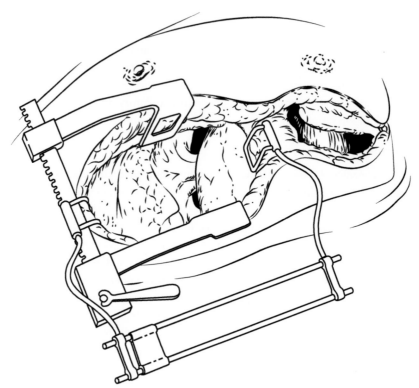

Figure 13.4 Bilateral anterolateral thoracotomy with two retractors placed at right angles.

Reproduced from From Meyers BF, Patterson GA: Technical aspects of adult lung transplantation. Semin Thorac Cardiovasc Surg 10: 213– 220, 199 with permission from Elsevier

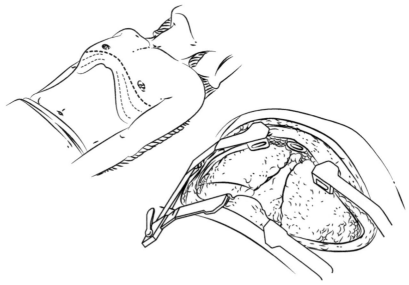

Figure 13.5 The sternum has been divided for a clamshell incision providing excellent exposure to the thorax.

Reproduced from Lau CL, Patterson GA. Technical considerations in lung transplantation. Chest Surg Clin N Am 13: 463–483: 2003 with permission from Elsevier

Median sternotomy is used if the recipient is undergoing concomitant cardiac surgery or in women with large breasts which compromise the exposure via anterolateral thoracotomy.

A small antero-axillary thoracotomy has been found comparable to the more conventional incisions in terms of operating times and ability to go on central cardiopulmonary bypass (CPB).[39,40]

Prior to excision of the recipient lungs bilateral hilar dissection and adhesiolysis should be completed and donor lungs should be prepared. The lung with the poorer function, based upon a preoperative ventilation perfusion scan, is transplanted first as the other lung will better support single-lung ventilation.

The phrenic, vagus, and recurrent laryngeal nerves must be protected. The right PA is transected about 1 cm beyond the truncus anterior branch and the left PA beyond the second branch to the left upper lobe. This downsizes the recipient PA and may provide better donor-recipient size match and the first branch (ligated) of the recipient PA provides an anatomic landmark for orientation during the anastomosis. Next, the pulmonary veins are divided at secondary branch points and the pericardium opened widely. The peribronchial tissue is divided, and bronchial arteries controlled with cautery or ligatures. The bronchus is divided just proximal to the upper lobe origin and the lung removed. All posterior mediastinal and posterior chest wall bleeders are controlled as this is the only opportunity to access this area safely. We set up hilar exposure by gently retracting the PA and pulmonary veins anteriorly, ready for the bronchial anastomosis.

The donor lung is covered with a cold sponge and placed in a bed of ice slush into the thoracic cavity. The bronchial anastomosis is performed in an end-to-end fashion using two strands of 4-0 PDS stitch in running fashion. The anastomosis is started on the membranous part and carried around over the anterior cartilaginous part with the second suture (Figure 13.6). If there is a significant size mismatch, we modify the anastomosis by approximating the cartilaginous part with simple interrupted 3-0 vicryl sutures. The peribronchial tissue on the donor and recipient sides is used to cover the anterior aspect of the anastomosis to offer some protection to the overlying vascular anastomoses in case of bronchial anastomotic breakdown. End-to-end airway anastomosis has been found to be superior to the telescoped anastomosis technique.[41]

Next, a vascular clamp is placed on the recipient PA, the donor and recipient PAs trimmed, and an end-to-end anastomosis performed using a continuous 5-0 polypropylene stitch (Figure 13.7).

The vein stumps are then retracted laterally and a Satinsky-type clamp is placed centrally on the recipient's left atrium. The recipient pulmonary venous stumps are amputated and the two openings connected to create the atrial cuff. The anastomosis is fashioned with continuous 4-0 polypropylene. Stitches are placed in a mattress technique, which achieves intima-to-intima apposition and excludes potentially thrombogenic atrial muscle (Figure 13.8.).

The last few sutures are left loose, the lung partially inflated, and the PA clamp is released momentarily. This maneuver flushes out air and perfusate from the lung. The left

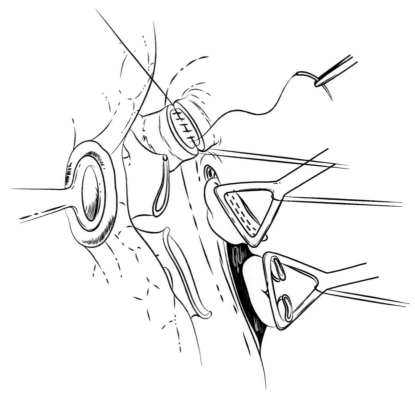

Figure 13.6 Retraction on the pulmonary artery and pulmonary vein stumps provides exposure for bronchial anastomosis. The anastomosis being performed with 4-0 PDS suture.
Reproduced from Meyers BF, Patterson GA: Technical aspects of adult lung transplantation. Semin Thorac Cardiovasc Surg 10: 213–220, 1998 with permission from Elsevier

atrial clamp is then opened to completely de-air the atrium. The atrial suture line is pulled up tight and tied down. All clamps are removed.

The pleural spaces are usually drained with two drains in each pleural space, one placed apically and one along the diaphragm. The ribs are reapproximated with heavy interrupted figure-of-eight monofilament non-absorbable suture.

A flexible bronchoscopy is performed after exchanging the double lumen tube for a single lumen tube to evaluate the airway anastomoses and remove blood and secretions.

We employ cardiopulmonary bypass selectively in our patients. It is indicated in children, small-statured patients in whom a double lumen tube cannot be placed, lobar transplants, concomitant intracardiac procedures, and most patients with pulmonary hypertension. CPB is also indicated for refractory hypoxemia, hypercarbia, pulmonary hypertension, or hemodynamic instability. Difficult exposure may necessitate CPB too. This is typically seen with a small pleural space in patients with IPF with the heart shifted to the left, thus making exposure of the left hilum difficult.

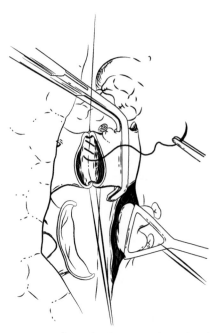

Figure 13.7 The PA anastomosis is performed using a running 5-0 polypropylene suture.

Reproduced from Meyers BF, Patterson GA: Technical aspects of adult lung transplantation. Semin Thorac Cardiovasc Surg 10: 213–220, 1998 with permission from Elsevier

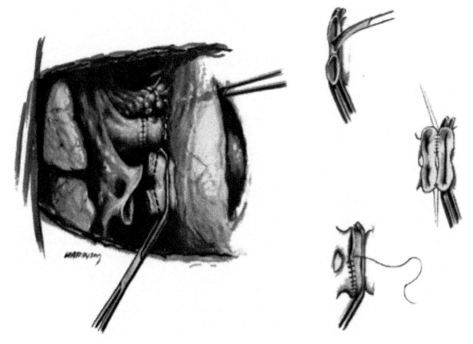

Figure 13.8 A large Satinsky is placed centrally across the left atrium. Both vein stumps are amputated and the bridge between connected to create a left atriotomy suitable for anastomosis.

Reproduced from Patterson GA: Bilateral lung transplant: Indications and technique. Semin Thorac Cardiovasc Surg 4:95–100, 1992 with permission from Elsevier

Recently, we have used the Urchin heart positioning device to elevate the heart (Medtronic, Inc, Minneapolis, MN) to improve exposure and avoid CPB.[42]

Lungs that are larger than the recipient's thoracic cage are downsized by performing a lobectomy on the back table, or bilateral wedge resections (lingula and the right middle lobe) after implantation.

At the conclusion of the operation, if the patient is unstable or shows continuous oozing due to a coagulopathy, we prefer to close skin only and resuscitate the patient in the ICU with closure planned in 24–48 hours. This strategy does not increase wound complications.[43]

Postoperative management and selected complications

Routine care

The patients are transported to the ICU and ventilated. Extubation is performed in accordance with standard parameters within 24–48 hours. After single-lung transplantation for emphysema, preventing hyperinflation of the native lung and compression of the freshly implanted lung are the main concerns.[44] This is accomplished by avoiding the use of PEEP and using lower tidal volumes. In single-lung recipients with pulmonary vascular disease, we use a prolonged period (48 hours) of elective ventilation. The patient is positioned to keep the native lung dependent to maintain inflation and appropriate drainage of the transplanted lung. Tidal volumes are standard, but a higher PEEP of 7.5–10 cm H_2O is applied. Postoperatively, a quantitative lung perfusion scan to assess for adequate patency and graft flow is usually performed.

Vigorous chest physiotherapy, postural drainage, inhaled bronchodilators, and frequent clearance of pulmonary secretions are required in the postoperative care, with early involvement of the physiotherapy team ensuring ambulation as soon as possible.

Immunosuppression

Postoperative induction therapy is controversial. Potential benefits include lower rates of acute rejection, protection from nephrotoxicity due to the delayed introduction of a calcineurin inhibitor, and a decrease in the occurrence of BOS (bronchiolitis obliterans syndrome). Disadvantages are the higher risk of infectious complications and post-transplantation malignancies. About 40% of patients undergoing lung transplantation receive induction immunosuppression.[3] Agents used include polyclonal antilymphocyte or antithymocyte preparations, monoclonal OKT3, and IL-2 receptor antagonists. All of the agents used in induction are generally associated with a decrease in the number of episodes of acute rejection, however their true impact on the incidence of BOS or overall survival remains to be determined. IL-2 receptor antagonists block activated T lymphocytes and may be associated with a lower risk of infectious complications and possibly post-transplantation lymphoproliferative disease.[45,46] Other studies however indicate that no single induction agent is superior to the other.[47]

For maintenance therapy we rely on triple-agent therapy for consisting of corticosteroids, a calcineurin inhibitor, and a cell cycle inhibitor. About 75% of lung transplant recipients are receiving a calcineurin inhibitor and a purine synthesis inhibitor at 1 and 5 years after transplantation, respectively.[3]

Cyclosporine and tacrolimus are calcineurin inhibitors which suppress the transcription of IL-2 and inhibit proliferation of T lymphocytes. Azathioprine inhibits de novo purine synthesis and suppresses proliferation of both T and B lymphocytes. Mycophenolate mofetil (MMF) is a prodrug of mycophenolic acid, which produces inhibition of de novo purine synthesis. Despite the lack of evidence for the superiority of MMF over azathioprine in lung transplantation, its use now exceeds that of azathioprine in lung transplant recipients.[48,49] Recently, a randomized, placebo-controlled, double-blind, multicenter trial on efficacy of inhaled cyclosporine in lung transplant recipients under a conventional triple immunosuppressive regimen was published.[50] Although the study had some limitations, and did not reach its primary efficacy endpoint (prevention of acute rejection), both survival and freedom from chronic rejection were significantly increased in the cyclosporin (CsA) arm, compared to placebo.[50] The same group has presented data on 30 transplanted patients, where aerosolized CsA in addition to conventional immunosuppression significantly preserved FEV1, versus placebo and historical controls.[51]

Sirolimus and its derivative everolimus, have been recently introduced into clinical lung transplantation. These agents block growth factor-driven cell cycle progression and proliferation of lymphocytes and other non-hematopoietic cells such as vascular smooth muscle cells. In an international, randomized multicenter study enrolling 213 BOS-free lung transplant recipients, efficacy was evaluated between azathioprine and everolimus. Although at 12 months the everolimus group showed a significantly smaller decline in FEV1 and had experienced less acute rejections, at 24 months only the incidence of acute rejection episodes still differed significantly between arms.[52] The interested reader may refer to a recent review of immunosuppression in lung transplantation.[53]

Primary graft dysfunction

Primary graft dysfunction (PGD) develops in up to 25% of lung transplant recipients.[54] The ISHLT has issued a grading system for primary graft dysfunction based on the Pao2/Fio2 ratio and findings on chest radiographs[55] (Table 13.1). Ischemia-reperfusion injury likely accounts for most cases of PGD. Levels of IL-8, a potent chemoattractant for neutrophils, increase during reperfusion of lung grafts, and correlate with the duration of the ischemic time, and negatively correlate with early lung function.[56]

PGD is managed with aggressive cardiopulmonary support in the intensive care unit. Appropriate ventilatory strategies, inhaled nitric oxide,[57] and aerosolized prostacyclin[58] are employed. In most patients, PGD resolves over several days of intensive care support.

Extracorporeal membrane oxygenation (ECMO) support is employed if conservative management appears to be unsuccessful. In a review of our experience with 983 lung transplant recipients, ECMO was used in 9.7% of the pediatric and 2.8% of adult

Table 13.1 Grading system for primary graft dysfunction

Grade	PaO$_2$/F$_{IO2}$	Radiographic infiltrates
0	>300	Absent
1	>300	Present
2	200–300	Present
3	<200	Present

Reproduced from Christie *et al.* (2005) Report of the ISHLT Working Group on Primary Lung Graft Dysfunction Part II: Definition. A Consensus Statement of the International Society for Heart and Lung Transplantation, The Journal of Heart and Lung Transplantation 24(10):1454–9. Copyright © 2005 International Society for Heart and Lung Transplantation with permission from Elsevier.

recipients. Only 38% of patients who received ECMO survived to discharge from the hospital.[54] The Duke University group advocates the use of venovenous ECMO due to much fewer complications encountered.[59]

The use of controlled reperfusion in combination with leukocyte depletion has been proposed as a preventive strategy. Lick and colleagues have published their original technique for the same.[60] We do not routinely employ this method, as PGD likely contributes to chronic rejection.[54]

Infections

Details of infection prophylaxis are beyond the scope of the current chapter. In brief, we routinely employ broad-spectrum antibacterial chemotherapy for several days post-transplantation. For the first year after transplantation we routinely give acyclovir for herpes simplex prophylaxis. In patients at high risk for cytomegalovirus (CMV) infection we use 12 weeks of IV ganciclovir starting 7–14 days post-transplantation. For transplants we use CMV-negative or leukocyte-reduced blood products. Lifelong *Pneumocystis carinii* prophylaxis is employed.

Bacterial infections are common in the early post-transplant period and remain the primary cause of mortality in the early post-transplant period.[61] Wound infections are generally due to conventional bacteria such as staphylococci. CMV disease is the most commonly noted postoperative infectious complication. It occurs in 13–75% of transplant patients depending on definitions of CMV disease and use of CMV prophylaxis.[62] Most programs match seronegative donors with seronegative recipients. Prophylactic regimens include oral or IV ganciclovir, with or without CMV IV immunoglobulin. Valganciclovir, an oral prodrug of ganciclovir, has been used as a prophylactic agent.[63] Although CMV infection is uncommon during prophylaxis, the rate of CMV disease increases after cessation of prophylactic therapy. Candidal infections are most commonly associated with airway anastomotic complications.[61] The most frequent cause of significant fungal infection after transplantation is *Aspergillus*. Invasive infection is the most feared complication and carries a high mortality. More commonly, however,

Aspergillus growing in sputum or bronchoalveolar lavage (BAL) cultures represents colonization.

Airway complications

Anastomotic complications resulting from airway ischemia include infection, dehiscence, stenosis, and malacia. The reported incidence of these complications is 7–14% of patients.[61-63] In a review of our experience, the rate of airway complications was during the initial period of the lung transplantation experience from 1988 through 1993, was 16%; this decreased to less than 10% during later time periods. Airway complications did not seem to have an adverse impact on overall survival.[54]

From a technical standpoint, a shortened donor bronchial length (one ring proximal to the upper lobe takeoff) reduces the length of donor bronchus dependent on collateral flow. Peribronchial tissue on the donor bronchus is preserved during preparation of the lung.

Occasionally, patchy areas of superficial necrosis of donor bronchial epithelium are observed. These areas are of no concern and ultimately heal. Membranous wall defects typically heal without airway compromise, whereas cartilaginous defects usually result in some degree of late stricture. Massive dehiscence of the airway with uncontrolled leak or mediastinal contamination requires retransplantation. Lesser degrees of dehiscence can be managed expectantly. Necrotic tissue at the bronchial anastomosis is an ideal medium for the growth of fungi. Nunley and colleagues found that saprophytic fungal infections involving the bronchial anastomosis occurred in 25% of recipients. In 47% of those patients with fungal involvement of the anastomosis, airway complications occurred.[64]

Chronic airway stenoses result from surgical stenosis, granulation tissue, infection, or bronchomalacia, with ischemia as the universal common denominator. Bronchoscopic balloon dilation and stent placement are the usual options.[65,66] Treatment of the granulation tissue consists of a combination of laser or forceps debridement, dilatation, and stenting.[66] Recurrent airway stenosis have been managed with topical application of mitomycin C[67] and high-dose brachytherapy.[68] If lesser approaches fail, sleeve resection and retransplantation are other options.

Chronic rejection—bronchiolitis obliterans (BO)

Because of the difficulties in documenting BO histologically, a clinical deterioration in lung function (termed bronchiolitis obliterans syndrome, or BOS) has been adopted as its surrogate and current diagnostic criteria have been outlined.[69] By 5.6 years post-transplantation, 51% of patients will have developed BOS.[15]

Many reports have shown an association between viral respiratory infections and the development of BOS.[70,71] Also, it has been postulated that chronic aspiration of gastric contents damages the lung allograft and contributes to chronic allograft dysfunction and that a fundoplication performed early after lung transplantation may reduce the incidence of BOS.[72]

Standard treatment protocols consist of augmenting immunosuppression in an attempt to stabilize the disease process. Regimens such as high-dose corticosteroids, cytolytic therapy, substitution of mycophenolate mofetil for azathioprine, and conversion of cyclosporine to tacrolimus have on occasion been successful in preserving pulmonary function at a stable level.[73,74] Recently mTOR inhibitors have been used in several single-center programs to stabilize lung function after the diagnosis of BOS.[75,76]

Other therapeutic strategies have included inhaled cyclosporine, inhaled high-dose corticosteroids, and photopheresis.[53] Rapamycin, azithromycin, and clarithromycin,[77] statins,[78] and IL-2 receptor antagonists[45] may hold promise in altering the outcomes from BOS. Retransplantation may be an option in carefully selected patients with BOS.[79]

Results

Generally speaking, patients are off supplemental oxygen and have significantly improved exercise tolerance by 4–6 weeks after transplantation. Registry data on overall survival for recipients of lung transplants from 1994[12] demonstrated unadjusted survival of 89% at 3 months, 79% at 1 year, 64% at 3 years, 52% at 5 years, and 29% at 10 years. Compared with data beginning in 1988, overall survival has consistently improved by era. The improvement in survival in the more current era is largely driven by improvements in 1-year survival. Among patients surviving at least 1 year, those with diagnoses of cystic fibrosis, primary pulmonary hypertension, sarcoidosis, and Alpha 1 antitrypsin deficiency had significantly better survival at 10 years after transplantation (48%, 45%, 44%, and 41%, respectively) than those with COPD (28%) and IPF (30%), most likely because COPD and IPF patients are older with more comorbidities.[12]

The major identified causes of death in the first 30 days are graft failure and non-CMV infections. After the first year, BOS and non-CMV infections were the predominant causes of death. Death caused by malignancies rises consistently until the 10-year mark, accounting for 12% of all deaths between 5 and 10 years after transplant.[12]

Conclusions

Lung transplantation is well established as a viable therapy for end-stage lung disease. Appropriate patient and donor selection, meticulous attention to technique, and continued improvement in the postoperative care of these patients will lead to optimal outcomes. Research to increase the donor pool and to prevent or manage BOS is the key to the future of lung transplantation.

References

1. **Toronto Lung Transplantation Group** (1986). Unilateral lung transplantation for pulmonary fibrosis. *N Engl J Med*, **314**, 1140–5.
2. **Maurer JR, Frost AE, Estenne M,** *et al.* (1998). International guidelines for selection of lung transplant candidates. *J Heart Lung Transplant*, **17**, 703–9.

3. Trulock EP, Christie JD, Edwards LB, *et al.* (2007). Registry of the International Society for Heart and Lung Transplantation: twenty-fourth official adult lung and heart-lung transplantation report-2007. *J Heart Lung Transplant*, **26**, 782–95.

4. Etienne B, Bertocchi M, Gamondes JP, *et al.* (1997). Successful double-lung transplantation for bronchioalveolar carcinoma. *Chest*, **112**, 1423–4.

5. Zorn GI, McGiffin DC, Young KR Jr, *et al.* (2003). Pulmonary transplantation for advanced bronchioloalveolar carcinoma. *J Thorac Cardiovasc Surg*, **125**, 45–8.

6. Organ Procurement and Transplantation Network. How Organ Allocation Works. Available at: https://optn.transplant.hrsa.gov/learn/about-transplantation/how-organ-allocation-works/

7. Davis SQ, Garrity ER Jr (2007). Organ allocation in lung transplant. *Chest*, **132**, 1646–51.

8. Iribarne A, Russo M, Davies R, *et al.* (2009). Despite decreased wait-list times for lung transplantation, lung allocation scores continue to increase. *Chest*, **135**, 923–8.

9. Hadjiliadis D, Ahya VN, Christie JD, *et al.* (2006). Early results of lung transplantation after implementation of the new lung allocation score [abstract]. *J Heart Lung Transplant*, **25**, S173.

10. Hachem RR, Trulock EP (2008). The new lung allocation system and its impact on waitlist characteristics and post-transplant outcomes. *Semin Thorac Cardiovasc Surg*, **20**, 139–42.

11. Organ Procurement and Transplantation Network. Home page. Available at: https://optn. transplant.hrsa.gov/

12. Christie JD, Edwards LB, Aurora P, *et al.* (2009). The Registry of the International Society for Heart and Lung Transplantation: twenty-sixth official adult lung and heart-lung transplantation report—2009. *J Heart Lung Transplant*, **28**, 1031–49.

13. Mason DP, Rajeswaran J, Murthy SC, *et al.* (2008). Spirometry after lung trasnplantation: how much better are two lungs than one? *Ann Thorac Surg*, **85**, 1193–201.

14. Anyanwu AC, McGuire A, Rogers CA, Murday AJ (2001). Assessment of quality of life in lung transplantation using a simple generic tool. *Thorax*, **56**, 218–22

15. Christie JD, Edwards LB, Aurora P, *et al.* (2008). Registry of the International Society for Heart and Lung Transplantation: twenty-fifth official adult lung and heart/lung transplantation report—2008. *J Heart Lung Transplant*, **27**, 937–83.

16. Meyers BF, Patterson GA (2001). Lung transplantation versus lung volume reduction as surgical therapy for emphysema. *World J Surg*, **25**, 238–43.

17. Meyers BF, Yusen RD, Guthrie TJ, *et al.* (2001). Outcome of bilateral lung volume reduction in patients with emphysema potentially eligible for lung transplantation. *J Thorac Cardiovasc Surg*, **122**, 10–7.

18. Kerem E, Reisman J, Corey M, Canny GJ, Levison H (1992). Prediction of mortality in patients with cystic fibrosis. *New Engl J Med*, **326**, 1187–91.

19. Aris RM, Routh JC, LiPuma JJ, *et al.* (2001). Lung transplantation for cystic fibrosis patients with Burkholderia cepacia complex. Survival linked to genomovar type. *Am J Respir Crit Care Med*, **164**, 2102–6.

20. Chaparro C, Maurer J, Gutierrez C, *et al.* (2001). Infection with Burkholderia cepacia in cystic fibrosis: outcome following lung transplantation. *Am J Respir Crit Care Med*, **163**, 43–8.

21. Organ Procurement and Transplantation Network. 2008 data files. Available at: https://optn. transplant.hrsa.gov/news/report-identifies-2008-transplant-trends/

22. McLaughlin VV, Genthner DE, Panella MM, *et al.* (1998). Reduction in pulmonary vascular resistance with long-term epoprostenol (prostacyclin) therapy in primary pulmonary hypertension. *N Engl J Med*, **338**, 273–7.

23. McLaughlin VV, McGoon MD (2006). Pulmonary artery hypertension. *Circulation*, **114**, 1417–31.

24. **Sundaresan S, Trulock EP, Mohanakumar T, Cooper JD, Patterson GA** (1995). Prevalence and outcome of bronchiolitis obliterans syndrome after lung transplantation. *Ann Thorac Surg*, **60**, 1341–7.

25. **Couetil JA, Tolan MJ, Loulmet DF,** *et al.* (1997). Pulmonary bipartitioning and lobar transplantation: a new approach to donor organ shortage. *J Thorac Cardiovasc Surg*, **113**, 529–37.

26. **Barbers RG** (1998). Cystic fibrosis: bilateral living lobar versus cadaveric lung transplantation. *Am J Med Sci*, **315**, 155–60.

27. **Steen S, Sjoberg T, Pierre L,** *et al.* (2001). Transplantation of lungs from a non-heart-beating donor. *Lancet*, **357**, 825–9.

28. **Puri V, Scavuzzo M, Guthrie T,** *et al.* (2009). Lung transplantation and donation after cardiac death—a single center experience. *Ann Thorac Surg*, **88**, 1609–14.

29. **Mason DP, Murthy SC, Gonzalez-Stawinski GV,** *et al.* (2008). Early experience with lung transplantation using donors after cardiac death. *J Heart Lung Transplant*, **27**, 561–3.

30. **Snell GI, Levvey BJ, Oto T,** *et al.* (2008). Early lung transplantation success utilizing controlled donation after cardiac death donors. *Am J Transplant*, **8**, 1282–8.

31. **Steen S, Ingemansson R, Eriksson L,** *et al.* (2007). First human transplantation of a nonacceptable donor lung after reconditioning ex vivo. *Ann Thorac Surg*, **83**, 2191–5.

32. **Cypel M, Yeung JC, Hirayama S,** *et al.* (2008). Technique for prolonged normothermic ex vivo lung perfusion. *J Heart Lung Transplant*, **27**, 1319–25.

33. **Pêgo-Fernandes PM, de Medeiros IL, Mariani AW,** *et al.* (2009). Ex vivo lung perfusion: initial Brazilian experience. *J Bras Pneumol*, **35**, 1107–11.

34. **Barr ML, Schenkel FA, Bowdish ME,** *et al.* (2005). Living donor lobar lung transplantation: current status and future directions. *Transplant Proc*, **37**, 3983–6.

35. **de Antonio DG, Marcos R, Laporta R,** *et al.* (2007). Results of clinical lung transplant from uncontrolled non-heart-beating donors. *J Heart Lung Transplant*, **26**, 529–34.

36. **Oto T, Rabinov M, Negri J,** *et al.* (2006). Techniques of reconstruction for inadequate donor left atrial cuff in lung transplantation. *Ann Thorac Surg*, **81**, 1199–204.

37. **Serra E, Feltracco P, Barbieri S, Forti A, Ori C** (2007). Transesophageal echocardiography during lung transplantation. *Transplant Proc*, **39**, 1981–2.

38. **Meyers BF, Sundaresan RS, Guthrie T,** *et al.* (1999). Bilateral sequential lung transplantation without sternal division eliminates posttransplantation sternal complications. *J Thorac Cardiovasc Surg*, **117**, 358–64.

39. **Pochettino A, Bavaria JE** (1997). Anterior axillary muscle-sparing thoracotomy for lung transplantation. *Ann Thorac Surg*, **64**, 1846–8.

40. **Toyoda Y** (2008). Lung transplantation through minimally invasive approach. *J Heart Lung Transplant*, **27**, S197.

41. **Aigner C, Jaksch P, Seebacher G,** *et al.* (2003). Single running suture—the new standard technique for bronchial anastomoses in lung transplantation. *Eur J Cardiothorac Surg*, **23**, 488–93.

42. **Lau CL, Hoganson DM, Meyers BF, Damiano RJ Jr, Patterson GA** (2006). Use of an apical heart suction device for exposure in lung transplantation. *Ann Thorac Surg*, **81**, 1524–5.

43. **Force SD, Miller DL, Pelaez A,** *et al.* (2006). Outcomes of delayed chest closure after bilateral lung transplantation. *Ann Thorac Surg*, **81**, 2020–4.

44. **Davis RD Jr, Trulock EP, Manley J,** *et al.* (1994). Differences in early results after single lung transplantation. *Ann Thorac Surg*, **58**, 1327–35.

45. **Brock MV, Borja MC, Ferber L,** *et al.* (2001). Induction therapy in lung transplantation: a prospective, controlled clinical trial comparing OKT3, anti-thymocyte globulin, and daclizumab. *J Heart Lung Transplant*, **20**, 1282–90.

46. Burton CM, Andersen CB, Jensen AS, *et al.* (2006). The incidence of acute cellular rejection after lung transplantation: a comparative study of anti-thymocyte globulin and daclizumab. *J Heart Lung Transplant*, **25**, 638–47.

47. Snell GI, Westall GP (2007). Immunosuppression for lung transplantation: evidence to date. *Drugs*, **67**, 1531–9.

48. Corris P, Glanville A, McNeil K, *et al.* (2001). One year analysis of an ongoing international randomized study of mycophenolate mofetil (MMF) vs azathioprine (AZA) in lung transplantation. *J Heart Lung Transplant*, **20**, 149–50.

49. Palmer SM, Baz MA, Sanders L, *et al.* (2001). Results of a randomized, prospective, multicenter trial of mycophenolate mofetil versus azathioprine in the prevention of acute lung allograft rejection. *Transplantation*, **71**, 1772–6.

50. Iacono A, Johnson BA, Grgurich WF, *et al.* (2006). A randomized trial of inhaled cyclosporine in lung-transplant recipients. *N Engl J Med*, **12**, 141–50.

51. Galazka M, Groves T, Corcoran T, *et al.* (2008). Preservation of pulmonary function by inhaled cyclosporine in lung transplant recipients. *J Heart Lung Transplant*, **27**, S206.

52. Snell G, Valentine VG, Glanville AR, *et al.* (2006). Everolimus versus azathioprine in maintenance lung transplant recipients: an international, randomized, double-blind clinical trial. *Am J Transplant*, **6**, 169–77.

53. Korom S, Boehler A, Weder W (2009). Immunosuppressive therapy in lung transplantation: state of the art. *Eur J Cardio Thorac Surg*, **35**, 1045–55.

54. Meyers BF, de la Morena M, Sweet SC, *et al.* (2005). Primary graft dysfunction and other selected complications of lung transplantation: a single-center experience of 983 patients. *J Thorac Cardiovasc Surg*, **129**, 1421–9.

55. Christie JD, Carby M, Bag R, *et al.* (2005). Report of the ISHLT Working Group on Primary Lung Graft Dysfunction part II: definition. A consensus statement of the International Society for Heart and Lung Transplantation. *J Heart Lung Transplant*, **24**, 1454–9.

56. De Perrot M, Sekine Y, Fischer S, *et al.* (2002). Interleukin-8 release during early reperfusion predicts graft function in human lung transplantation. *Am J Respir Crit Care Med*, **165**, 211–5.

57. Date H, Triantafillou AN, Trulock EP, *et al.* (1996). Inhaled nitric oxide reduces human lung allograft dysfunction. *J Thorac Cardiovasc Surg*, **111**, 913–9.

58. Fiser SM, Cope JT, Kron IL, *et al.* (2001). Aerosolized prostacyclin (epoprostenol) as an alternative to inhaled nitric oxide for patients with reperfusion injury after lung transplantation. *J Thorac Cardiovasc Surg*, **121**, 981–2.

59. Hartwig MG, Appel JZ, Cantu E, *et al.* (2005). Improved results treating lung allograft failure with venovenous extracorporeal membrane oxygenation. *Ann Thorac Surg*, **80**, 1872–80.

60. Lick SD, Brown PS, Jr., Kurusz M, *et al.* (2000). Technique of controlled reperfusion of the transplanted lung in humans. *Ann Thorac Surg*, **69**, 910–2.

61. Avery RK (2006). Infections after lung transplantation. *Semin Respir Crit Care Med*, **27**, 544–51.

62. Gutierrez CA, Chaparro C, Krajden M, *et al.* (1998). Cytomegalovirus viremia in lung transplant recipients receiving ganciclovir and immune globulin. *Chest*, **113**, 924–32.

63. Humar A, Kumar D, Preiksaitis J, *et al.* (2005). A trial of valganciclovir prophylaxis for cytomegalovirus prevention in lung transplant recipients. *Am J Transplant*, **5**, 1462–8.

60. Hadjiliadis D, Howell DN, Davis RD, *et al.* (2000). Anastomotic infections in lung transplant recipients. *Ann Transplant*, **5**, 13–9.

61. Chhajed PN, Malouf MA, Tamm M, *et al.* (2001). Interventional bronchoscopy for the management of airway complications following lung transplantation. *Chest*, **120**, 1894–9.

62. **Griffith BP, Hardesty RL, Armitage JM**, *et al*. (1993). A decade of lung transplantation. *Ann Surg*, **218**, 310.

63. **Shennib H, Massard G** (1994). Airway complications in lung transplantation. *Ann Thorac Surg*, **57**, 506–11.

64. **Nunley DR, Gal AA, Vega JD**, *et al*. (2002). Saprophytic fungal infections and complications involving the bronchial anastomosis following human lung transplantation. *Chest*, **122**, 1185–91.

65. **Santacruz JF, Mehta AC** (2009). Airway complications and management after lung transplantation. *Proc Am Thorac Soc*, **6**, 79–93.

66. **Chhajed PN, Malouf MA, Tamm M**, *et al*. (2001). Interventional bronchoscopy for the management of airway complications following lung transplantation. *Chest*, **120**, 1894–9.

67. **Erard AC, Monnier P, Spiliopoulos A**, *et al*. (2001). Mitomycin C for control of recurrent bronchial stenosis: a case report. *Chest*, **120**, 2103–5.

68. **Halkos ME, Godette KD, Lawrence EC, Miller JI Jr** (2003). High dose rate brachytherapy in the management of lung transplant airway stenosis. *Ann Thorac Surg*, **76**, 381–4.

69. **Stewart S, Fishbein MC, Snell GI**, *et al*. (2007). Revision of the 1996 working formulation for the standardization of nomenclature in the diagnosis of lung rejection. *J Heart Lung Transplant*, **26**, 1229–42.

70. **Billings JL, Hertz MI, Savik K**, *et al*. (2002). Respiratory viruses and chronic rejection in lung transplant recipients. *J Heart Lung Transplant*, **21**, 559–66.

71. **Khalifah AP, Hachem RR, Chakinala MM**, *et al*. (2004). Respiratory viral infections are a distinct risk for bronchiolitis obliterans syndrome and death. *Am J Respir Crit Care Med*, **170**, 181–7.

71. **Keenan RJ, Konishi H, Kawai A**, *et al*. (1995). Clinical trial of tacrolimus versus cyclosporine in lung transplantation. *Ann Thorac Surg*, **60**, 580–4.

72. **Cantu E 3rd, Appel JZ 3rd, Hartwig MG**, *et al*. (2004). J. Maxwell Chamberlain Memorial Paper. Early fundoplication prevents chronic allograft dysfunction in patients with gastroesophageal reflux disease. *Ann Thorac Surg*, **78**, 1142–51.

73. **Ross DJ, Lewis MI, Kramer M**, *et al*. (1997). FK 506 'rescue' immunosuppression for obliterative bronchiolitis after lung transplantation. *Chest*, **112**, 1175–9.

74. **Ross DJ, Waters PF, Levine M**, *et al*. (1998). Mycophenolate mofetil versus azathioprine immunosuppressive regimens after lung transplantation: preliminary experience. *J Heart Lung Transplant*, **17**, 768–74.

75. **Groetzner J, Wittwer T, Kaczmarek I**, *et al*. (2006). Conversion to sirolimus and mycophenolate can attenuate the progression of bronchiolitis obliterans syndrome and improves renal function after lung transplantation. *Transplantation*, **81**, 355–60.

76. **Ussetti P, Laporta R, de Pablo A**, *et al*. (2003). Rapamycin in lung transplantation: preliminary results. *Transplant Proc*, **35**, 1974–7.

77. **Fietta A, Meloni F** (2008). Lung transplantation: the role of azithromycin in the management of patients with bronchiolitis obliterans syndrome. *Curr Med Chem*, **15**, 716–23.

78. **Johnson BA, Iacono AT, Zeevi A, McCurry KR, Duncan SR** (2003). Statin use is associated with improved function and survival of lung allografts. *Am J Respir Crit Care Med*, **167**, 1271–8.

79. **Novick RJ, Stitt LW, Al-Kattan K**, *et al*. (1998). Pulmonary retransplantation: predictors of graft function and survival in 230 patients. *Ann Thorac Surg*, **65**, 227–34.

Index